THE
Body Bible

The essential companion for all women

SUZI GODSON

WITH PHOTOGRAPHS BY HARRIET LOGAN

MICHAEL JOSEPH
an imprint of PENGUIN BOOKS

Thanks

Published by the Penguin Group

Penguin Books Ltd,
80 Strand,
London WC2R 0RL,
England

Penguin Group (USA) Inc.,
375 Hudson Street,
New York,
New York 10014, USA

Penguin Books Australia
Ltd, 250 Camberwell Road,
Camberwell,
Victoria 3124, Australia

Penguin Books Canada Ltd,
10 Alcorn Avenue, Toronto,
Ontario, Canada M4V 3B2

Penguin Books India (P)
Ltd, 11 Community Centre,
Panchsheel Park,
New Delhi -110 017, India

Penguin Group (NZ),
cnr Airborne
and Rosedale Roads,
Albany, Auckland 1310,
New Zealand

Penguin Books (South
Africa) (Pty) Ltd,
24 Sturdee Avenue,
Rosebank 2196,
South Africa

Penguin Books Ltd,
Registered Offices:
80 Strand,
London WC2R 0RI, England
www.penguin.com

This book could not have been produced without the help of an enormous number of people, in particular, the hundreds of women who painstakingly responded to the online questionnaires at www.suzigodson.com. To ensure their privacy, once they had emailed me I had no way of getting in touch with them again, so this is my only opportunity to say a big **THANK YOU** to everyone who provided a quote and made this book such an illuminating insight into the hearts and minds of 'normal' women. **THANK YOU** also to the amazing and inspiring women who volunteered to be photographed. Each one had a unique story to tell and Harriet Logan's pictures of these extraordinary 'ordinary' women create a powerful and sympathetic counterbalance to the airbrushed unreality that the media promotes as 'beauty'. Harriet and her eternally cheerful assistant Becky made everyone feel relaxed and the smiles in the photos are as much a testament to Harriet's exuberant character as they are to her photographic skill. In the end there simply weren't enough pages to get everyone in, so apologies to those women whose quotes or pictures ended up on the cutting-room floor.

Throughout the course of my research I have pestered many clever and important people, and without exception they have been incredibly generous with their time and their advice. A big **THANK YOU** to Professor Steve Bloom at the Division of Investigative Science at Hammersmith Hospital who has been a real inspiration. His work on the PYY3-36 hormone to suppress appetite is now globally renowned, but he still found time to help me with my project. Without his assistance I would not have had the help of his colleagues; Dr Alison Wren, Wellcome Clinical Research Fellow (and Supermum); Professor Tony Chu, Head of Dermatology, Dr Kevin Murphy at the Department of Metabolic Medicine and Gary Frost PhD SRD, Head of Service Nutrition & Dietetics. Thanks also to cosmetic surgeon Dai Davies for sharing the delights and horrors of his practice with me, to Clinical Psychologist Dr Louise de Haro for her insight into body dysmorphic disorders, to Steve Bloomfield at the Eating Disorders Association, to Caroline Bennett at Moshi Moshi Sushi and to Jan Petherick at Fighting Fit for all her help with the fitness chapter.

On a professional level I am indebted to my agent Felicity Rubenstein for believing in me, to Kate Adams, Louise Moore and everyone at Michael Joseph who helped this book take shape and to Hilly Janes for her encouragement at the Saturday *Times*. I am also enormously grateful to Jon Summerill, Leah Speakman, Kevin Edwards and everyone at NMI for all their support over the years. On a personal level I would like to thank my family, my friends and my partner Tim, who now knows more about female body image than any man has a right to.

The Body Bible. The essential companion for all women.
Suzi Godson

Michael Joseph, an imprint of Penguin Books

MICHAEL JOSEPH

Set in Gill Sans, Bank gothic and Snell. Printed in Spain by Artes Graficas Toledo, S.A.U.
A CIP catalogue record for this book is available from the British Library
isbn 0-718-14663-8

Contents

Introduction

For most women, fat is not a 'feminist issue', it's a four letter word, and we'd probably all turn back the ageing clock if it wasn't such a frightening physical and financial commitment. Self-confidence and self-consciousness are so closely linked for women that 'the female condition' is better described as constant state of mild paranoia. I can't pretend to be any different. How I look frequently, if not always, determines how I feel about myself, and over the years I have searched for my fair share of quick fixes in an effort to shift the ten pounds, or the ten years, that I believed to stand between myself and my self-esteem. But despite copious quanti-ties of good advice, every time I have tried a new way to to 'quit, lose or improve' something in the past, my initial enthusiasm has been swiftly followed by intimida-tion and disillusion. And I have rarely succeeded in changing anything.

Determined to find out whether my continued efforts at self improvement were just a recurrent triumph of hope over experience, I decided to investigate the elusive mysteries of health, fitness, diet and 'celebrity style' grooming for myself. When I started my research I realised one thing straight away. Wellbeing, health, fitness, beauty, weight, how well you age, how long you live and even how happy you are, are entirely interconnected. For me, this was the key to change. Once I understood the conflict between my short term goals and my long term health, I realised that there is no point doing any diet if you don't address your overall eating patterns and, as Marlene Dietrich once said, 'careful grooming may take 20 years off a woman's age, but you can't fool a long flight of stairs'.

That simple realisation was the begining of *The Body Bible*, an encyclopedic look at the bigger picture. It examines every aspect of the female body – from biological and physical differences to historical and cultural influences, in an effort to find out where women have come from, and where we should be trying to get. It takes a holistic view and questions all aspects of our emotional relationship with our physical selves. And it presumes that although the spirit is usually willing, the flesh is generally weak and, well, pretty out of shape. It demonstrates how gradual lifestyle changes, such as eating properly and taking some regular exercise, can have a cumulative and beneficial effect on your skin, your weight, your bone density and your self-esteem (issues that are as relevant to a 16-year-old girl as they are to a 65-year-old woman). And it tries to keep things simple. There is no point in proposing the unsustainable to the easily diverted. Although we are all full of good intentions, at the end of the day what woman has the time or the inclination to find the 16 ingredients required to cook 'Gourmet Rock Cornish Hen à l'Orange' for her Zone diet supper?

To support my research, over a period of 18 months, a Body Bible website gathered quotes and tips from women around the world. These perspectives form the backbone of the book and provide a unique insight into how 'normal' women feel about themselves, their lives and their bodies. The responses highlighted fundamental differences between women who have positive body image and those who do not. In general, when a woman has a good relationship with herself, self-improvement is a plus, but problems arise when women with damaged self-esteem are buffeted from one diet/fitness/beauty 'promise' to another in search of self-worth. Without doubt, the women who were most positive about themselves were those who had participated in sport as children because they viewed fitness as recreation rather than a tool for weight loss.

Though aspects of my research highlighted how much women have been, and still are, exploited by a myriad of industries with a vested interest in keeping them dissatisfied with themselves, it didn't make me want to bin my Manolos and slip into a hair shirt. The information I gathered suggested to me that although the majority of women are conscious of the external pressures placed upon them, and do strive to be thinner, fitter, younger and more beautiful, in reality, most are not really trying to impress others, they are simply trying to be the best they can.

The fairer sex are, by nature, very competitive about appearance. And the more educated and aware women become, the more emphasis they choose to place on physical attractiveness because they believe that maximising their potential brings positive benefits, firstly, in terms of personal self-esteem and, secondly, in terms of how others react to them. This is not a bad thing and certainly does not demonstrate that as a gender, women are being manipulated. Rather it illustrates that women can, and often do, make the most of their assets.

Though *The Body Bible* began as a personal project, it has ended up providing a platform for a whole community of women and I hope that the voice it gives to female concerns about body image will draw attention to the fact that good looks have little to do with happiness and wellbeing, but negative self-image disturbs both.

For me, thinking in terms of 'health span' as opposed to 'life span' was the kick up the butt I had always needed. Last year I finally quit smoking for good. And then I ran the London Marathon.

Suzi Godson

I was a size 16 and over 14st [89kg] about a year and a half ago. I hated myself so much and I had developed a very unhealthy relationship with food. I was always on the go with work, travelling at ridiculous times, and I was bingeing on junk so the pounds piled on. I have a pressured life, but I figured, I can fit 12 meetings in a day but I can't find time to look after myself. It took Weight Watchers, the gym, and an education in healthy eating to help me develop a good relationship with food. I kept a food diary which highlighted my snacking, but I don't need to now as the diary is always in my head. Now I make sure I have the time to check the scales, eat healthily and keep fit. It was hard at first but Weight Watchers is great as you can eat what you want and once you have learned the language of points you can scratch cook your own recipes, which makes it an easy to maintain lifestyle. Now when I feel low I go to the gym and release some happy endorphins and then eat whatever I want because I have earned it. I am now a size 10, 10st [63.4kg] and 5'11' and I feel great.
Aimee, 29, UK

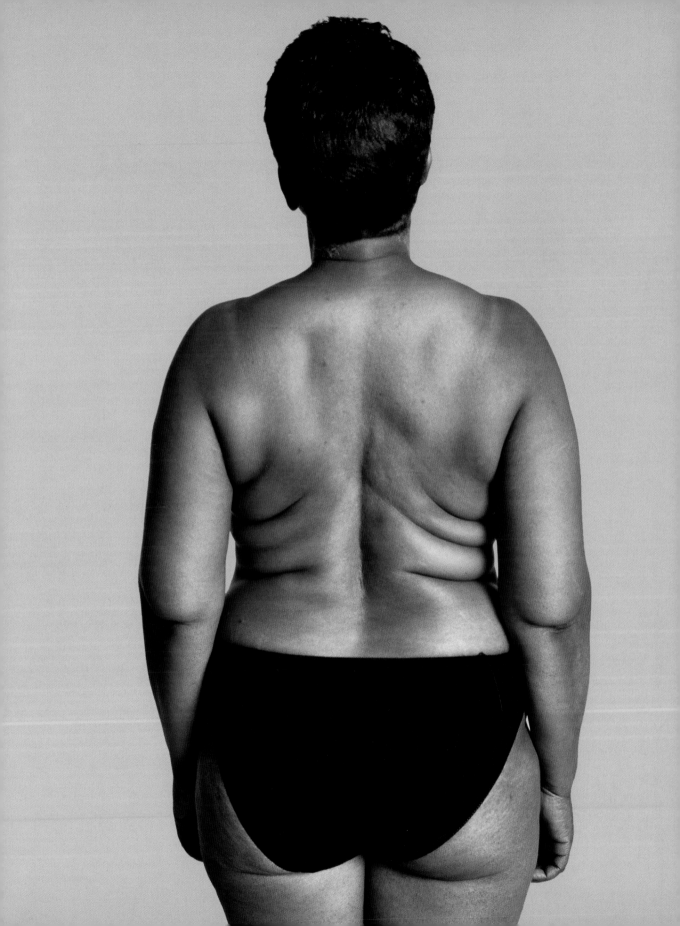

THE Body CHAPTER

From Titian to Aniston

Before the invention of photography, art was the only method of visually documenting beauty. But although the paintings of Titian (1485–1576), Rubens (1577–1640) and Rembrandt (1606–69) celebrate voluptuous women sporting body mass indexes that would have the 21st-century fat police out in force, by the beginning of the 18th century a fuller female figure was no longer considered to be a sign of prosperity, fertility and good health. In fact, Rubenesque ripples were already seen as indelicate, overindulgent and a sign of working class origins.

Though it is difficult to believe that the dictate of thinness predates media of any kind, long before photography established itself, poets such as Keats (1795–1821) and Shelley (1792–1822) had romanticized the notion that beauty, sensitivity and creativity were linked to physical frailty (in fact, it is suggested that Byron starved himself to look more poetic) while Rossetti (1828–82) and the Pre-Raphaelites created a new aesthetic with their paintings of big eyed, pale skinned women with angular bony bodies. In an ironic parallel with the anorexic appearance of the contemporary catwalk model, the thin tubercular woman with a consumptive gleam in her eye, pale skin and a feverish glow, came to embody the 19th-century ideal of beauty. Women dieted and tied their whalebone corsets ever tighter in an effort to ape the fashion for frail. Even Royalty could not escape. By the time Queen Victoria came to the throne in 1837, aged just 18, she was obsessed with the idea that she was too stout. Indeed, her diaries reveal that her own mother had already warned her that she was in danger of being mistaken for a milkmaid.

When Louis Daguerre invented photography in 1839, he changed the course of visual history. But being able to capture reality did not mean the media would choose to present it so. As photographic techniques have improved, photographers and directors have employed liberal quantities of artistic licence to stretch, graft, trim, tuck and smooth a beautiful but wholly unrealistic image of what now constitutes female physical perfection. Ironically, in an effort to sustain the art director's fantasy, real models have had to become thinner and thinner. In the mid-70s, the average model weighed 8% less than the average woman. Today, the average model is 23% below average weight and the anorexic androgyny of Twiggy (5' 8'', 44kg/97lb) which was shocking in the 1960s, is now the norm. Though the models that grace the covers of magazines represent the body type of approximately 5% of the female population, women, particularly high achieving or fashion conscious women, have been trying to hit a constantly decreasing target body weight for the past 50 years. Though they are the human equivalent to a needle in a haystack, the power of media magnification has projected the few fat-free into public consciousness with such force that this fractional minority now set the standard by which 95% of women judge themselves.

As a result, 95% of the female population have dieted at some time and 50% of women are on a diet at this very moment. Viewed in the context of studies which show that calorific deprivation induces depression, anxiety and irritability, these statistics would suggest that right now, half of all women are too hungry to be happy or healthy.

Although research repeatedly shows that high levels of exposure to fashion magazines leave women feeling depressed, the number of new titles crowding the newsagents' shelves suggests that female masochism is alive and well and fuelling the market. Women have always been encouraged to transfer their anxieties into actions (buying clothes, using beauty products, dieting, joining a gym) and for the last 50 years magazines have been the medium of choice for anyone selling a promise 'guaranteed' to make a woman look or feel better. As a form of immediate therapy, it half works. If a woman wears a new dress, does a diet or applies a new perfume, and gets paid a compliment, she smiles, inside and out. But if no one notices any change, she feels that her efforts have failed. Though she remains the same person either way, she allows her perception of herself to either escalate or plummet as a result of how other people react to her. Since her feelings about herself and the choices she makes are not supported by self-belief, she is at the mercy of other people's likes, dislikes, moods or emotions. Negative feedback, regardless of accuracy, destabilizes her, and she then expends more time and energy searching for another way to 'improve' herself so that she can conform more closely to someone else's idea of attractive.

The media has created such a currency out of appearance that many women now believe good looks pay greater and more immediate dividends than hard work or intelligence. Jennifer Aniston is a good example. At approximately 5' 6'' in height and weighing 50kg (110lb), she has gone from girl-next-door good looking to international superstar who wakes up next to Brad Pitt. How did she do it? Simple. She lost 13.5kg (30 pounds), nearly a third of her current bodyweight. Aniston says 'I wasn't fat, I was just Greek. Greeks are round, with big asses and boobs', but she was told by her agent in no uncertain terms that she was too big to get parts so she dieted. It becomes increasingly difficult to present a convincing argument that says self-respect is more important than self-flagellation when the evidence against this statement appears to be so overwhelming. A recent survey revealed that nearly half of all women in the UK feel they derive greater happiness from being the 'right weight' than anything else in life. Is that progress? Our 18th-century sisters didn't have the vote but they didn't have to flaunt their belly buttons either. In a devil's pact 21st-century women are free to wear hipsters and crop tops but they are imprisoned by an all consuming, and seemingly incurable, body consciousness.

My mother worked in the fashion industry all her life. She started out as a model and she went on to design her own clothing label. I spent my childhood surrounded by people who were either modelling her clothes, coming for fittings or buying her label. I was simultaneously fascinated and repulsed. The women that she worked with were all, and I mean all, absolutely tiny — anorexic really. I was a cute kid but as I grew into a big-boned adolescent I felt more and more awkward. As a child I adored dressing up in the beautiful dresses my mother made. As a teenager I couldn't fit into them. I became increasingly withdrawn and by the time I was 20 I had been both bulimic and anorexic for seven years. Ironically, when I was at my most anorexic I modelled for my mother's label, a fact which did nothing but confirm to me that I will spend my life fighting my genetic build.
Anon, 34, US

I start the day by starving myself, which feels really good for a while, but then I get so hungry that I gorge on anything and everything until I sicken myself.
Lucia, 29, Brazil

Little women

SOMETIMES IT'S HARD TO BE A ... At first glance the advantages to being born female are not automatically apparent. Bar being first off a sinking ship and having a nicer wardrobe, women, by virtue of their biology, have a lot to contend with. It all starts at puberty, the humiliating transition from 'child' to 'reproductive being'. Anyone who has come out the other side can look back and laugh, but from a 12-year-old's perspective, it's hard to put a positive spin on the impending, and very public, arrival of spots, weight gain, breasts, pubic hair, hormonal chaos, mood swings and monthly bleeding. And there is no doubt that the experience has an impact on confidence. Until puberty, tests on physical and mental health show girls to be more focused, more socially competent, tougher and less likely to injure themselves than boys. However, as soon as puberty begins, these advantages disappear and between the ages of 11 and 16 young women are statistically more likely to suffer from unexplained depression than boys of the same age.

TOO MUCH TOO YOUNG It goes without saying that the younger a girl is when puberty starts, the more difficult she is likely to find it. So the fact that the average age at which girls begin puberty has fallen continually for the last 200 years is bad news. In 1830 it was about 17, in 1962 it was 12.8 and now it is 12.5. Recent research indicates that there is a biological floor beyond which the age of first menstruation will not fall – the baseline of nine or ten years has remained the same for about 30 years. However, the appearance of secondary sexual characteristics, such as breasts and pubic hair continues to drop. By the age of eight, 48% of African American girls and 15% of Caucasian girls show clear signs of puberty.

There are a number of reasons why earlier puberty poses a problem for young girls. In the long term, it is thought that girls who reach puberty early have an increased risk of developing breast cancer as adults. And paediatricians are also worried because bone growth slows after menstruation, girls who hit puberty early may not reach their full adult height. In the short term, the one in eight girls in UK primary schools who are already menstruating face many practical problems. The vast majority of them have no support, no access to information, no bins to put used sanitary towels in and, most of the time, no toilet roll. However, the most difficult issue facing girls who develop early is that young girls who look grown up tend to be treated in a more adult way, whether it is appropriate or not. Physical and emotional growth are not synchronized, but a girl who looks 14 is rarely expected to behave like the ten-year-old she really is. As such, she is more likely to attract attention that she is not ready to deal with, more likely to be exploited and more likely to have sex that she does not want, sooner rather than later. Hardly surprising, then, that young girls who experience early puberty are statistically more likely to suffer from depression, substance abuse and self-harm.

Puppy fat

FAT CELLS Fat cells are only formed in the body twice. Once in the developing foetus during the last three months of pregnancy and again at puberty. After puberty no new fat cells are created but, as a girl grows, if she takes in more calories than she requires, her existing fat cells expand and she gains weight. Likewise, if she consumes fewer calories than she requires, her fat cells deflate and shrink. Girls and boys have very similar body compositions during infancy and childhood, but during adolescence boys add more lean muscle mass while girls, much to their chagrin, lay down stores of body fat on their breasts, hips, waist, thighs and buttocks.

BODY FAT AND ACCELERATED PUBERTY There are several different theories as to why puberty is occurring earlier in girls. These include hormones in food; exposure to pesticides; chemicals such as phthalate esters in toys, vinyl flooring, detergents, and cosmetics; a sedentary lifestyle; global warming and even watching too much sex on TV. Though the jury is out on chemicals, climate and carnal knowledge, the correlation between accelerated puberty and increased body fat has been accepted for some time. Fat cells manufacture leptin, a hormone thought to be involved in triggering puberty, and when a girl lays down a big enough store, menstruation begins. However, the body is incapable of differentiating between accelerated weight gain caused by a diet of cream buns and burgers and normal weight gained through skeletal growth and physical maturity. As a result, the 13% of eight-year-old UK girls currently classified as obese are more than likely to experience early puberty and all its associated difficulties.

VITAMINS AND MINERALS Teenage girls have greater nutritional needs than any other age group in terms of calories, protein, vitamin and mineral requirements. It's a crucial time for building bone mass, getting taller and creating muscle. A good diet as a teenager will encourage bone growth and limit the risk of osteoporosis and coronary heart disease in later life (p.279) but studies show that young girls are not getting the right nutritional balance. On average, girls only get 60% of their recommended iron intake and one in four is anaemic. Iron is vital to compensate for menstrual blood loss and it may also be linked to intelligence. IQ tests in a 1997 trial showed that iron-deficient girls scored almost ten points lower than those with normal iron levels. This difference was levelled out after the girls were put on a ten-week course of iron supplements. Folic acid is essential for reproductive health but tests on a group of 15-year-olds in Ireland found that only one quarter had healthy levels in their system because they were dieting. Girls aged 15–18 also tend to be deficient in vitamin D, zinc, potassium iodine and magnesium because their diet isn't varied enough. In the UK, 19% of teenagers are vegetarian. Though it's perfectly feasible to be a healthy vegetarian, many girls don't know how to balance their diet and compensate for lost protein, iron and folate (p.84).

I was overweight when I hit puberty. I gained a lot of weight and I have had a hang up about my body ever since. I lost a lot of weight when I was around 16 or 17 by simply starving. I was at boarding school and I would skip meals and chew Bovril cubes. It is revolting but it puts you off food. It took six months to lose the weight and I was very happy. I turned from an ugly duckling into a reasonable looking young woman and my life changed hugely as a result. I became much more confident. However, I have literally been on a diet since 1966. I put on weight incredibly easily so I have to constantly monitor what I eat. I have pretty much cut out carbohydrates. I don't eat pasta, potatoes, sugar, or bread, though I eat cheese. I try to live by the Hay diet so I food combine. If I have the occasional sandwich, it will be a tomato or cucumber sandwich. Maybe I didn't eat enough in the past because now anything I eat stays. I have put on at least 9lb [4kg] since I gave up smoking, but I am not even aware that I am eating any more.
Annabel, 51, UK

DIET If a young girl is to reach her full height and grow healthily she requires an adequate intake of useful calories. But a high fat, high sugar diet means many teenage girls are consuming empty calories and as a result they are simultaneously overweight and undernourished. Most just don't understand that it is possible to eat well without gaining weight and food and calories are often judged in terms of quantity, rather than quality. A girl who eats a small burger and fries with a fizzy drink and doesn't feel full afterwards probably considers her meal modest compared to a dinner of sirloin steak with baked potato, broccoli and salad. However, the more substantial meal is considerably healthier and less likely to cause weight gain because it contains less fat and sugar. Educating young girls about the benefits of eating for health will help them to make better dietary choices. And as young girls often have strong moral and political views, explaining what awful rubbish goes in to junk food and how exploitative the production process is can help them break fast food habits (p.30).

INACTIVITY Most children don't take enough exercise but the problem is generally worse for young girls than it is for boys because concerns about safety mean they have less freedom than ever. They don't get to walk to school and their social life centres around sedentary activities such as ... well, eating, using computers and watching TV. Research shows that young people consume up to 25% of their daily calories in front of the television set. Besides the fact that eating while concentrating on watching TV makes everyone less aware of how full they feel, 50% of the advertisements broadcast during 'youth' TV are for processed snack foods like chips, crisps, biscuits and sweets, none of which are balanced by adverts for fruit or veg.

BODY IMAGE Since practically every teen magazine and TV show focuses on how to look slim and sexy, it's hardly surprising that studies reveal 53% of American 13-year-olds to be unhappy with their bodies. By the age of 17, 78% of girls are dissatisfied. Exacting ideals of physical perfection have created a crisis of confidence amongst teenage girls who, from a very early age, battle their preoccupation with body shape, often in the company of mothers who are doing exactly the same thing. Research by UK nutritionists suggests that almost three-quarters of pubescent girls are attempting to lose weight at any given time. Emerging research now suggests that anxieties about weight and shape develop in late childhood and into puberty, before the typical age for the development of eating disorders, but dieting has also been shown to increase the risk of developing an eating disorder. The current popularity of crash diets that involve cutting out whole food groups, such as carbohydrates, meat or dairy products, can have seriously detrimental effects on long-term physical health, but future consequences seem very unimportant to a sensitive teenage girl who can't do her zip up.

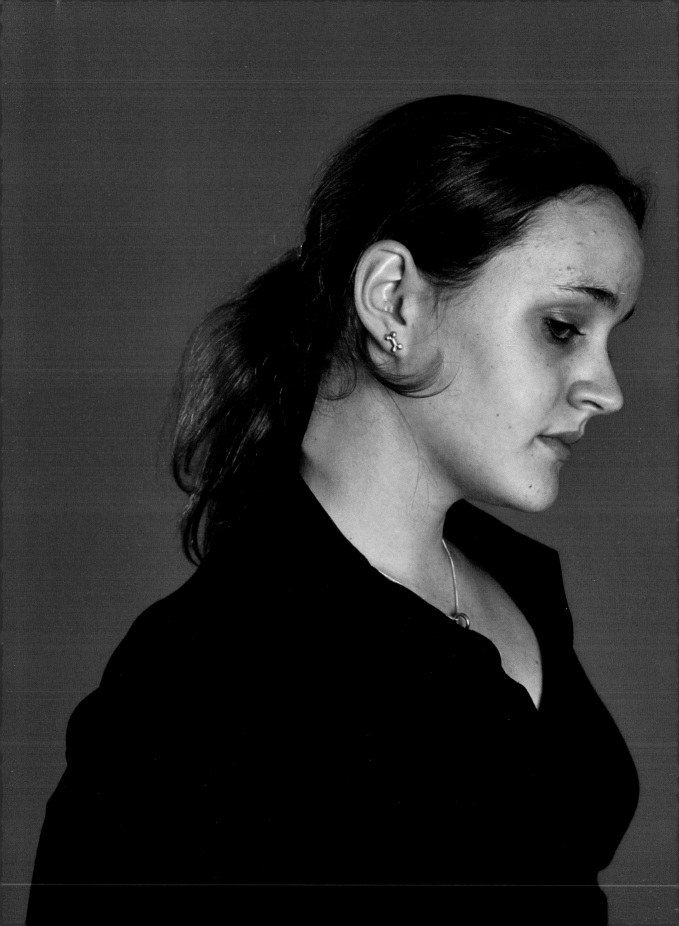

Fat puppies

WHO BUYS THE HAPPY MEALS? Parents. And they bear responsibility for the fact that the proportion of overweight and obese children has rocketed since the mid-1980s. One in five children in the UK and the US is now overweight and one in ten is obese. Fat accumulated prior to and during puberty won't disappear without a great deal of effort and the reality is that at least 50–80% of these children will grow up to be obese as adults. Overweight teenagers are susceptible to emotional problems. They suffer continual negative assumptions about both their character and their appearance. They are often teased at school and excluded by their peer groups. These feelings of isolation then create a vicious circle where an excluded girl feels the only place she can seek solace is by eating.

WHO SETS AN EXAMPLE? Parents. If parents don't eat properly and don't exercise, they can hardly expect their children to. Most experts agree that it is inactivity rather than diet that has exacerbated the problem of childhood obesity. Studies show that teenage girls eat half as much as boys, but they are still becoming overweight in increasing numbers because they do too little exercise. Of girls aged two to seven, 38% are already not meeting the recommended daily activity levels, while 64% of 15-year-old girls are classed as 'inactive', which means they do absolutely no exercise at all.

WHO SUFFERS THE CONSEQUENCES? Children. Fat kids are storing up health problems for the future, but they also face serious health problems while they are young. The first cases of type-2 diabetes, a condition that normally only affects adults, have now been found in children. Children and teenagers who are obese can also suffer from raised levels of cholesterol, triglycerides and lipoproteins in the blood. They also tend to have higher levels of harmful low-density lipoproteins (LDL) and lower levels of helpful high-density lipoproteins (HDL). This pattern is strongly associated with heart disease in later life. Hypertension or high blood pressure is very uncommon in children, but it occurs nine times more frequently in obese children and teenagers than in those who are a normal weight. Untreated, it can lead to stroke, heart, eye and kidney disease.

Bones and cartilage in children stretch slightly but they are unable to cope with excess weight, which can cause orthopaedic and joint problems, such as bow legs or abnormalities in bone growth. Recently, US researchers have found that obese children are also 77% more likely to have asthma, possibly because they are less likely to participate in sport because of the extra effort involved, but it may also relate to the greater respiratory effort required to move a ribcage covered in excess fat. Obese children can also suffer from obstructive sleep apnoea (stopping breathing while asleep), leaving them too tired to concentrate at school.

Body types

BODY TYPES Women come in all shapes and sizes, but there are three basic body types and everything else is a variation on a theme. Those three broad categories of body types, or 'somatypes', were defined in the early 1940s by American psychologist William H. Sheldon (1898–1977), who studied 4000 photographs of college students and divided them into endomorph, a system centred on the abdomen, and the digestive system; mesomorph, a system focused on the muscles and the circulatory system, and ectomorph, a system focused on the brain and the nervous system.

Sheldon's real goal was actually to establish whether body type was in any way connected to temperament. After several hundred in-depth interviews he came up with three personality categories that appeared to correspond with body type. He called them; endotonia, a love of relaxation, comfort, food and people; mesotonia, an assertive personality and a love of action; and ectotonia, private, restrained with a highly developed self-awareness. While his connection between personality and physical shape plays only a minor role in modern psychology, his body types have endured to influence, in part at least, how many people exercise, body build and manage their weight.

ENDOMORPHS Oprah Winfrey, Marilyn Monroe or Kate Winslet are endomorphs. They have softer, rounder bodies, a higher than average body fat percentage and their muscle mass may be proportionally lower. Endomorphs should take plenty of aerobic exercise such as swimming, walking or running, though it can take them longer to achieve more defined muscle tone.

ECTOMORPHS Kate Moss, Naomi Campbell and Jodi Kidd are classic ectomorphs. They have a tall, thin, delicate build and are often flat chested. Their shape gives them a young appearance and they are often tall, lightly muscled and tend to be a little stoop-shouldered. Ectomorphs can improve their muscle profile with weight training and are suited to sports like long-distance running and basket-ball where limb length and light weight are an advantage. Ectomorphs who overeat are more likely to gain weight around the abdomen.

MESOMORPHS Brigitte Neilson, Cindy Crawford or Serena Williams are mesomorphs. They are well built, muscular and athletic and they tend to have a higher muscle to body fat ratio. Mesomorphs are good at most sports, but their power gives them an advantage at sprinting, gymnastics and team sports like volley-ball or hockey. Mesomorphs see results in the gym very quickly and extra muscle makes for a faster metabolism. However, in mid-life, or if they stop training, their muscle will turn to fat.

My body is a mystery to me. I have tiny bones obviously because my fingers and wrists and ankles are minute but I have absolutely bloody enormous hips. I literally treble in size around my arse and then I get small again around the waist. I can't seem to change my shape, no matter what I do, so I try not to let it bother me. But I am confined to A-line skirts for life.
Eleanor, 25, UK

Unfortunately, due to starting my periods early, I also gained my womanly figure (with big hips and bum). In fact, one of my nick-names at age 11 was big bum! I had noticed it myself but I felt worse about it after I was teased. I have tried different types of exercise but it's really not my thing and no matter how much I do, I will still be the same shape.
Kellie, 30, UK

According to my mother I was born prematurely. As a result I was a very skinny child and even when I hit puberty I always had very narrow hips and didn't gain weight like the other girls in my high school. Over the years I have gradually put on weight around my waist mainly but I guess I just never caught up.
Olga, 29, US

Body mass index

Body mass index (BMI) is one of the quickest and easiest ways of gauging weight in adults. It's better than jumping on weighing scales because it takes height into account, but it should only be viewed as a broad measure of your weight and any associated health risks. See the chart opposite to work out your BMI.

A BMI of 30+ means you are obese and increasing your risk of death from any cause by 50–150 per cent. If you also have a waist circumference of over 89cm (35in) (see opposite), you are considered to be at an especially high risk of developing heart disease, diabetes or high blood pressure and you should take immediate steps to lose weight and avoid ill health.

A BMI between 18.6 and 24.9 is considered normal, though certain ethnic groups should aim for lower rather than higher figures. Women who are planning to get pregnant should aim to have a BMI within this range.

A BMI of less than 18.5 means you may be underweight, though measuring your waist circumference (p.20) may place you back in the normal category.

Though a BMI of 24 or less is considered to be healthy, experts from the world health community believe this figure should be revised down because the tables do not adequately reflect variation in the population. The charts were originally developed by US life insurance companies in 1951, but health experts argue that people who bought life insurance at that time tended to be more affluent and so were more likely to live longer, be healthier and weigh less than the general population.

New research now suggests that because the scale was worked out for a Caucasian population, up to one out of four people may be misclassified by BMI. Differences in body composition and a greater fat to bone and muscle ratio amongst other ethnic groups mean that even though they appear to fall within the existing 'normal' BMI range, they are at a higher risk of developing conditions such as diabetes. The study calculated BMIs for 2626 Aborigines in 15 remote areas in Australia and looked at levels of impaired glucose tolerance and diabetes. Results show that the risk of developing diabetes was four times higher for those with BMIs of 22 or more even though that score falls well within the normal range. The study concluded that if gains in BMI beyond 22 were actively discouraged, they could prevent an estimated 46% of diabetes cases and 34% of impaired glucose tolerance cases.

In the UK, Asian and Afro-Caribbean people are up to five times more likely to have diabetes than white populations and doctors believe this figure would decrease substantially if a lower 'healthy BMI' range could be encouraged.

Find your body mass index

Find your height in the column down the left hand side. Read across to find your weight in pounds and then read up to the the the column along the top. The white number is your BMI.

	19	20	21	22	23	24	25	26	27	28	29	30	35	40
4'10"	91	96	100	105	110	115	119	124	129	134	138	143	167	191
4'11"	94	99	104	109	114	119	124	128	133	138	143	148	173	198
5'0"	97	102	107	112	118	123	128	133	138	143	148	153	179	204
5'1"	100	106	111	116	122	127	132	137	143	148	153	158	185	211
5'2"	104	109	115	120	126	131	136	142	147	153	158	164	191	218
5'3"	107	113	118	124	130	135	141	146	152	158	163	169	197	225
5'4"	110	116	122	128	134	140	145	151	157	163	169	174	204	232
5'5"	114	120	126	132	138	144	150	156	162	168	174	180	210	240
5'6"	118	124	130	136	142	148	155	161	167	173	179	186	216	247
5'7"	121	127	134	140	146	153	159	166	172	178	185	191	223	255
5'8"	125	131	138	144	151	158	164	171	177	184	190	197	230	262
5'9"	128	135	142	149	155	162	169	176	182	189	196	203	236	270
5'10"	132	139	146	153	160	167	174	181	188	195	202	207	243	278
5'11"	136	143	150	157	165	172	179	186	193	200	208	215	250	286
6'0"	140	147	154	162	169	177	184	191	199	206	213	221	258	294
6'1"	144	151	159	166	174	182	189	197	204	212	219	227	265	302
6'2"	148	155	163	171	179	186	194	202	210	218	225	233	272	311
6'3"	152	160	138	176	184	192	200	208	216	224	232	240	279	319
6'4"	156	164	172	180	189	197	205	213	221	230	238	246	287	328

Metabolism

BURN BABY BURN Metabolism is the rate at which your body burns up energy. Though a 'slow metabolism' (and big bones) is often used as an excuse for weight gain, bar rare cases of serious illness, it is not possible to blame your metabolism for obesity. Metabolism does vary, but research shows that obese people actually have a faster metabolism than skinny people.

Metabolism is measured by a system called Basal Metabolic Rate (BMR), which works out the number of calories you'd burn if you stayed in bed all day – what you might call your tick-over speed. As a very rough guide, the average person's BMR is about half a calorie per pound of body weight, per hour. So, if you weigh 63kg (140lb) you will use up about 70 calories an hour or 1680 calories per day doing absolutely nothing. And the more you weigh, the higher your BMR will be.

The metabolic rate of very fat women is about 25% higher than that of thin women and the higher your BMR, the easier it is to lose weight. The more energy your body needs to tick over, the more food you can eat without gaining weight – or, conversely, a smaller reduction in food is required in order to lose weight. The good news is that this makes dieting and weight loss easier for women who are overweight. The bad news is that your BMR gradually decreases as you lose weight. When you consume fewer calories than normal your body thinks there is a famine and your metabolism 'slows down' in order to conserve energy. Hence the 'plateau' effect during dieting.

People with a higher proportion of muscle to fat have a higher BMR, but people with less muscle can speed up their metabolism by taking exercise because it preserves lean body tissue. Many diets claim to increase metabolic rate with special fat-burning foods but exercise is the ONLY effective way to increase BMR. Excercise burns up calories and increases BMR for several hours after you stop exercising. Even a modest increase in physical exertion can help women who are 'plateauing' on a diet to counteract the body's tendency to decrease BMR when cutting calories. Women's metabolic rates increase during pregnancy and are even higher when breastfeeding, but drop sharply when they go through menopause, which is why a lot of women find they gain weight then. As you get older, your BMR drops by about 5% every ten years unless you exercise and maintain your lean muscle mass.

STOP BABY STOP So why, if they have a higher metabolic rate, do fat people find it hard to lose weight? The answer is actually nothing to do with how fast their body releases energy from food and everything to do with the fact that their brain fails to recognize when they are full. Stories abound of women who eat

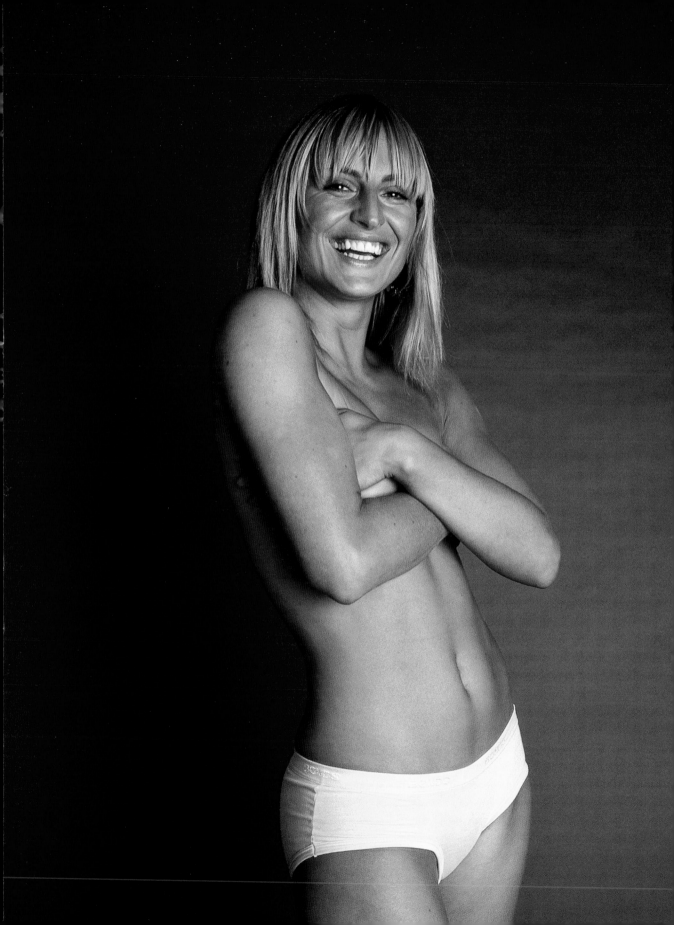

all they want and stay thin while others eat like a bird and stay fat but this isn't because of metabolic variation, it is because the mechanisms that tell a fat person that they are full kick in later than they do for thin people. Kate Moss can eat all the chips she wants, because all the chips she wants is six, whereas all the chips Kirstie Alley wants is 60. With ketchup and mayo. Chubbies have to do by willpower what mother nature automatically does for skinnies, and most of the time they don't succeed because their brain doesn't tell them to stop so they keep eating more than they need. Research on hormones that turn appetite on and off may soon solve this problem though pharmaceutical solutions are a long way off (p.92).

APPLE OR PEAR The World Health Organisation states that excess fat around the stomach, which gives a woman a large waist circumference and an 'apple'-shaped body, is more associated with risk factors for serious conditions such as heart disease, raised blood pressure, diabetes and some types of cancer. Although women often moan about being pear-shaped, excess fat around the bottom, hips and thighs, which gives a woman a smaller waist circumference and a bigger bum and thighs, is considered far less dangerous than weight carried around the stomach. These findings are based on a long-term, ongoing study that began in 1986 and followed the health of 44,000 middle-aged women. All were free of heart disease, stroke and cancer when they submitted their waist and hip measurements to the researchers. Over the next eight years, several hundred of the women had non-fatal heart attacks or fatal coronary artery disease and researchers began to realize that the most apple-shaped women had more than twice the risk of heart disease than the most pear-shaped women. The differential applied to those who weren't particularly overweight and those who were obese.

It is now generally accepted that a waist circumference over 80cm (31½in) indicates a slight health risk to a woman while a waist circumference over 88cm (34½in) indicates a substantially increased risk. Check your own waist measurement at www.ashwell.uk.com/shape

THE BATTLE OF THE BULGE Metabolic changes mean weight is put on more easily in later years. After the age of 25, the average woman gains approximately 450g (1lb) in weight every year, which adds up to a total of 13.5kg (30lb) of excess weight by the time she is 55 years old. Between the ages of 25 and 70, the average woman also loses 5kg (11lb) of muscle. As muscle cells burn more energy than fat, your metabolism slows in proportion to the amount of muscle tissue you lose. As less than 20% of middle-aged and older adults are sufficiently active for health, we currently have a situation where millions of baby boomers are heading into a flabby, unhealthy and inactive old age.

The shape of things to come

FIT FOR 40 Since women hitting 40 have had at least two decades of fantastic advice about diet, health and fitness rammed down their throats, they should all be rubbing their hands with glee as they anticipate a zimmerframe-free old age. Not. Most spent their 'youth' doing what they wanted, not doing what they should. And the two are generally pretty incompatible. By the time most women hit middle age, their behaviour patterns are so well and truly ingrained that it is virtually impossible to find the motivation to change, but the painful reality is that our bodies will treat us as well as we have treated them. Years of celebratory bingeing and complacent nothingness, punctuated by New Year's resolutions, panic diets and expensive gym memberships may be the habits of a lifetime, but if women are to stand any chance of enjoying life into their 80s, there needs to be a fundamental shift in attitude. When it comes to long-term health, short-term reactive masochism is about as effective as sticking an elastoplast on an amputation.

WEIGHT If the proportion of older people who are overweight and obese continues to rise at current rates, more elderly people will be prone to degenerative diseases and mechanical disorders such as arthritis of the knees and hips. In a recent survey, only 39% of the over-50s were considered to have a healthy weight while 68% of women aged 55–64 were classified as either overweight or obese. In later life, nutritional needs are not significantly different but a slower metabolism and increased inactivity means fewer calories are required. A 65-year-old woman should be eating 1900 nutritionally balanced calories a day or less, while a 75-year-old woman should be eating 1800 nutritionally balanced calories or less.

Research from three different trials in the UK and the US indicates that the best way to increase lifespan is to reduce calorie intake by about 30%. Tests on animals fed a third less food than normal showed a slowing of the biological markers of ageing and better general health. A study on humans is underway, but scientists realize that recommending such an enormous calorie reduction would be pointless. Their intention is to find out why undernutrition without malnutrition extends lifespan so they can develop a pharmacological equivalent.

DIET Many women pay less, rather than more, attention to diet as they get older. People over 65 currently eat twice the amount of sugar younger adults do. They consume more cakes, biscuits and sweet drinks and eat less fish, fruit, veg, meat and cheese than younger adults. This is partly to do with cost – processed foods that are high in sugar, salt and fats are generally cheaper – but it is also to do with the fact that lugging heavy fruit and veg home and preparing and cooking it is both exhausting and pretty pointless for someone who is elderly, living alone and cooking for one.

As I get older, I find myself finding ways to conserve my energy and not move if I don't have to. I feel I am slowly shutting down.
May, 79, UK

I don't think I appreciated my body until it started to age. Then I thought bugger, should have flaunted it more.
Caroline, 40, Aus

My doctor tells me I am overweight and that I ought to take more exercise but I tell him I am too old to start changing the way I live my life. My mother never took any exercise and she lived until she was 86 on a diet of tea, biscuits and cigarettes.
Betty, 68, UK

I am diabetic now. I don't really know why, but it does seem to be age related. I can monitor it if I watch my diet very carefully and stay away from anything that pushes my blood sugar up. It's not that difficult because I know that I will get very sick if I don't. However, when I was younger there was no way I could have stuck to a diet – though God knows I tried. I think that the fact that it is a medical condition makes it easier, though I do miss certain things.
Sandra, 60, UK

In this respect, diet is one area where the over-60s can learn a couple of things from their cash-strapped, body-conscious grand-daughters. Single girls with no interest in cooking, but a wholehearted obsession with weight have some top tips on easy, low cost, low calorie nutrition. The 20-something

breakfast of porridge, All Bran, Fruit and Fibre or Weetabix (great sources of vitamins and fibre) topped with half a chopped banana and skimmed milk or soya milk is great at any time of day. Bread (try soya and linseed or sunflower and barley) freezes well, so economy-conscious chicks divide out a loaf and freeze a few slices at a time in separate bags or toast a slice or two straight from the freezer. For a quick. nutritious meal they make low salt, low sugar baked beans on wholemeal toast or fresh soups to boost their veggie intake with no boring peeling. Canned tuna with fried onion in tinned plum tomatoes makes a passable pasta sauce, while canned chopped tomatoes with a cup of canned broad beans, some chopped ham and a handful of cooked pasta makes a decent Tuscan bean soup. They then boost their calcium intake with low fat yogurt bulked up with chopped apple, pear and seeds.

Supermarkets now offer a huge range of fresh pre-prepared meals, salads, soups and fruit boxes but they are more expensive and there is some concern that the preparation process and preservative chemicals decrease their nutritional value. It's cheaper to buy small quantities every day from local markets and an opportunity to get some exercise too. Balancing a bag in each hand as you walk means you'll get a bit of weight training in on the way home.

VITAMINS AND MINERALS As women get older, their absorption of some vitamins and minerals decreases, particularly in those who are on prescription drugs. A 1998 survey of people aged 65+ revealed that the majority were deficient in vitamin D, which is vital to bone health. As women are four times more likely than men to suffer from osteoporosis, ensuring an adequate supply of vitamin D and calcium is very important. Vitamin D is naturally generated through exposure to sunlight but as women get older, absorption through the skin becomes increasingly less efficient (p.138). Eggs or fatty fish are good dietary sources but it's difficult to achieve the recommended daily dose through diet alone, so it's better to take a supplement or a spoonful of cod liver oil every day. Low levels of B vitamins, folate, magnesium, potassium, vitamin C, iron, zinc and beta carotene can be boosted by eating plenty of fruit, vegetables, fibres, plant oils, oily fish, nuts, seeds, pulses and some dairy products. Of new cancers, 64% occur in people over 65. Including antioxidant foods (p.43) in your diet can decrease the risk of cancer, coronary heart disease and stroke.

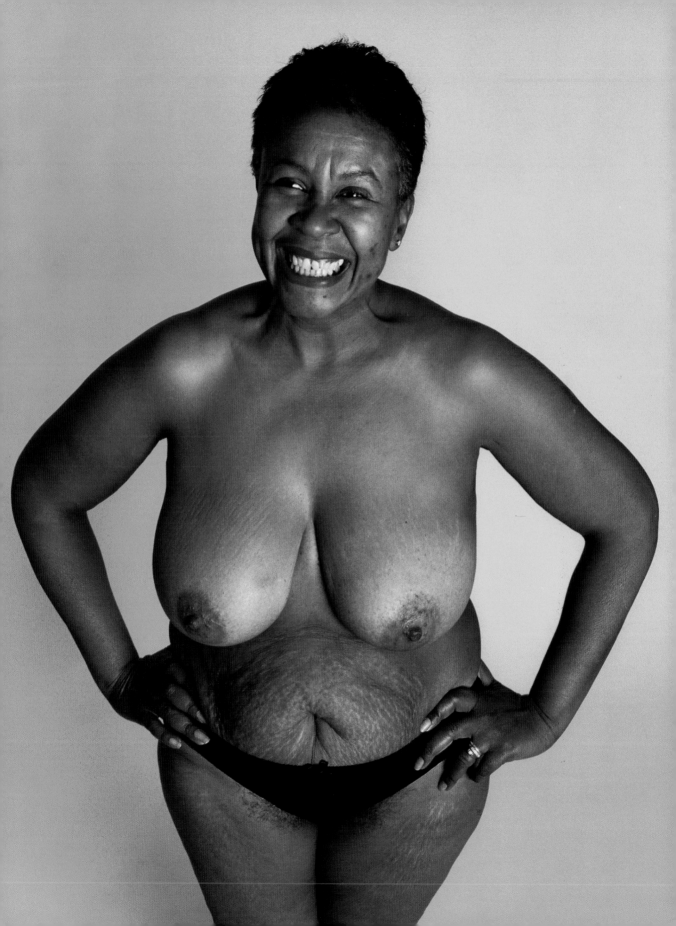

THE E WORD Only one in four women take regular exercise so it's fair to say that most women don't enjoy it very much. Arguably they are just not used to it. In the past, it was taken for granted that boys would climb trees and play team sports like football and rugby, while girls sat at home and played dollies. As adults, many men carry on playing team sports at weekends, affirming the link between fitness, fun and fresh air, whereas women – one in four women to be precise – squeeze into lycra and jump on and off a step in an airless gym to fight a solo battle against their body. 'Sport' is fun. Fitness for the sake of it generally isn't. That said, when the subtle psychological battle against wrinkles, flab and menopause begins, the women that bothered with yoga, Pilates, or whatever else was the flavour of the millennium, will have a distinct advantage over those who didn't.

The benefits of being physically fit are enormous. Women who exercise regularly are less likely to gain weight and one study shows that the chances of a 12kg (26lb) weight gain over a ten-year period are seven times higher in sedentary women than their active sisters. An exercise programme involving daily walking or three or four sessions of exercise per week will produce a weight loss of approximately 900g (2lb) per month in people who are overweight, but viewing exercise as a means of losing weight rather than improving health is missing the point. Excercise improves physical and psychological wellbeing. It reduces the risk of coronary heart disease, high blood pressure, osteoporosis, arthritis, diabetes, bowel cancer and breast cancer. And as the fit few enter into their 60s they will challenge stereotypical perspectives of old age as a time of ill health and immobility by remaining active and independent.

IT'S NEVER TOO LATE TO START If you make an effort to exercise in middle age and old age, you will start to see dramatic results very quickly. Studies show huge improvements in cardiovascular fitness amongst 70-year-old women following an exercise programme for the first time and one group of men aged between 60 and 72 doubled their muscle strength within 12 weeks of regular weight training.

One of the most common mistakes is assuming that exercise has to involve hard-core running or aerobics. It doesn't. Walking a mile improves fitness and burns as many calories as running a mile – it just takes a bit longer. And exercise can take any form. Whether it is climbing stairs, cleaning floors, gardening or golf, as long as you exert yourself for between thirty minutes and an hour a day, five times a week (sorry, we're all so lardy now that health experts have revised the half hour three times a week upwards) you will be increasing your fitness and stamina.
Resistance or strength training activity has been proven to benefit overall health and

fitness for older people because it preserves muscle and bone mass and decreases the likelihood of coronary heart disease, hypertension, osteoporosis, type-2 diabetes and obesity. It also increases endurance and improves lung capacity, both of which make daily tasks such as climbing stairs, walking and carrying shopping much easier. T'ai chi and yoga are particularly good for people over 65 as they are gentle on joints. A brisk walk for 30 minutes a day or three hours a week can reduce heart attack and stroke by 45%, which is why women who have dogs tend to be fitter and healthier than women who don't.

Before embarking on a fitness programme, talk to your doctor about how hard you should push yourself, particularly if you have any ailments or have been ill recently. Get some professional advice at a gym to ensure that you avoid injury and don't push yourself too hard at first. Build up slowly. (p.113)

HEALTH Traditionally, women have always lived longer than men. Though that ratio is now shifting as women fall prey to illnesses previously associated with male pursuits, such as smoking, drinking, eating business lunches and having a terrible day at the office. Most women in developed countries can still expect to live seven to ten years longer than the average man because a lifetime of exposure to doctors telling us how not to get pregnant, how to have babies, how to vaccinate, how to have smear tests and how to get through the menopause, means we are twice as likely as men to seek medical help and therefore, are more likely to nip potential health problems in the bud.

Physical competence is one of the strongest predictors of psychological wellbeing in old age, however research shows that happiness and the perception of good health can actually be a better predictor of mortality and depression than true health status. In other words, if you think you feel well, you are well. A 1997 study reported that while older men living alone have a higher risk of death than those who don't, the same is not true of women because they are significantly better at maintaining social contact and less likely to become isolated and depressed.

That's the good news. The bad news is that although people who took risks with their health in the past didn't generally live long enough to to regret it, we probably will. But as the number of men and women entering into old age increases, so too will the drain on healthcare resources. Sustaining an increasingly ageing population costs money and the National Health Service is already predicting financial crisis. Still, although we can't avoid getting old, it is reassuring to know that we can avoid becoming ill and incapacitated. Every time we are physically active and eat healthily we exercise a choice about how fit, healthy and happy we plan to be in later life.

When I get older I would either like to live in a small community such as a village or I would like to get together with some friends and buy a big house where we could all grow old together and club together for care if necessary. I don't know why more young people don't think seriously about old age and set something up for the future while they have money and energy. It seems so short-sighted because you can live for thirty years and more after you retire so you should do what you can to ensure that those years are comfortable and happy. I look at my gran and I am determined not to end up like her, isolated, lonely and quite bitter really. She gave her life to my Grandpa and when he died she had nothing. No friends, no social life, no career, nothing. She has literally shrivelled up since then.
Marsha, 23, US

When I was 8 stone I thought I was fat, then I had kids and I was 15 stone. I really was fat but sometimes I liked myself a lot more than ever before. My mother began me dieting at 13 and the pattern stayed for a long time. I think it is the hardest of all issues to deal with.
Bernie, 45, UK

BODY IMAGE No matter how iron-clad your self-esteem, growing older and broader in the beam in a culture that idolizes 'young' and 'skinny' presents problems. And the notable absence of middle-aged women in advertising and the media leaves older women feeling totally ignored. We see very few positive images of women who have allowed themselves to age naturally, but surgical celebrities such as Cher and Joan Rivers – women who refuse to pass the baton of youth to the generation that rightfully owns it – are omnipresent.

The exponential rise in the number of anti-ageing treatments and cosmetic surgery procedures is testament to a generation of overachievers who will go to any lengths to stay young looking. And with so many promised miracles in pill, diet or surgical applications, it has never been easier for women to divert their unease about ageing into a mission to keep the inevitable at bay.

But although cosmetic or surgical treatments are temporarily effective in a physical sense, women who wage war on the ageing process are usually fighting a losing psychological battle. It is inevitable that if you look for flaws, you will find them. And the cumulative effect of finding faults and trying to fix them is an enormous drain on female energy, intellect and finance. A tendency to focus on the potentially perfect future (once I've had the op) stops women enjoying the perfectly pleasant present.

EVERY WALL IS A DOOR The more useful older women feel to society, the higher their self-esteem. The scrapping of the retirement age suggests that the government now realizes that many people over sixty five are fit, healthy and functioning well past their previous use-by date, and this should eventually provide greater opportunities for women who wish to bridge the gap between full employment and full retirement with less pressurized jobs.

Women over 60 who are healthy and active tend to view growing older as a kind of liberation. They report feeling a great sense of freedom – freedom from parental responsibilities; freedom to ignore society's excessive emphasis on appearance; freedom to pursue new interests, and freedom to speak their minds more frankly. They regret the amount of time and energy they wasted worrying about what they looked like when they were younger and say that retrospectively they can't see what they were worried about. The last word has to go to Blanche, aged 76, who sends this important message to younger women, 'you should value your looks while you have them and stop being so hard on yourself. You are much more beautiful than you give yourself credit for and don't wait until you get to my age to appreciate the fact.'

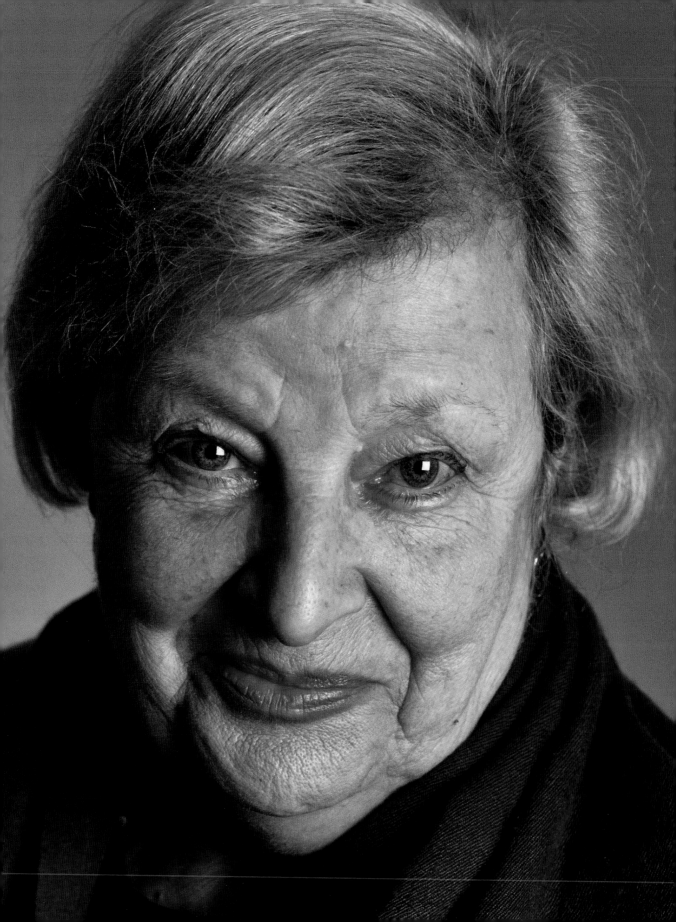

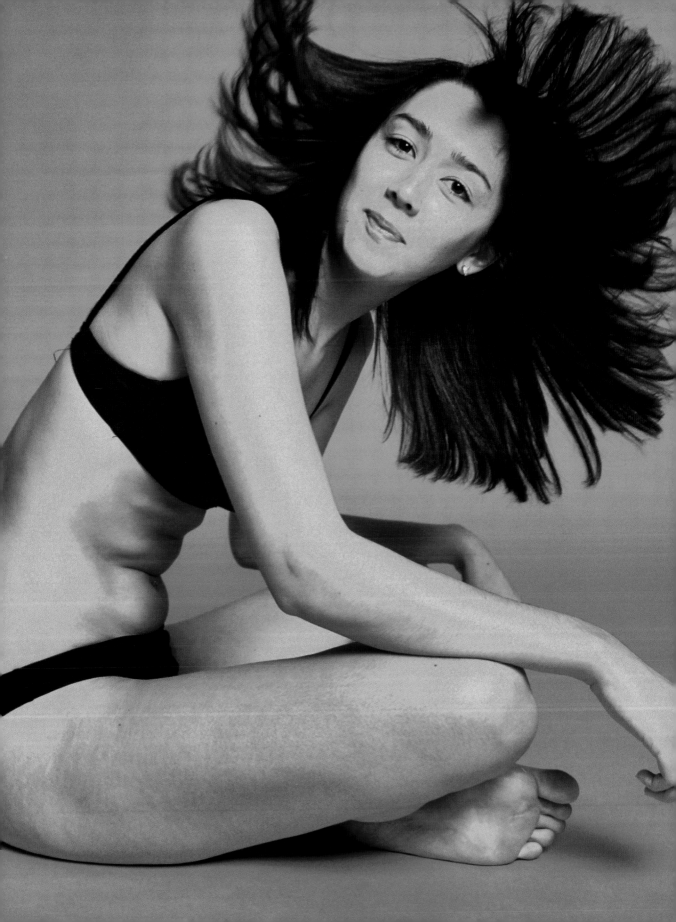

THE *Food* CHAPTER

From quality to quantity

In the 18th century it took an unskilled labourer two hours to earn enough money to buy 1kg (2lb) of grain. At today's minimum wage, it takes about five minutes. Since the agricultural revolution, technological advances and the growth of the agro food industry have increased yields, production and preservation techniques so dramatically that food has never been so plentiful or so cheap. But unfortunately, quantity has not necessarily equated to quality. In the last 50 years food producers have increasingly chosen to transform simple ingredients into chemical concoctions loaded with fat, sugar or salt. And we, the people, have grown inexorably fatter.

Health experts first began to draw attention to the implications of an increasingly processed diet back in the 1970s. Though the link between a diet high in fat, sugar and salt and illnesses like coronary heart disease (the leading cause of death for US and UK women), stroke, cancer, obesity and diabetes was well established, the incidence of these illnesses had increased dramatically. Experts warned the public that death rates would continue to climb unless fats, sweets and alcoholic beverages were consumed in moderation, but the message fell on deaf ears. In 1977, the average woman in the US chomped her way through about 57kg (125lb) of fat, and 45kg (100lb) of sugar. Fruit and vegetable consumption was half what it was in the 1900s, making up only 20% of the daily diet, and soft drink sales had more than doubled in 20 years. As a result, six of the ten leading causes of death in the US were diet related. And Europe was not far behind.

In 1988, the US Department of Agriculture (USDA) devised their famous food pyramid. Widely publicized by health and education authorities, it soon became, and still remains, the globally accepted guideline for healthy eating (in the UK it is called the Balance of Good Health Plate Guide). Designed in a triangular shape, the tiny peak of the pyramid represents fats, oils, sugars and salt, which people are advised to use sparingly. The body of the pyramid is made up of three to five servings of vegetables a day, two to four servings of fruit, two to three servings of milk, yogurt or cheese, two to three servings of meat, fish, poultry, eggs, pulses or nuts. And the base, or bulk, of the pyramid is made up of six to eleven servings of carbohydrates, such as bread, rice, cereal, pasta and noodles daily (p.39).

The pyramid was designed around the principle that an excess of any calories makes a person gain weight, but a diet based on carbohydrates is less likely to because, while a gram of fat contains nine calories, a gram of carbohydrate or protein only contains four calories. Nutritionists concluded that if people could be persuaded to fill up on carbs instead of fats, they would automatically cut their calorie intake in half, and lose weight. Scientists also knew that the body finds it easier to burn carbohydrate for energy and stores fat for later, so in theory, a high carb diet would satisfy energy needs and prevent people getting fat too. The dietary guidelines were widely publicized, though women were the primary target because wives and mothers are usually responsible for shopping, cooking and feeding their family. Since their preferences, and their understanding of what constitutes a healthy balanced diet, heavily influence the diet of their household, it is vital that women are educated about nutrition. However, many women following the US food pyramid found themselves, and their families, getting fatter rather than thinner because nutritionists had failed to anticipate that decreased fat consumption and increased carb consumption would inadvertently lead to a huge increase in sugar intake. As families replaced their traditional breakfast of eggs and bacon with Frosted flakes and a low fat blueberry muffin, the only thing that got healthier was the bank balance of the processed food manufacturer.

Between 1972 and 2000, annual grain consumption increased from 50kg (110lb) to 64kg (141lb) per person, most of it in the form of cereals, bread, muffins, bagels, pancakes, waffles, croissants, crumpets, cakes and biscuits (with butter and jam on top). Then, in 1971, Japanese food scientists found a way to produce high fructose corn syrup (HFCS), a cheaper alternative to sugar, but six times sweeter. This enabled manufacturers to sweeten their grain products more effectively without incurring any extra cost. And as grain was relatively cheap, HFCS enabled food producers to add 'perceived' value by increasing product sizes. However, because the amount of pre-prepared and packaged foods that we consume has increased exponentially in the last thirty years, these increased portions have now become accepted serving sizes. Bagels and croissants are three times larger than they were in the 70s. Muffins, which used to weigh 25g (1oz) now weigh as much as 225g (8oz) and cookies are 700% bigger.

And it gets worse. In the 70s, the fast food industry embarked on another equally dangerous chemical collaboration. The introduction of palm oil, which contains 45% saturated fat, has been a disaster for the global waistline. Fat calories in fried foods shot up overnight, but consumers had no idea because the products still looked and tasted the same. In 1960, a serving of french fries contained 200 calories. By the mid-90s the same portion contained 450 calories. Today, it contains 610 calories – more than 25% of your daily calorie allowance. Because the palm oil revolution came hand in hand with the Americanization of portion sizes, its impact has been particularly significant. In 1955, a single order of French fries weighed in at 60g (2.4oz). Today, an average single serving is 205g (7.1oz) – nearly three times bigger – and all cooked to a crisp in 45% saturated fat. For a genereration of couch potatoes, food technology developments have made obesity less of a possibility and more of an inevitability.

I think it's sickening that GOOD food, vegetables, fruits, whole grain stuff, non processed goods and the like are so expensive and fast food places are so cheap. I work above a large commuter train station with a huge food court and you can't buy a salad for under $6 but you can get a cheeseburger for the change in your pocket. When I was little going to McDonald's or Carvel was a treat – a reward...now there are so many families where parents are working two jobs or there is only one provider in the family working their ass off to keep the family afloat. Junk food is a fast, cheap dinner / breakfast/ lunch option because there is very little other choice.
Jen, 27, USI

I mainly eat junk food when I am sad or out of control with my emotions. I guess it attracts me because it is like the forbidden fruit. I know it is bad for me yet I eat it when I am unhappy.
Sarah, 24, UK

I would like to see more organic fast food places. Organic is the way forwards! There is always a point in eating something good.
Kelly, 24, NZ

As health experts tried to flag up the heinous health implications of saturated fat, the food industry was, as ever, ten paces ahead. 'Fat' became public enemy number one as governments, nutritionists, dieticians, health professionals and the media drummed the 'less-fat-lose-weight' message into public consciousness. But where others saw calamity, manufacturers spied opportunity. Though the key to good health was, and still is, a diet largely based on fresh fruit and vegetables, manufacturers realized that they couldn't push for profit out of produce so they took advantage of public paranoia and began producing thousands of reduced-fat food products such as low fat meats, cheeses, snacks, spreads, sauces, crisps, yogurt, cookies, chocolate and ice cream. Their primary market was the weight-conscious woman. She wouldn't get too excited about a banana, but put the reassuring words low fat on the label and she would happily tuck into a plastic packaged long-life banana muffin with vanilla icing on top. Manufacturers conspired to create a nutritional illusion, a fantasy world where it was possible to eat low fat sweet food and not put on weight. And women bought into it wholesale.

Predictably, the west now finds itself in the midst of an obesity epidemic and unfortunately, women are more negatively affected than any other group. In the US, 34% of adult women are obese compared to 28% of men and, in the UK, 21% of women are obese compared to 17% of men. And obesity related health conditions afflict more women than men. Women who are severely obese are 50 times more likely to develop diabetes. Obesity is implicated in 20% of cancer deaths in women and women who gain about 20kg (45lb) or more after age 18 are twice as likely to develop breast cancer after menopause than women who maintain a healthy body weight. Women are already three times more likely to suffer from osteoarthritis than men. But women who are obese are four times more likely again to develop osteoarthritis than non-obese women. They are three to four times more likely to develop endometrial cancer and gall bladder disease. Obesity has also been found to effect ovulation, response to fertility treatment and pregnancy rates, though infertile women who are obese increase their chance of becoming pregnant if they lose weight. High pre-pregnancy weight is also associated with an increased risk of hypertension, gestational diabetes, Caesarean section delivery and toxaemia.

It is difficult to visualize just how huge the obesity problem is, but if it remains unchecked, it is predicted that almost all Americans will be overweight by 2050. People have tried to lower the amount of fat in their diet (from 40 to 33% in the US), but with so many more hidden calories, the average daily intake of calories has increased from 1854 to 2002 per day. That's only three chocolate biscuits which doesn't sound like a lot, but over a year, those bickies add up to a weight gain of 6.8kg (15lb) which is 300 wobbly pounds of fat over 20 years!

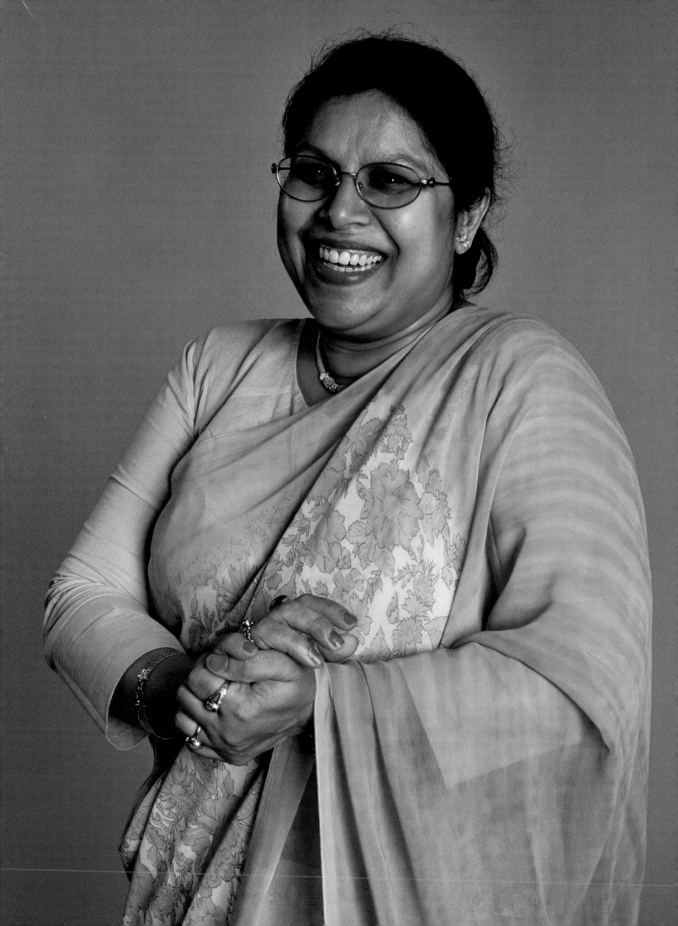

Good fats, bad fats

Though fat gets a lot of bad press we all need some fat in our diet. It helps us store energy, insulates our bodies, cushions organs, helps to make hormones, maintains blood pressure, keeps skin and hair healthy and helps to transport vitamins A, D, E and K through the bloodstream. It is also thought, like sugar, to have an effect on mood. In studies, monkeys fed on high fat diets to study the effects of heart disease became more sociable and groomed themselves and their mates more. And a study of people put on cholesterol lowering drugs and diets found that although it cut deaths from heart disease, it produced a marked increase in deaths from suicides, accidents and fights.

Many fats can be manufactured in the body, but the ones that can't have to be sourced from food and these are called essential fatty acids (EFAs). Understanding the differences between fats can make it easier to decipher labels and work out whether the fat content is helpful or harmful. Helpful fats such as polyunsaturated fats and monounsaturated fats create high-density lipoprotein (HDL), or 'good' cholesterol, which helps to remove low-density lipoprotein (LDL), or 'bad' cholesterol, from the tissues and deliver it to the liver for excretion. Studies show that high levels of HDL cholesterol reduce your risk of heart attack. Fat currently makes up about 39% of our daily calorie intake, but the problem is that most of it is saturated fat and trans fats. Fat has a large, round, smooth molecule, making it very pleasing on the tongue but it doesn't actually taste of much by itself. Fat's real talent is releasing flavour from other foods and giving a great feeling of satiety. Unfortunately, however tasty they are, saturated fats and trans fats cause high levels of LDL, which clog up your arteries, increasing your risk of coronary heart disease, heart attack and stroke.

LOVE POLYUNSATURATED FATS Most polyunsaturated fats are liquid (except nuts) at room temperature, eg. vegetable oils such as corn oil, sunflower oil, safflower oil and walnut oil. These oils are very high in omega-6 polyunsaturates and work to lower levels of bad cholesterol or LDL. They are a rich source of vitamin E, and more importantly they contain EFAs such as linoleic acid (omega-6) and alpha linoleic acid (omega-3), which we need but can't make in our bodies. Sunflower oil, safflower oil, sesame oil, sesame seeds, brazil nuts, pumpkin seeds, almonds, cashew nuts, pistachio nuts, oatcakes and hazelnuts are good sources of omega-6. Evening primrose oil, linseed oil, walnut oil, olive oil, walnuts and pine nuts are good sources of both omega-6 and omega-3. Other EFAs – gammalinolenic acids (GLA) – can be found in starflower oil and evening primrose oil. These can help ease symptoms of PMS and menopause and aid motor coordination. Eicosapentaenoic acid (EPA) and docosahexaenoic acid (DHA) are found in fish and fish oils, which also contain omega-3 and omega-6. Fish and fish oils are particularly beneficial in reducing the stickiness of the blood and its ability to clot. They are also thought to improve intelligence and reduce the risk of depression. In a UK study on the impact of fish oils, violent offences by young prisoners given a course of fish oil supplements fell by 40% and both depressives and manic depressives felt better. In fact some scientists suggest that the phenomenal rise in depression over the last 50 years is directly related to the fall in oily fish consumption. European guidelines suggest one small portion of tuna, mackerel, herring, salmon or trout a week will give you all the EFAs you need.

LOVE MONOUNSATURATED FATS

These fats are usually liquid at room temperature though they can solidify when cooled. Mostly found in olive oil, rapeseed oil (aka canola oil), groundnut oil and sesame oil. They are also present in reasonable quantities in eggs, fish and meat. Mono fats improve or raise levels of HDL (good cholesterol), lower levels of LDL (bad cholesterol) and are rich in vitamin E. A diet rich in mono fats is associated with increased longevity and a lower risk of cancer. Other good sources are olives, avocados, macadamia nuts, hazelnuts, almonds, brazil nuts, bacon, hummus, mackerel and lean minced beef.

HATE SATURATED FATS

These fats are solid at room temperature and are found in the largest quantities in meat, cream, cheese, eggs, butter, lard, milk chocolate, pies, pastry, cakes, biscuits and basically anything that you quite fancy snacking on right now. A diet high in saturated fat has been proven to raise levels of the bad blood cholesterol LDL and is a major risk factor in heart disease, cancer and obesity. Currently, saturated fat makes up about 15% of our total calorie intake and that figure needs to be cut by a third to substantially reduce the risk of coronary heart disease. Natural saturated fats such as butter and cheese are not as harmful as the saturated fats found in processed foods because although they raise levels of bad LDL, they also raise levels of good HDL simultaneously.

DESPISE TRANS FATS

Trans fats are even worse for you than saturated fats. They are unsaturated fats that have been modified or hydrogenated during food processing making them hard at room temperature. A large USA trial has shown that trans fats are the only type of fat that not only raise the levels of bad cholesterol LDL, but also lower the levels of good cholesterol HDL. The amount of trans fat in a product is sometimes listed on the label but in general hard margarines and cooking fats contain the highest concentrations. Trans fats are mainly consumed in mass-produced baked goods such as digestive biscuits, cakes, puddings, sweets, chocolate bars, soft margarines, and take away foods like fish and chips. Even some 'health' foods contain trans fats. If you see the words 'partially hydrogenated' in the ingredients, the product contains trans fat.

How to reduce fat

- Avoid fried foods.
- Use olive oil instead of butter. The calories are similar but olive oil has only 1.8g of saturated fat per tbsp; butter has 7g.
- Use fish or skinless poultry instead of meat. Removing the skin from 100g (4oz) of cooked chicken removes nearly 5g of fat (1.3g saturated).
- Cut the fat off meat. Use extra lean mince meat. 75g (3oz) raw fatty hamburger meat can have nearly 23g (1oz) of fat (9g saturated). 91% lean beef contains only 8g of fat (3g saturated).
- Switch to skimmed milk. 225ml (8fl oz) of whole milk contains close to 8g of fat (5g saturated). 225ml (8fl oz) of skimmed milk has less than 0.5g fat.
- Use non-fat plain yogurt instead of sour cream. 225ml (8fl oz) contains 40g (1¼oz) fat (32g (1½oz) saturated), and 200mg of cholesterol. 225ml (8fl oz) skimmed-milk plain yogurt contains 0.5 g fat and only 4mg of cholesterol.
- Use natural peanut butter. Regular peanut butter is made with hydrogenated oils.
- Choose Parmesan or extra-sharp Cheddar. 1tbsp of Parmesan contains only 2g fat (1g saturated).

The sugar rush

I think laziness and lack of personal motivation has a lot to answer for. As people have made it to affluence, they declare their children will never, 'Suffer the hardships they had to.' Those hardships include going without takeaways, sugar and getting everything they want.
Ashling, 28, US

I have two kids who are incredibly skinny. I do my best trying to get them to eat healthy food and their basic diet is not bad but my problem is that in between meals they will eat whole packets of biscuits and sweets and because they really are so thin I don't stop them. I wish I could get them to fill up on bananas but they won't.
Justine, 42, UK

I think I am a carb addict. If I try and cut them out I end up dreaming about big thick slices of crusty white bread and butter or a moist chocolate cake with filling. Mmm.
Laura, 28, Ireland

My partner has recently been diagnosed as diabetic. The doctor believes that years of drinking too much alcohol has destroyed his capacity to control his blood sugar levels.
Patricia, 64, UK

Like fats, all carbohydrates are not the same either. They can be broken down into two different compounds; sugars, which are known as simple carbohydrates, and starches, which are known as complex carbohydrates.

SUGARS Sugars are called simple carbohydrates because your body digests them quickly and easily. They are usually sweet, e.g. biscuits, sweets, cakes, fizzy drinks. The sugars from simple carbohydrates are absorbed into your bloodstream much faster, and while they provide energy very quickly they are often combined with lots of fat and don't have much nutritional value. The World Health Authority (WHO) recommends that sugars should only form 10% of our diet, 11% if you don't drink alcohol. For an average woman that adds up to two chocolate biscuits (24g sugar) and one can of coke (36g of sugar) per day, so, not much. Fruits contain natural sugars (fructose) and they are a better bet if you need an energy boost because they don't contain fat and also provide lots of essential vitamins and minerals.

STARCHES Starches are known as complex carbohydrates. Unrefined starches take longer to digest and provide a more balanced source of energy. Wholegrains and unrefined cereals, such as brown rice, wholegrain bread, oats, barley, fresh vegetables, fruits, nuts and pulses, are 'intact' carbohydrates, which means they contain fibre, vitamins, minerals and phytochemicals. Refined carbohydrates, such as white flour, white bread and white rice, are a less healthy option because the healthy bran and germ layers are removed during production, and with them go many nutrients, like vitamins, minerals, and fibre. 'White' starches such as white flour, white bread, rice, noodles, pasta and potatoes behave in a very similar way to sugars once they are in the bloodstream.

CARBOHYDRATES AND BLOOD SUGAR When you eat carbohydrates your body breaks them down into glucose, a form of sugar that is transported to the cells in your body via the bloodstream. Glucose gives your body an immediate rush of energy, but your cells can only use a small amount of it at one time. When the levels of glucose or sugar in your blood get too high, your pancreas secretes the hormone insulin. This regulates your blood sugar levels and shunts any excess glucose away to the muscles and the liver where it is stored as glycogen.

Glycogen is your back-up fuel reserve. It can be called on as an energy source when the glucose in your blood stream runs out. When there is enough glycogen stored in the muscles and the liver, insulin turns any excess energy into fat, which can be turned back into energy if necessary. When insulin levels are high it means there is too much sugar in the blood. It is only when insulin levels are low or depleted, i.e. energy from the blood, liver and muscles has been used up, that our bodies actually begin to burn the reserves we store as fat as fuel for energy. The fatter we get, and the more carbohydrates we eat, the more insulin our pancreas has to pump out per meal in an effort to get rid of the sugar in our blood. Because we eat so regularly, insulin levels and blood sugar are rarely allowed to get low enough, so we never get around to burning fat as fuel. As we gain weight, the extra insulin our pancreas has to produce makes it easier to store fat and harder to lose it. Because ever greater amounts of insulin are required to keep blood sugar in check, our cells eventually become less sensitive to its action. Over time, these powerful surges of insulin exhaust the pancreas to the point where diabetes can develop.

THE SNACK ATTACK Insulin also has a significant effect on hunger and tiredness. It works in the brain to suppress hunger – when insulin levels are high, your brain realizes that your body doesn't need any more energy. However, if your brain loses its sensitivity to insulin, just as your cells do when they are flooded with it, then the higher insulin production that comes with getting fatter no longer compensates by suppressing your appetite. So, although insulin is meant to suppress appetite, too much of it actually has the opposite effect. After two or three hours, large amounts of insulin bring blood sugar levels crashing down. At this point, people feel tired and get a strong urge to snack in an effort to boost their flagging energy levels.

After a snack, blood sugar rises again, insulin levels increase, more fat is stored but then insulin levels drop and tiredness and hunger set in. The problem with carbohydrates, particularly sugars and starches like cakes, biscuits, white bread, white rice, potatoes, pasta and noodles, is that they seem to have a much bigger impact on insulin levels and blood sugar than was previously thought. They are known as high glycaemic index carbohydrates, which means they are absorbed quickly into the blood and as a result, they cause a spike of blood sugar and a surge of insulin within minutes but within a few hours your blood sugar is lower than it was before you ate. Your body effectively thinks it has run out of fuel, but the insulin levels are still high enough to prevent you from burning your own fat. The result is hunger and a craving for more carbohydrates.

HOW TO BALANCE YOUR BLOOD SUGAR Eat regularly and exercise. If you eat three balanced meals a day you are less likely to snack and if you avoid processed, refined and sweet foods and concentrate on wholegrains, you will release the energy from your food more slowly. Exercise helps to balance your blood sugar by using up reserves of glucose and glycogen, thereby decreasing the amount of insulin your body is required to make.

I eat too much fat and too much chocolate and sugar. I dislike most fruits and veg so I have little choice of healthy eating alternatives. Because I don't eat a lot of fruit and veg, I take a multi-vitamin. I also go to the gym, which raises my immune system and energy levels. I think they allow me to lead an active lifestyle without getting sick.
Kelly, 24, NZ

If I am really tired, I will have a coffee and some chocolate or biscuits to boost my energy levels. I don't normally eat sweet things but I do find sugar, particularly chocolate, is a great way of picking myself up. I try to choose better quality chocolate with 70% cocoa because I know it contains less sugar.
Erika, 28, UK

When I need something sweet I choose a diet soda or something like diet Kick which is a stimulation drink. It gives me the buzz and the sweet taste too.
Parki, 28, UK

I always feel incredibly sleepy after I eat. It happens when I am at work a lot, which is bad because I have to do so many business lunches. I have to have double espressos to keep going.
Laura, 25, UK

The glycaemic index

Scientists have known for decades that sugary foods are quickly digested and lead to a rapid rise in blood sugar, but until relatively recently it was thought that starches such as potatoes, rice and pasta elevated blood sugar levels more gradually. However in 1981, Dr David Jenkins, a professor of nutrition at the University of Toronto, discovered that this was not necessarily true. While trying to establish the type of foods that were best for people suffering from diabetes he found that foods such as potatoes actually led to a very rapid rise in blood sugar, while some foods high in sugars appeared to elevate blood sugar more slowly. This led to the development of the glycaemic index (GI), a scale that determines the immediate rise in blood sugar that occurs after you eat a food high in carbohydrate. Foods that digest rapidly and lead to a fast release of glucose are known as high glycaemic index foods. Foods that digest more slowly are known as low glycaemic index foods.

The original index was based on measuring levels of sugar in the blood after drinking 50g (2oz) of pure glucose. Volunteers were then fed one food at a time and their blood sugar rise was measured and a value was placed on the food related to the rise caused by glucose. The results were weird. Baked potatoes, the dieter's staple, turned out to have a higher glycaemic index than table sugar while brown rice had a glycaemic index of 55 compared to a Mars bar, which had a rating of 40. Obviously you'd have to be two Scotch eggs short of a picnic to believe that a sugar-laden Mars bar is healthier than brown rice with its high fibre, vitamin and mineral content, so the scientists went back to the drawing board. They soon worked out that the readings were incorrect because they didn't factor in serving sizes. The system was updated and is now known as the glycaemic load (GL). Though it still evaluates how much sugar-raising carbohydrate there is in a serving of a particular food, it gauges levels by the amount you are likely to eat too. This means that foods like watermelon, which has a high GI because the starches and fruit sugars push blood sugar up quickly, gets a low GL because the reality is that there is only a very small amount of those sugars in a serving. Diets filled with high glycaemic index foods have been linked to an increased risk for both diabetes and heart disease, so the WHO recommends a diet based on low GI/low GL foods.

CHOOSING LOW GL AND LOW GI FOODS There are a few simple ways to avoid the sugar rush, sugar crash. In general, carbohydrates that are high in fibre tend to have a lower GI than their more highly processed counterparts. Choose a wide variety of non-starchy vegetables such as greens, beans, pulses, salads and tomatoes. Replace refined foods such as white bread, white rice, pasta and noodles with wholegrain products such as wholegrain bread, brown rice, oats and barley. Limit starchy vegetables such as potatoes or combine them with lean proteins and fibre, which release energy more slowly.

Healthy eating pyramid

A NEW APPROACH The indications of the glycaemic index have led many experts to question the wisdom of a food pyramid which places such an enormous emphasis on carbohydrates (p.30). Chief spokesperson for this new way of thinking is Professor Walter Willets of Harvard Medical School. He believes that for up to 30–40% of the population, low fat, high carbohydrate diets are counter-productive and actually make people gain weight. After decades of research, Professor Willets has developed an alternative called the Healthy Eating Pyramid. The quantities below are per day. Look in the side columns for a guide to servings.

USE SPARINGLY Eat potatoes, white bread, pasta and white rice in minimal quantities. Use red meat and butter sparingly. They contain more saturated fat than other proteins. Avoid processed or preserved meats, which contain high levels of salt, preservative and saturated fat. Alcohol can be drunk in moderation as it has been shown to reduce the risk of heart disease and stroke.

TWO SERVINGS OF FIRST-CLASS PROTEINS Protein is a combination of chemicals called amino acids, which help to make haemoglobin, which oxygenates the blood. Protein also makes antibodies that fight infection. It builds and repairs body tissue so it is essential for good skin, glossy hair, creating muscle and healing wounds. First-class proteins such as meat, fish, poultry, eggs and dairy contain all the essential amino acids your body needs. Oily fish (kipper, mackerel, salmon, sardine, fresh tuna) are low fat, low calorie and contain omega-3 polyunsaturated fatty acids. Just one portion of fish a week helps to prevent heart disease, stroke, certain cancers and arthritis and may ward off depression. Shellfish contain zinc, iodine, magnesium and B vitamins but prawns are relatively high in cholesterol and salt and only crabmeat and mussels contain significant amounts of omega-3 fats and fatty acids. Most fish also contain the antioxidant selenium. Choose wild, organic and undyed fresh fish and avoid smoked varieties, which may be carcinogenic. The UK Department of Health recommends a daily protein intake of 1.5g per kilo of body weight (95g for a woman who weighs 64kg (10st)). However, the recent popularity and low cost of high protein diets (p.87) means many women are consuming three to five times that amount despite the fact that an excess of animal protein has been linked to kidney damage and osteoporosis.

THREE SERVINGS OF SECOND-CLASS PROTEINS Second-class proteins such as nuts, seeds and pulses (adzuki, broad beans, chick-peas, haricot beans, brown and green lentils and soya beans) don't contain all the essential amino acids your body needs. Pulses need to be combined with grains, nuts or seeds, e.g. hummus with pitta bread or beans on toast, to form a complete protein block. Plant proteins should be eaten one to three times per day. They are

What is a serving?

Carbs
1 slice of bread
½ hamburger bun
½ English muffin
6 small crackers
½ cup cooked cereal
¾–1 cup dry cereal
½ cup rice, pasta or potatoes.

Veg
½ cup of cooked or chopped raw vegetables
1 cup leafy raw vegetable

Fruit
1 whole medium fruit
2 small fruits
e.g. plums, satsumas
½ a larger fruit
e.g. mango, papaya
Large slice of a big fruit
e.g. pineapple, melon
½ cup fresh berries
½ cup canned fruit
125ml (4fl oz) juice
⅓ cup dried fruit
1 tbsp dried fruit
3 tbsp stewed or canned fruit

Dairy
225ml (8fl oz) milk
225ml (8fl oz) yogurt
25–50g (1–2oz) hard cheese

Protein
50–75g (2–3oz) lean meat
50–75g (2–3oz) lean fish or poultry

For vegetarians
1 egg
= 25g (1oz) meat
= ½ cup cooked dry beans
= 25g (1oz) meat

rich in heart-healthy nutrients and unsaturated fats. Pulses are low in fat, high in complex carbohydrate, low on the glycaemic index and a rich source of soluble fibre, which lowers blood cholesterol, iron and vitamin B. They are also a valuable source of vitamins, minerals and zinc for vegetarians or people who are non-dairy eaters. Soya beans are one of the few plant proteins that contain all the essential amino acids. They also contain phyto-oestrogens, which are thought to lessen symptoms of menopause (p.275). Dried pulses need lengthy soaking but tins of low salt, low sugar pulses need no preparation. Nuts contain iron, zinc and magnesium and have been shown to lower the risk of developing heart disease. They have a high fat content and are high calorie, but it is mostly unsaturated fat. Sunflower and pumpkin seeds are full of minerals and polyunsaturated fats.

THREE SERVINGS OF VEG AND THREE OF FRUIT

Vegetables and fruits decrease your risk of heart attack or stroke, protect against cancer, lower blood pressure and guard against certain intestinal and eye diseases. Most nutrients are found in dark green, leafy vegetables and yellow, orange and red fruits. The cancer-fighting component lycopene enters the bloodstream more easily from cooked tomatoes. Variety is important because veg and fruit contain different micronutrients. Some prepared salads itemize how many servings of fruit and vegetables they contain. A glass of juice counts as one serving of fruit. A multivitamin pill is recommended, but it is not a substitute for fresh produce.

OILS AS NECESSARY
Plant oils (olive, canola, soy, corn, peanut and vegetable) provide monounsaturated fats, essential fatty acids and vitamin E.

UP TO FIVE SERVINGS OF WHOLEGRAIN FIBRE

Intact or coarsely ground wholegrains provide more nutrients and fibre than refined grains and should be eaten at most meals. Women consume an average of 13g (½oz) of fibre a day but UK health authorities recommend 24g (1oz) a day (approximately 3.5 servings of All Bran). Wholegrains, brown rice, corn, vegetables, pulses, beans, barley, bran, wholemeal bread, peas, prunes, shredded wheat, mango, papaya, Brussels sprouts and apricots are good sources. Fibre comes in two different forms. Insoluble fibre (cellulose) is mainly found in plants (wheat, corn, rice, vegetables and pulses) and cannot be digested. It passes straight to the bowel where it bulks up stools, speeds their passage through the bowel and helps prevent constipation, haemorrhoids, bowel cancer, diverticulitis and irritable bowel syndrome. Because it swells in the stomach it can also help you feel full. Soluble fibre, which comes from apples and citrus fruits, helps to control blood sugar levels by slowing absorption and studies show that it can also decrease levels of LDL, the bad cholesterol.

AND EXERCISE FOR ONE HOUR EVERY DAY!

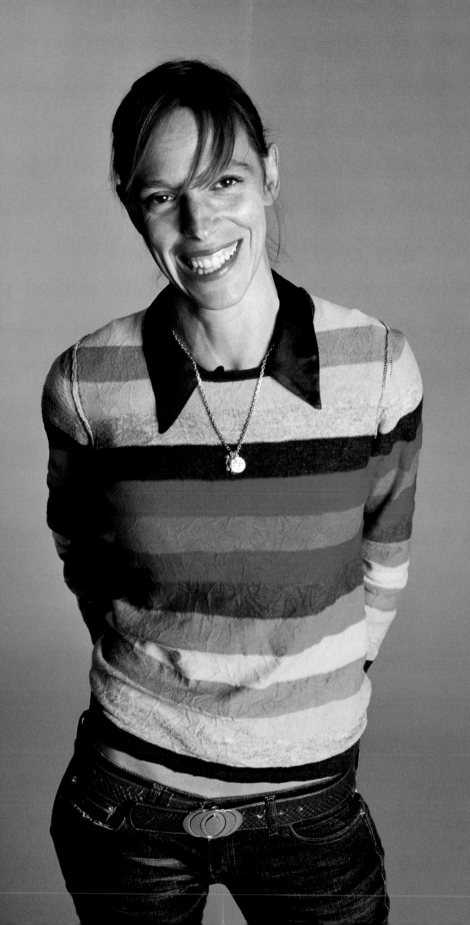

Vitamins from food

Preserving nutrients

• If stored at normal temperatures, concentrations of some vitamins can decrease by 50% within seven days of harvesting. If you consider how long it takes for produce to be harvested, imported, stored and eventually bought, you can understand why leaving it for another week before you eat it doesn't make much sense. Vegetables such as broccoli, turnip greens and salad greens, retain nutrients best when refrigerated at near-freezing temperatures in moisture-proof bags which maintain some humidity.

• Steaming vegetables retains nutrients best. If cooking in liquid use less than 60ml (2fl oz), cover the pot with a tight fitting lid and cook till tender, not soggy. Leave the lid off the cabbage family for the first 5–10 minutes to allow the sulphur to escape. If you cook cabbage in ⅓ water to the amount of cabbage, 90% of the vitamin C will be retained. When you use large amounts of water, retention of vitamin C drops to below 50 per cent.

Since our bodies can't make vitamins we have to get them from food. There are two types: fat soluble and water soluble. *Fat-soluble* vitamins like A, D, E and K are stored in the fat tissues and in your liver until you need them. Some last a few days, others last up to six months. *Water-soluble* vitamins travel through the bloodstream and any excess not required gets passed in urine so they need to be replaced more often. Vitamin C, the big group of B vitamins and pantothenic acid are all soluble.

VITAMIN A (Fat-soluble) Also known as Retinol, Vitamin A aids eyesight, growth and skin condition. Pregnant women should not take vitamin A supplements as they risk damaging their baby and they should avoid liver, which is rich in vitamin A. Sources: liver, cod liver oil, carrots, mangos, sweet potatoes, apricots and milk.

THE B VITAMINS (Water-soluble) The B vitamins help make energy and set it free when your body needs it. They are also involved in making red blood cells, which carry oxygen throughout your body and stop your skin looking dull. They are important for people who smoke, drink or suffer from stress (that's just about everyone then). As the 16 different B vitamins can't be made or stored in the body you need to include some of the following foods in your regular diet: pork, nuts or bacon for vitamin B1 (thiamine); offal, dairy or breakfast cereal for vitamin B2 (riboflavin); meat, fish or cereal for vitamin B3 (niacin); eggs, meat, fish, wholegrains or cereals for vitamin B6 (pyridoxine); offal, meat, dairy or seaweed for vitamin B12. Vitamin B6 is thought to ease the symptoms of PMS but in 1997 supplements containing over 10mg were banned because of a link with nerve damage.

VITAMIN D (Fat-soluble) Vital for strong bones and teeth, it also helps calcium and phosphorus absorption. Deficiency is linked to osteoarthritis. Ten minutes sunlight a day helps your skin to manufacture vitamin D but women who veil their faces or are confined indoors may need to increase D in their diet. Sources: milk, cod liver oil, salmon, herring fillet, fresh tuna, bran flakes and eggs.

VITAMIN K (Fat-soluble) This vitamin helps your blood to clot. Sources: dark green vegetables like broccoli, spinach, lettuce, cabbage and cheese.

FOLIC ACID (Water-soluble) Folate is one of the B-group vitamins. Vital for the formation of blood cells and physical development. Because 47% of UK women are folate deficient, flour is now fortified with it. Women planning a pregnancy should take a 400mg supplement of folic acid (= six servings of broccoli) every day up until the 12th week of pregnancy, to help prevent neural tube defects, or spina bifida, in an unborn baby. Sources: yeast extract, chicken livers, purple sprouting broccoli, green leafy veg, wholegrains, nuts, pulses and breakfast cereals.

Antioxidants from food

Antioxidant vitamins and minerals protect our bodies from 'free radical' (p.139) tissue damage, help maintain healthy organs and good skin, decrease the risk of cancer, lower blood pressure, protect against heart disease and heart attack.

BETA CAROTENE (Water-soluble) A class of yellow to red pigment that can be converted to vitamin A in the body. It is an anti-cancer anti-inflammatory, which protects the skin. Women who smoke should not take beta carotene supplements as they have been linked to an increased cancer risk. Sources: carrots, sweet potato, mango, cabbage, tomatoes, apricots, nectarines, cantaloupe, broccoli, spinach, curly kale and spring greens.

SELENIUM Necessary for growth and development, regulates thyroid hormones, preserves tissue elasticity, slows down ageing and hardening of tissues and helps treat dandruff. Increased intake decreases the risk of breast, colon, lung and prostate cancer but if you take it with the plant-derived chemical sulfurophane seleniums cancer prevention properties become 13 times more powerful. Selenium sources: Brazil nuts, tuna fish, sunflower seeds and lamb's liver. Sulfurophane sources: broccoli, sprouts, cabbage, watercress and rocket salad.

VITAMIN C (Water-soluble) Helps build connective muscle tissue, aids bones, teeth and gums, increases iron absorption and helps your body resist infection. If you are stressed, a smoker, a heavy drinker, have bad skin, or work in a polluted environment, you should boost vitamin C intake by an extra 35mg a day. Sources: oranges, tangerines, lemons, grapefruit, honeydew melon, watermelon, strawberries and raspberries, broccoli, tomatoes, peas and green peppers.

VITAMIN E (Fat-soluble) Helps store vitamin A. Aids vitamin K with blood clotting. It is great for your complexion and can reduce osteoarthritis pain. A 1997 UK trial found vitamin E intake between 268mg and 537mg reduced the risk of non-fatal heart attack by 77 per cent. People on anti-coagulant drugs like warfarin should not take vitamin E supplements as they thin the blood. Buy vitamin E labelled as D alpha-tocopherol, the active natural compound. Synthetic versions are less effective. Current RDA is thought to be too low, so boost your intake of vegetable oils, nuts, avocados, sun-dried tomatoes, almonds, sunflower seeds and cereals.

ZINC An antioxidant mineral necessary for protein synthesis, wound healing, reproductive development, tissue function, blood stability, digestion and metabolism of phosphorus. Lack of zinc can result in delayed sexual maturity, stretch marks, fatigue, decreased alertness, susceptibility to infections, prolonged healing and those mysterious white spots that appear on your fingernails. Sources: meat, shellfish.

- *Microwaving destroys most nutrients. Spinach has 60% vitamin C retention when cooked in water and 25% vitamin C when microwaved. If you microwave veg, use little or no water to conserve nutrients.*

- *Most frozen veg is frozen immediately after harvest when nutrient concentrations are at their highest. Studies show that the vitamin C content in cooked frozen peas is comparable with raw peas. Frozen vegetables stored at 0° lose from ⅓ to ¾ of their vitamin content if stored for a year.*

- *When preparing foods for the freezer, cook thoroughly, cool quickly, then freeze when cold. When defrosting foods, thaw at room temperature or defrost overnight in the fridge. Reheat foods thoroughly and throw away anything not used within 24 hours.*

- *Fruit and vegetables can be kept in the freezer for a maximum of six months. Store soups or purées with milk or cream for two months max. Store fish for three months max. Store meat/poultry (either raw or made up into dishes) for three months max.*

The A to Z of vegetables

ASPARAGUS Contains vitamin E and anti-inflammatory glycosides, which may ease arthritis. A natural diuretic. Can help with premenstrual bloating.

AVOCADO A very complete food, a great source of vitamin E and many other minerals and vitamins. It is high in monounsaturated fats and is great for your skin.

BROAD BEANS Packed with vitamins and minerals, they are a great source of soluble fibre, which helps lower blood cholesterol. They also contain the flavonoid quercetin, which helps lower cholesterol and improves lung function.

BROCCOLI High in fibre. Contains beta carotene, vitamin c, sulfurophane and is rich in folate. It also contains phytochemicals, which reduce the risk of cancer.

BRUSSELS SPROUTS Contain fibre, folate, vitamin C, sulfurophane and phytochemicals as do the dark green leaves of savoy cabbage.

CARROTS A rich source of beta carotene and vitamin A.

CHILLIS Contain high levels of capsaicin, a natural pain killer. They also appear to stimulate metabolic rate, lower cholesterol, relieve congestion and aid digestion.

FRENCH BEANS French and runner beans contain the antioxidants beta carotene and vitamin C and are a good source of fibre.

GARLIC Contains allicin, which has antibiotic and antifungal properties. It also contains sulphides, which may prevent cancers, and an antioxidant that lowers cholesterol and prevents clotting.

GREEN PEPPERS One of the best sources of vitamin C. Red peppers are higher in beta carotene and rich in vitamin C. They also contain capsaicin, which may be useful for people with arthritic pain(see chillis above).

KALE/SPRING GREENS A good source of beta carotene, vitamin C and vitamin E and high in phytochemicals which reduce the risk of cancer.

ONIONS Thought to help lower cholesterol, blood pressure and prevent clotting. Helps ward off colds and flu. Also contains quercetin which helps prevent coronary heart disease. The green portion contains folate and beta carotene.

PEAS Frozen or fresh, peas are a good source of vitamin C.

SPINACH Contains lutein, which protects the eyes and may help reduce the risk of colon cancer. Rich in folate, which reduces the risk of neural tube defects in unborn babies. In traditional medicine, it was used to treat constipation, high blood pressure and anaemia. Excellent source of carotenoids, iron, vitamin K, oxalic acid, folates, vitamins C and E, calcium, potassium and magnesium.

SQUASH Butternut squash, pumpkins and orange-fleshed sweet potatoes are rich in carotenoids and antioxidants and contain vitamins C and E.

TOMATOES Rich in lycopene, the antioxidant phytochemical that helps prevent heart disease and cancers. Lycopene is more potent in cooked and canned tomatoes than it is in fresh tomatoes. Also contains beta carotene, vitamin C and E.

WATERCRESS Contains antioxidants, minerals, sulfurophane and phenethyl isothiocyanate, which, in large amounts, fights tobacco-induced lung cancer.

The A to Z of fruits

APPLES Low on the glycaemic index so they give a more balanced and more sustained energy boost. A good source of vitamin C when fresh. Contain quercetin which helps lower cholesterol and improve lung function.

APRICOTS Dried or fresh, high in beta carotene, low on the glycaemic index.

BANANAS Bananas are rich in potassium and an excellent source of vitamin B6, which is needed to make serotonin in the brain. Serotonin helps to reduce pain, depress appetite and make you feel more relaxed. Traditionally used to treat stomach ulcers. Rich in carbohydrate, so high in calories – 1 banana = 95 calories.

BLACKBERRIES Contain vitamin E and ellagic acid. which has been shown to halt tumour growth in the lungs, oesophagus, breast, cervix and tongue.

BLACKCURRANTS 100g (4oz) of blackcurrants contain 200mg of vitamin C – five times the RDA for adults. Also contains the antioxidant lutein.

CHERRIES Contain ellagic acid and anthocyanins which relieve pain.

CRANBERRIES Known to prevent and treat cystitis and urinary tract infections. Recent research indicates that drinking three glasses of cranberry juice a day can cut the risk of coronary heart disease by up to 40 per cent.

GRAPES Contain ellagic acid and polyphenols, which reduce heart disease.

KIWI FRUIT Contains a pigment called chlorophyll, which may reduce the risk of cancer. One fruit has more than the adult's daily requirement of vitamin C.

MANGOES Rich in soluble fibre and vitamins E and C. The best source of antioxidant carotenoids, so may protect against some cancers, such as colon and cervical. A study looking at the diets of a large group of women showed a link between those eating a carotenoid-rich diet and a reduced risk of cervical cancer.

MELONS Cantaloupe or orange- or red-fleshed melons contain vitamin C and beta carotene and carotenoids, which, besides being able to protect body cells against damage from free radicals, can also be converted into vitamin A in the body. Vitamin A is needed to maintain a healthy immune system, healthy skin and good vision in dim light. Watermelons contain lycopene, which has been shown to act as an anti-cancer agent. A slice of watermelon is equivalent to a glass of water.

ORANGES One orange contains your entire daily vitamin C allowance. Also contain phytochemicals called hesperidin, which protect against damage from free radicals. A good source of pectin, which can lower blood cholesterol. Rich in folate.

PAPAYAS Rich in beta carotene, soluble fibre and enzymes that aid digestion.

PLUMS Contain a phytochemical called ferulic acid, which reduces the risk of colon cancer. Rich in fibre and potassium.

RASPBERRIES One of the best fruit sources of fibre. Contain vitamin C.

STRAWBERRIES Full of vitamin C and ellagic acid. Usually eaten quickly before vitamin C is lost. Eight strawberries a day provide a fifth of a woman's folate requirement. A US study showed that strawberries reduced the effects of carcinogens in tobacco smoke. Thought to have anti-bacterial properties.

As you get older you become more aware of what your body needs. As you hit 40 you realize that what you have now may be it. You start weighing up what you have in your hands right now. I think I have become more conscious of my health in the last couple of years. I am aware of the creaks beginning and I am trying to pay more attention to nutrition.
Alison, 42, UK

At my school there is just nothing that I want to eat at lunchtime. It all looks so manky. The salads are covered in salad cream and if there is any fruit it is all bruised. They manage to make it so unappetizing that I usually end up eating biscuits.
Scarlet, 13, UK

When I eat salad, vegetables and fruit for lunch at work I feel virtuous and clean. Then I go outside with the girls and have a cigarette and a coffee and ruin it all.
Camilla, 26, UK

I pay so little attention to the vitamins, minerals and proteins in my diet that it is ridiculous. Occasionally I have an apple but hardly ever. I just can't be bothered but I am fit as a fiddle as I do a lot of sport.
Ant, 37, UK

Minerals from food

CALCIUM Helps build strong bones and teeth. Assists in blood clotting and nerve function. You should get all the calcium you need from your daily diet (700 mg a day) but menopausal women should boost their intake with fish or dark green leafy veg. If you take calcium supplements you should also take magnesium. Sources: milk, cheese and yogurt (but try to choose skimmed milk or low fat versions).

COPPER Helps produce red and white blood cells and triggers the release of iron to form haemoglobin – the substance that carries oxygen around the body. It is thought to be important for infant growth, brain development, the immune system and for strong bones. Sources: green vegetables, fish and liver

FLUORIDE Supports bone mineralization and protects against dental decay. Very large amounts can cause mottled and crumbling teeth and changes to the bones (fluorosis). Found in few foods but routinely added to toothpaste and some water supplies, where the fluoride content is low (about 1 part per million).

IODINE Used to make thyroid hormones, which control many metabolic activities. Insufficient iodine is rare but can make you feel lethargic and lead to swelling of the thyroid gland in the neck. Too much depletes zinc and is toxic. Sources: milk and seafood.

IRON Required for the formation of haemoglobin in red blood cells, which transports oxygen around the body. Too little can lead to anaemia. Vitamin C aids iron absorption. Phytate (in cereals and pulses), fibre, tannins and calcium can reduce absorption. Sources: red meat, liver and dried beans, baked potato with skin, apricots, enriched or wholegrain breads, cereals and raisins.

MAGNESIUM Helps regulate heart rhythm and is present in all tissues including bone. Necessary for calcium and Vitamin C metabolism. Helps convert blood sugar to energy. Sources: wholegrains, nuts, seeds, green veg, instant coffee.

PHOSPHORUS An essential component of all cells, present in bones, teeth and the skeleton. Sources: milk, cheese, meat, fish and eggs.

POTASSIUM Found in body fluids and essential for the functioning of cells and nerves. Sources: in almost all fresh fruit (bananas in particular) and vegetables.

SODIUM Helps regulate body water content. Involved in energy utilization and nerve function. Routinely added to processed foods so the average woman's intake is 7.6g per day. It should be 6g. Too much salt can cause high blood pressure.

Dietary supplements

TOO MUCH OF A GOOD THING As our awareness of healthy eating has grown, so too has our consumption of dietary supplements. In the UK, 12 million people use some form of herbal supplement and the over-the-counter market is currently worth about £277 million a year (not including sales from health food shops and mail order). In the US, a survey developed with the US Food and Drug Administration (FDA) estimated that 158 million consumers spend approximately $8.5 billion per year on dietary supplements. Yet there is very little evidence that taking supplements actually works. Labelling restrictions mean vitamins, minerals and herbal supplements can't make actual health claims. Since these products can't even say what they are supposed to treat, and since most consumers don't have the PhD in chemistry required to really read the labels, it would be fair to say that the sucess of this industry has to be a reflection of public paranoia about health. Naturally, adult women, the most weight conscious, health conscious, self-conscious strand of our society are both the biggest consumers and the primary target for advertising.

Because most of these products are bought on impulse, they are generally positioned by the till or on the counter in pharmacies or supermarkets where a woman who feels a bit run down will make a spontaneous decision to add a jar of iron to her basket. But women who routinely use herbal cures without getting advice from a nutritionist or doctor are often unaware that boosting consumption of one nutrient can interfere with others. For example, iron supplements can impede the absorption of zinc and vitamin E. Taking high levels of zinc may mean you also need to take copper, and calcium supplements need to be taken with magnesium as they work together. The Department of Health in the UK says that supplements should only be taken after medical advice has been sought because long-term use of substances, particularly vitamin B6, beta carotene, niacin, zinc, manganese and phosphorus, are thought to pose a serious health risk, particulary to anyone who smokes or is on prescription medication.

THE EXCEPTION TO THE RULE Doctors recommend that women who are trying to get pregnant or who are pregnant should take folate, and iron is prescribed for anaemia. Menopausal women may be advised to take calcium and women over 65 can sometimes need vitamin D too. Doctors will also consider recommending supplements to women who have a disease of the liver, gall bladder, intestine or pancreas; who have had surgery on their digestive tract; who have a poor diet or are on a very low calorie diet; who suffer from severe food allergies; are vegetarian or vegan; are on large amounts of antibiotics, laxatives or diuretics that interfere with nutrient absorption; who smoke or drink alcohol excessively; or who don't get 15 minutes of sun each day on their skin.

I have every vitamin and mineral under the sun in my bathroom but I only take them sporadically. I don't think I have ever finished a whole box and some of them must be ten years old. I haven't got a clue if they stop working after a while.
Morgan, 28, UK

I went to see a diet therapist and she said that every weekend I should juice up seven days' supply of veg and fruit and drink a glass a day. I did it for a while and then I got lazy and started buying V6 and tomato juice but then I just gave up completely.
Allison, 25, UK

If you want to buy a multivitamin look at the label first and make sure the amounts don't exceed 100 percent of the recommended daily allowance. Your body will excrete an excess of water-soluble vitamins such as B and C as urine but fat-soluble vitamins dissolve in your fat and are carried into the bloodstream. Some vitamins are advertised as time release ie. they are supposed to release the nutrients over an extended period but I don't believe that they work at all.
Pharmacist, 38, UK

Supplements that work

Some food supplements like evening primrose oil are well tested and have proven benefits. Others remain a mystery to nutritionists and consumers alike. Because supplements are sold as food, manufacturers are not obliged to pay for large clinical trials, so scientific evidence of their effectiveness is scarce. This means that they can't claim to cure anything specific, but it also means that they are not subject to the rigorous medical testing that drugs have to go through before they are allowed onto the market. Whether they work or not is one issue. What goes into them is another. Without proper regulation, manufacturers can sell and promote products that contain substances that may be toxic. The British Dietetic Association believes that supplements should come under tighter regulations and be classed as medicines rather than foods. This would legally oblige a manufacturer to prove that its products were safe and effective. Preparations would also have to contain exactly the same dose or ingredient. At the moment the upper limits vary. Although supplements have the potential to do good, and many of the more popular herbs have been used in traditional medicine for centuries, they also have the potential to harm so always consult a doctor before taking them. For example, herbal supplements such as St John's wort can react dangerously with warfarin yet a recent UK study found that 1 in 5 patients on warfarin were also taking some form of herbal supplement and hadn't informed their GP. St John's wort also interferes with the effectiveness of antidepressants and the contraceptive pill; evening primrose oil can provoke epileptic attacks in susceptible patients; and echinacea may contribute to a range of allergic reactions. Certain Chinese remedies can cause renal failure and Ginkgo biloba has been linked to excess bleeding. Listed below are the ones that do work though http://www.nlm.nih.gov/medlineplus/herbalmedicine.html will give you more detailed information.

CO-ENZYME Q10 Our bodies make this enzyme naturally. Supplements are untested, but may strengthen the heart and act as an antioxidant.

COD LIVER OIL Full of vitamins A and D and essential fatty acids so they are a must for people who are not keen on eating fish. Said to relieve the pain of arthritis and aid the immune system. It is also believed to bring on labour close to term. Some bottled fish liver oils have been found to contain toxins but it is taken in very small quantities so they are harmless.

EVENING PRIMROSE OIL One of the richest sources of the omega-6 fatty acid, gamma linoleic acid (GLA). GLA minimizes symptoms of PMT and it is anti-inflammatory so it is good for people with arthritis. Its also very good for skin and may help eczema. There are no known adverse reactions nd the benefits are well documented, so a supplement is probably worth trying.

FLAX SEED OIL Provides a positive balance between omega-3 and -6 essential fatty acids. A good supplement for vegetarians. One 1000mg capsule will provide your daily requirement of alpha linoleic acid.

GARLIC Lowers cholesterol, is good for the heart and is thought to have anti-viral properties too. Cooking may destroy the active ingredients so it should be eaten raw or taken as a supplement. 600–900mg/day will give you the protection that you need.

GINGKO BILOBA Thought to improve mental alertness and increase blood supply to the hands and feet so it may be useful for the elderly or those suffering from Alzheimer's. Often used as an alternative to Viagra though it shouldn't be taken by anyone with angina or a heart condition. It should not be taken with aspirin as they are both anticoagulants and can reduce blood clotting.

GINSENG Used for thousands of years to help fight stress and stimulate the immune system. Classic ginseng (panax, Korean) may have antibiotic properties while Siberian ginseng is used to fight fatigue and improve athletic performance.

GLUCOSAMINE SULPHATE Involved in building cartilage, clinical trials have failed to show that supplements ease the pain and disability of diagnosed osteoarthritis (as opposed to other joint pains) but doctors support the use of 1500mg a day and a $6.6 million trial is now underway in the US.

GREEN-LIPPED MUSSEL Lyprinol, the active compound, has been shown to reduce swelling and pain in joints. Worth trying if you suffer from arthritis or rheumatism. It takes four to eight weeks to see results from supplements.

LEMON BALM UK research shows that dried lemon balm can improve secondary (not primary) memory and increase feelings of calmness.

MILK THISTLE Clinical efficacy is not clearly established but trials have shown some possible improvement in liver function.

FISH OILS These help the heart, skin and brain. Best from fresh fish but you need so much – 800mg+ a day – that a supplement is often easier.

STARFLOWER OIL A richer source of GLA than evening primrose oil.

VALERIAN Proven effective as a natural cure for insomnia and stress.

I live in a very hot and humid climate so I do regularly take supplements, i.e. vitamins, to increase my energy levels. They help to counteract tiredness and keep the energy levels up.
Carra, 31, La Réunion

I take a multi-vitamin every day as I think it helps me stay in balance. I used to take vitamin C tablets until I realized it didn't do anything for me.
Sari, 24, UK

I would love to believe that taking a pill every day would hep me to live a longer and healthier life but I know I am fooling myself. Apparently living in London is the equivalent of smoking 600 cigarettes a day, so how the hell would one tiny vitamin tablet have a chance of countering negative effects on that scale?
Charlotte, 34, UK

I take vitamins, minerals or food supplements when I have mouth ulcers or pimples. For these symptoms I think vitamin pills are effective. I know if your diet is healthy enough you don't get these irritations, then you don't need supplements. But who can ensure their diet is always good?
Junko, 41, Tokyo

And the jury is out on...

I was vegetarian for ten years but when I had Flora I started to eat chicken and now I eat sausage and pancetta, but I won't eat roast pork or beef because I am worried about what goes into them. I eat a lot of fruit and veg but I have left out wheat in the last few years as it gives me an upset stomach (I lose a lot of weight when I don't eat wheat). I take propolis supplements if I think I have a cold, and I do acupuncture every month – have done for 14 years.
Kate, 42, Flora, 6`
(Pictured right)

Vitamin supplements are a big con. If you have a healthy diet you don't need them but a healthy diet involves self-discipline and moderation. The issues that relate to poor eating habits stem from our psychological state of mind. We should be looking deeper into the reasons why we eat too much or too little and there should be much more education about healthy eating. There should also be more control over an industry that exploits female insecurity about health and diet.
Kathryn, 31, NZ

BLACK COHOSH Previously hyped as preventing menopausal symptoms, including number and intensity of hot flushes, there is increasing concern that it could cause breast cancer metastasis and liver failure

ECHINACEA Echinacea sales represent 10% of the dietary supplement market in the US. It is one of the most popular remedies for colds and flu and is also thought to have anti-inflammatory properties. The pure ingredient does have beneficial properties. Several clinical trials have shown positive results but others have shown no improvements. In one study, the control group taking echinacea took 6.27 days to recover compared to 5.75 days for those on dummy pills. However, the problem with echinacea is that it can cause allergic reactions and there is no guarantee as to the content, quality, variability or contamination in preparations. Of 59 samples tested in the US, 10% contained no measurable echinacea while only 43% met the quality standard described on the label.

KAVA KAVA Has psychoactive properties, and is sold as an antidepressant but recent reports of severe liver toxicity have led to restrictions on its sale in Europe.

KOMBUCHA Promoted as a cure-all for a wide variety of conditions, including baldness, insomnia, intestinal disorders, arthritis, chronic fatigue syndrome, multiple sclerosis, AIDS and cancer. There is no scientific evidence to support any of the claims though in April 1995, two women who had been consuming the tea daily for two months were hospitalized with severe acidosis – an abnormal increase in the acidity in the body fluids. One died of cardiac arrest.

PROPOLIS AND ROYAL JELLY When fed to an ordinary female bee, Royal Jelly extends her life 20-fold and enables her to produce twice her weight in eggs, but there is no scientific proof that benefit crosses over to humans. In fact although Propolis or bee pollen is meant to help fight infection, it actually helps feed invading germs and both products can trigger hay fever, asthma or allergies.

ST JOHN'S WORT In 1998, US sales of St John's wort were estimated at $210 million. Considered to be the natural Prozac for years, some trials show that it could prove effective for people who suffer from milder forms of depression. However, two US trials have now found that it scores lower than placebo and anti depressants in those suffering from serious depression. St John's wort shouldn't be taken by anyone on antidepressants, contraceptives or anticoagulants.

WHEAT GRASS No scientific studies in humans support any of the claims that suggest a wheatgrass diet can cure or prevent disease.

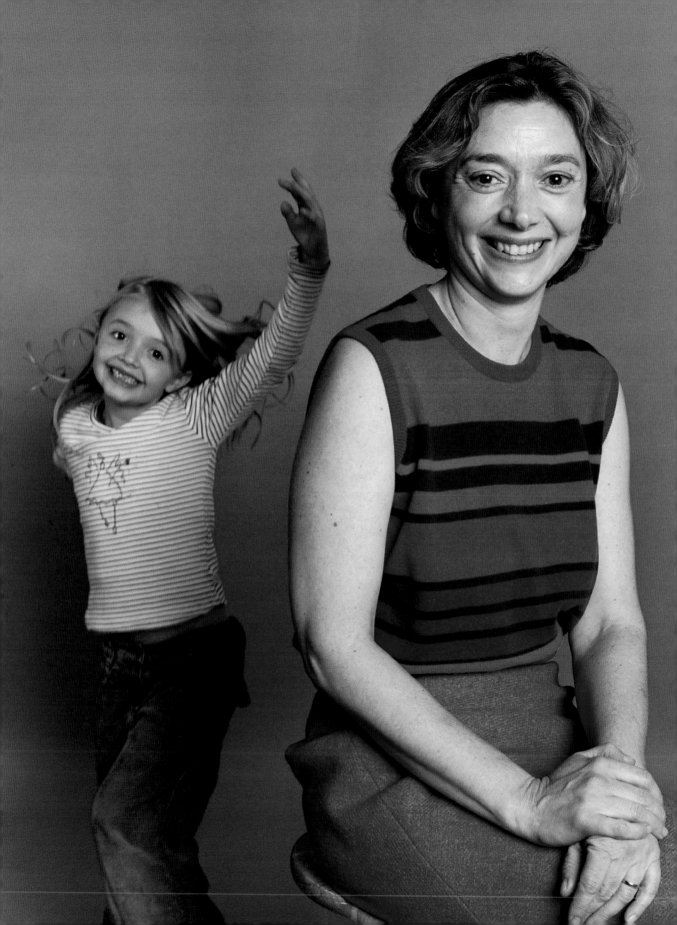

The food industry

For manufacturers to make a profit, food has to be cheap to produce. It has to travel well, have a long shelf life and maintain its visual appeal until it is bought. To achieve all this, manufacturers employ the help of a range of pesticides, chemicals, preservatives, additives, fillers, colours and sweeteners, which blur the boundaries between doing the shopping and taking a chemistry degree. When it comes to food you get what you pay for. Higher quality food costs more, but it is worth the investment. When it comes to long-term health, cheap food is a false economy.

MEAT AND POULTRY The animals that make up the bulk of the meat and poultry products in supermarkets have been reared indoors, fed on pellets of food made of anything from crops heavily sprayed with chemicals to cheap, genetically modified soya or, worse still, the ground-up remains of other animals. They are force fed a high calorie diet to encourage growth and antibiotics are routinely used to avoid the spread of diseases. The outcome of this intensive animal farming has been BSE, salmonella, food poisoning and increased human resistance to antibiotics. A recent survey by the Food Standards Agency (FSA) in the UK found that beef and pork proteins had been routinely injected into imported chicken. More than half of the chicken fillets they tested had been fraudulently bulked up with water by up to 50 per cent. And nearly half the samples of frozen chicken also contained DNA from pork even though they were labelled as Halal. The FSA describes these practices as a 'deliberate con' with a total disregard for Muslim communities. Labelling on processed meat products does not have to qualify what kind of 'meat' is included, so cheap sausages, burgers or chicken nuggets are likely to contain mechanically recovered meat, rind, gristle, sinew and the slurry retrieved from the machine. In 2004 it was discovered that the date stamp on fresh chickens is routinely changed by manufacturers before they leave the premises meaning that the fresh chickens bought in supermarkets may already be several weeks old.

ORGANIC MEAT AND POULTRY Consumer fears about quality have lead to enormous growth in sales of organic meat. However, many shoppers are not aware that imported organic meats are not subject to the same standards as organic meat produced in the UK so make sure you buy British. If you can't buy organic, opt for leaner cuts, as toxins tend to gather in the fatty tissues. Wild meats like game are less likely to be contaminated, and lamb can be a safer option than beef. Some experts say the standards for organic animal farming in the UK are still too low. Organic chicken can still be kept in cages and fed on a diet that is 20% non-organic and the vast majority of organic and free-range chickens are slaughtered in the same large plants as intensively reared ones. In 2003 researchers from Bristol University found that organic and free-range birds were twice as likely to carry the campylobacter food poisoning bug as chickens reared indoors.

EGGS Hens and chickens eat virtually anything they are given and, naturally, their eggs reflect the quality of their diet. Battery eggs come from battery farmed hens who have been fed on waste or animal carcass by-products. Barn hens have a little more space, but their diet is just as bad. Free range means the hens have had access to the outdoors and they may have been fed more natural foodstuffs – but to the minimum standard. Four-grain eggs means the hens have been fed on foods that are natural to hens and they have not been given hormones or antibiotics, though they may not have had outdoor access. In the UK, eggs with the Lion Quality mark account for 75% of the total market. The lion symbol, which appears on both the eggshell and egg box, shows that the hens have been vaccinated against salmonella and each egg is date stamped. In 2003 however, over 12% of eggs tested by UK government scientists contained residues of lasalocid, a toxic antibiotic.

Organic eggs are the best bet because the hens eat a diet that is at least 80% organic and live a more natural life, however one sample of organic eggs was also found to be lasalocid positive and growers standards can vary. Organic Farmers and Growers Association organic eggs come from flocks of 3000 or less while Soil Association-approved eggs come from flocks of 500 or less. Eggs should be transported and displayed in shops at a temperature below 20°C. Smaller shops may not be able to follow these guidelines and, as they tend to have a slower turnover of stock, the eggs may not be as fresh when you buy them. At home, store eggs in the fridge, preferably in the box to keep them away from other foods. Look for clean eggs and never use eggs that have been cracked in transit, even if you know it was you that broke them on the way home. Use eggs by the 'best before' date. Write the date of purchase on eggs that have no stamp and use within three. Eat cooked egg dishes as soon as possible after cooking.

MILK Virtually all milk is now pasteurized to destroy bacteria but UK scientists have found that a bacteria suspected of causing or contributing to Crohn's disease is capable of surving the pasteurising process. Crohn's disease causes chronic inflammation of the bowel, and affects about 50,000 people in the UK.

FISH Fish is a food we should all be trying to eat more of, but unfortunately intensive farming methods have also been applied to farmed fish. Irresponsible commercial fishing has left the seas depleted, while industrial pollutants such as polychlorinated biphenol (PCB) and dioxins have poisoned seas and rivers. In the North Sea, tests on the livers of fish found high concentrations of cadmium. One third of plaice tested had pollution-related skin complaints, and bacteria caused by sewage was found in shellfish. Recent research suggests that industrial chemicals mimicking the oestrogen hormone are causing up to 60% of male river fish to

I read the labels on foods and try to avoid E-numbers, colorants and monosodium gluta-mate. I think that it's particularly worrying that what is sold as fresh in the super-market is actually processed beyond recognition. I eat a lot of fresh fish and it really annoys me that it is generally dyed and processed before it even hits the shops, yet it is sold as fresh fish. I am very careful about the meat I eat. It is generally organic and can be traced right back to the field it originated from.
Clair, 36, UK

I eat fish and meat only occasionally and never eat animal food in large volume. I think vegetarianism is logical and reasonable, both economically and health-wise.
Yoko, 33, Japan

I love food and cooking and gathering round a table. I don't want to make food into an issue that contains guilt, sacrifice and punishment. I try to eat non-fat and cut down on sugar – but apart from that, I try to maintain a 'normal' relationship to food.
Guri, 40, Norway

change sex. Farmed fish such as salmon and trout suffer from lice that are killed with antibiotics and they are fed on a concentrated feed made from dead fish from polluted waters. White fish such as cod and haddock, which are fished in deeper waters, are less likely to be contaminated, though overfishing and the fact that netted babies don't get thrown back into the sea now means that previously plentiful fish such as cod are virtually an endangered species. Scallops, crabs, lobster and prawns are less likely to be affected by pollution than shellfish that live on the shoreline such as mussels, oysters and prawns.

Unfortunately, because toxins such as cadmium and dioxins are stored in the fat and the livers, oily fish, the fish that is best for us, are more likely to be affected. Though the FSA advises only one portion of farmed salmon a week, a recent US review of Scottish farmed salmon damned the product as dangerous and advised eating only four portions a year because of chemical links to birth defects and cancer. The UK food standards agency feels this is extreme and it suggests that it is safe for women of child bearing age to eat two portions of farmed salmon a week. The Marine Stewardship Council has produced a label that recognizes environmentally responsible fishery management. Better still, buy wild or organically reared fish. It is more expensive but seems to be the only way to ensure optimum quality and health. Though most fish is prepacked so you can't smell it, don't buy or cook fish that smells too 'fishy' or smells of ammonia.

FRUIT AND VEG A healthy diet calls for lots of fruit and veg, but pesticides and preservative are routinely used to keep them bug free and longer lasting. Residue levels in fruit and veg are monitored by the FSA but in random tests these levels are often exceeded. In 1999, 43% of produce tested contained chemical residues, 1.6% of them were over the safe limit. The cumulative effect of these chemicals is unknown, so limit your exposure by washing and peeling fruit and veg, discarding the outer layers of cabbages and lettuces and removing an inch from the green end of root vegetables like carrots and parsnips.

Because supermarkets will only buy fruit and veg that is large and uniform, farmers have to use chemicals to meet their exacting standards. However because the British climate is not conducive to such perfection, most of it ends up being imported from abroad anyway. Economy packs of fruit and veg that are more irregular in shape are more likely to have been grown in the UK, which means their journey to the supermarket shelf has been considerably shorter. This means they are likely to be more nutritious, cheaper and should taste better because imported produce is usually harvested before it is ripe and often comes from countries where chemicals and pesticides that are not approved in the UK are used routinely.

Though we are used to having everything we want all the time it makes much more sense to try and eat locally grown foods when they are in season because they provide us with the vitamins and minerals that we need at that particular time of year. Strawberries, for example, contain high levels of antioxidants – vital during the summer, when exposure to the sun increases. Similarly, root vegetables and onions, which grow in the autumn and winter, have more carbohydrate and give us more energy, which we need during the cold weather.

ORGANIC PRODUCE It is estimated that the levels of nutrients in fresh fruit and veg may have declined by up to 75% in the last 50 years thanks to pesticides, spraying and storage. Fears about the impact of chemicals and declining nutrients have lead to such a boom in sales that the UK, which does not have enough dedicated organic farmland to meet demand, has to import 65% of its organic produce from countries where standards are not as well monitored as they are in the UK. Fruit and vegetables are the most heavily imported and are likely to have travelled the furthest. Organic produce is more eco-sustainable than conventionally farmed food and is undoubtedly better for the environment in the long run but, arguably, its benefits for humans are undermined by flying the food around the world so the French for example import only 10% of their organic produce. Many argue that when you take these factors into account, there is limited evidence that organically produced fruit and veg is more nutritious, though researchers who tested the antioxidant content of corn found organically grown corn had almost 60% more flavonoids (which reduce the risk of cancer) than corn grown with pesticides. Plants produce flavonoids to defend themselves against pests and diseases but crops protected by pesticides have less need for them and so produce less of them. The organic market has grown exponentially in the past ten years and, including meat and poultry, it now accounts for 5% of all food sales in the UK. Most supermarkets now have organic sections but a 1999 UK study by a British newspaper found that supermarkets were charging nearly 170% premiums for organic produce. Playing upon consumers' fears to charge higher prices and produce greater profits on foods that they bill as 'safer' is a win-win situation for supermarkets.

GM FOODS Genetic modification involves taking beneficial genes from one species and implanting them into a new species so that it can develop the same positive attributes, e.g. genes from fish being implanted into tomatoes to give them greater resistance to the cold and to help them keep their shape when frozen. GM crops are currently grown commercially or in field trials in over 40 countries. In 2000, over 100 million acres were planted with herbicide and insecticide-resistant soybeans, corn, cotton and canola. Other crops grown commercially or field-tested are virus-resistant sweet potatoes, rice with increased iron and vitamins, tomatoes

I am prepared to pay a little more for organic food and as the organic farmer begins to gain market share, the prices will undoubtedly come down as we've already seen. Then organic produce will be far more freely available. Not everything can be organic but I feel a duty to myself to try to reduce the toxins in my food intake as much as possible. I haven't eaten in a fast food restaurant for ten years. The food is not only trash but the human rights' records surrounding the industry are appalling. I think that the book Fast Food Nation *should be put on the national curriculum as a compulsory read for all 12-year-olds. It would solve many of the wider social problems like childhood obesity and colonic cancer, and it may get people back to the dinner table, which was once and still is in my home, a nightly venue for conversation, communication and interaction.*
Clair, 36, UK

Two breasts of organic chicken costs £7. Two breasts of non organic chicken costs £2. I am a single mother of three on benefit. Which one do I choose?
Anita, 38, UK

that protect against cancer and a variety of plants able to survive weather extremes. On the horizon are bananas that produce human vaccines against infectious diseases such as hepatitis B; fish that mature more quickly; fruit and nut trees that yield years earlier, and plants that produce new plastics. GM promoters, the people that will make the most money from the technology, say that it will solve world hunger, make food stay fresh, taste better and contain more health giving properties. But studies show that at the moment pesticide usage is higher and yields are lower with GM crops. That said, the companies that make GM food ingredients are also the ones that make pesticides, so that's handy for them.

Some 60% of the soya in the world is now GM and up to 30% of animal feed can be made of GM foods. Avoiding GM foods means avoiding all products containing soya, maize and their derivatives, which is difficult, because soya is in practically everything: processed foods, confectionery, margarines, spreads, mayonnaise, cakes, breads, biscuits, gravy, soups, stock cubes, meat dishes, tomato purée. A US poll found that only 50% of women surveyed said they would eat genetically modified foods, compared to 71% of men, and over 60% of women said they would not give GM foods to their children. This poses a problem because nearly two-thirds of the food for sale in US supermarkets is already genetically modified. A UK review by the Wellcome/CRC Institute singles out the use of genetically modified soya in baby food as a cause for concern. Because babies are so small and formula is generally their major food source, any potential health problems are likely to be magnified.

The long-term consequences of monkeying around with mother nature are anyone's guess, but there are concerns that consumers of GM food may become resistant to antibiotics, because GM foods are engineered to be resistant. Likewise, crops could become pesticide-resistant and create mutant superweeds. Cross pollination is already a problem. The current distance between a GM crop and a non-GM crop is only 200m (210yd) so the more crops that are planted, the harder it will be to get rid of them if the 'experts' are proved wrong. In 1998, the UK passed a bill requiring all GM food to be labelled, but it is already virtually impossible for farmers to be sure that any crop is 100% GM free. Controversy over safety and labelling and continued consumer resistance has meant that nearly two-thirds of the EU's biotech companies have cancelled GM research projects in the last four years and in May 2004, Monsanto, the world's biggest seller of GM seeds, abandoned plans to introduce GM wheat on to the world market, despite spending seven years and hundreds of millions of dollars developing the crop. Though GM advocates sugest that their aim is to eliminate Third World hunger, they consistently miss one vital point. There is more than enough food in the world at the moment. It's just that half the global population is too poor to buy it.

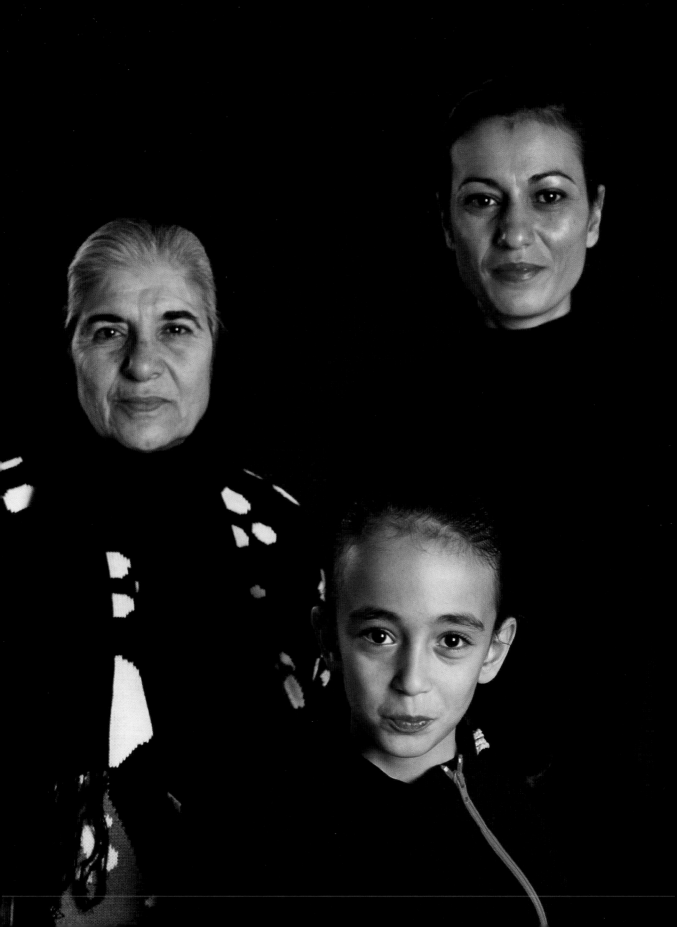

ADDITIVES It is estimated that each person eats about 2.3kg (5lb) of E-numbers and additives a year. Though having an E number means that an ingredient has passed certain EU safety tests, it doesn't mean that it is any good for you. Colours (E100–80) are used to make foods look more appetizing and more like they looked before they were processed. Preservatives (E200–285, E1105) are used to prevent bacteria building up and stop food from decaying. Sulphur dioxide, which causes allergies, is often used on dried fruits (E220). Antioxidants (E300–321) are used to stop foods going off. Emulsifiers, stabilizers and thickening agents (E322–495) are used to stop fats separating and give foods texture. Flavourings (E620–40) are used to give foods flavour. Glazing agents (E901–14) are used to add 'shine'. Bleaches and improvers (E920–6) are used in baking and breads to improve texture and whiteness. And sweeteners (saccharin, or E420/421, and E953–9) replace sugar with chemicals. Colours, preservatives, antioxidants, stabilizers, flavour enhancers, glazing agents and artificial flavouring have been associated with skin complaints, behavioural problems, asthma and allergies. Anyone who is vulnerable should avoid the following if possible: *dyes*: E104, E110, E122, E123, E124, E127, E128, E131, E132, E133, E142, E151, E154, E155; *colours*: E120, cochineal, annatto E160b; *preservative benzoates and sulphides*: E210–19 and E220–8, and *antioxidants*: E310, E311, E312, E320 and E321. Always read the label on packaged foods and go for products that contain a short list of identifiable ingredients. Avoid anything you don't recognize, i.e. acidity regulator, glucono delta-lactone or maltodextrin. You definitely don't need these in your diet.

SUGAR Sugar is the master of all disguises and creeps into foods under a range of other names, eg. sucrose, glucose, fructose, dextrose, glucose syrup and corn syrup. Fructose, the natural sugar present in fruit, is slowly absorbed as energy when eaten in fruit but if it is separated from the fruit fibre and turned into, say, a fruit-flavoured drink, it is absorbed like any refined sugar. Honey and brown sugar have healthier connotations but they are absorbed in exactly the same way as refined sugar and contain just as many empty calories. Labelling can be confusing. Products that state they have no added sugar may be sweetened with artificial sweeteners, syrup or concentrated fruit juices. Foods that do not contain artificial colours and preservative may well contain sugar, sweeteners or flavourings.

SALT Salt is added to nearly all processed savoury foods and is not necessarily listed on the label. There is strong evidence that high salt intake is linked to high blood pressure (the main cause of strokes) and heart attacks. It is also widely recognised that a diet high in salt can lead to osteoporosis, cancer of the stomach and asthma. A major UK campaign was launched in 2004 to encourage people to reduce their salt intake from 9g (our current average intake) to 6g per day.

Functional foods

Functional foods are ordinary foods that have ingredients incorporated into them to give them a specific medical or physiological benefit. In many cases it is possible to get the same ingredients more cheaply and more naturally from a healthy, balanced diet, but consumers respond to claims relating to heart disease, cancer prevention, osteoporosis, digestive health and obesity, whether therapeutic benefit is proven or not. The products invariably cost more and the UK market is already worth £239 million. Manufacturers are not allowed to make health claims but can and do imply health benefits using emotive wording or symbols such as hearts and bones. A product can legally state something like, 'provides calcium, which is important for strong bones' because it is a health claim, but it cannot state, 'provides calcium which helps prevent osteoporosis' because it is a medicinal claim. Frankly, not many consumers see the difference and worryingly, most believe that the government controls and monitors health claims on packaging. They don't.

CHOLESTEROL-LOWERING MARGARINES The most popular brands contain plant stanols and sterols, compounds that lower levels of LDL or 'bad' cholesterol by preventing it from entering the bloodstream. It is well worth switching to a cholesterol-lowering margarine because medical experts suggest that adding 2g of plant sterol or stanol to the average daily portion of margarine would reduce the risk of heart disease by about 25% – a larger effect than most people would manage to achieve by reducing their saturated fat intake.

FORTIFIED BREADS Bread containing soya flour and linseeds provides phyto-oestrogens, natural substances that mimic the hormone oestrogen. This can help alleviate symptoms of menopause and may protect against breast cancer but you need to eat at least six slices daily on a long-term basis for any health benefits.

PROBIOTICS Studies have linked probiotic bacteria to fewer respiratory infections in children and a lower incidence of eczema in babies of mums who took probiotics, however they have also shown that it is very difficult to keep the friendly bacteria alive long enough to reach the colon, where their usefulness begins. Sold as fermented skimmed milk drinks, yogurts, fruit juice, pills or powders, one brand claims to contain 6.5 billion 'friendly bacteria' in a 65ml (2½fl oz) bottle. However, a Belgian investigation into probiotics found that only 20% of 55 products tested contained all the organisms listed and nine products failed to contain any at all.

FORTIFIED DRINKS Drinks fortified with antioxidants, calcium and herbal extracts claiming to help overcome problems ranging from PMS to lack of energy don't work. According to the Food Commission, drinks containing caffeine to 'improve concentration and reaction speed' are no more effective than a cola.

When I look at all the options available to help me eat better, look better, be healthier I just get totally confused. I don't see how anyone could possibly process all that information and turn it into a lifestyle.
Vanessa, 31, UK

Surely someone can invent a pill that provides us with all the 'scientific' nutrition we need so we can get back to just enjoying our food.
Tonya, 21, UK

Vogel soya and linseed bread and sunflower and barley bread are absolutely delicious and I do feel that they do me a lot of good. I think more manufacturers should add value to their products by including seeds and soya. It's great for women.
Helga, 35, UK

My kids hate dairy products so I buy foods that are artificially fortified. I don't like the fact that they get their nutrients from someone dumping a bunch of vitamin tablets into the mix at the cornflake factory but what can I do? I recently bought calcium fortified water and juice but the kids just hated it. They said it tasted like sweet milk.
Gina, 40, UK

Drink to your health ...

WATER Boring but beautiful. Plain water has no calories, no artificial anything and is the best way to rehydrate everything from plants to congealed sauces. You could survive for weeks without food but without water you would die within a week. The average person needs to drink between six and eight glasses of water a day, more if it is hot, or you exercise and sweat a lot. Many women avoid drinking water because they are afraid that it will make them bloated. In fact, the majority of women are in a permanent state of dehydration and this can have a detrimental effect on metabolic rate. Dehydration can drop metabolic rate by up to 3%, resulting in a 450g (1lb) gain every six months. And if you have any doubt about the effect of water on your skin, put a grape and a raisin side by side. UK consumers get through 995 million litres (218 million gallons) of bottled water a year, though taste tests by the consumer group *Which?* gave top marks to filtered and unfiltered tap water. Sparkling waters generally contain lower levels of bacteria than still waters because carbonation makes it more difficult for bacteria to grow. If you are buying water (that you could otherwise get from the tap for free), make sure you are getting what you paid for. Look for the words 'spring', 'glacial', 'artesian', 'naturally sparkling' or 'natural'. Beware of water labelled as 'purified' or 'drinking water'. This is just water from a local tap that has gone through intensive processing. Processed water is often packaged with very misleading labels. Aquafina, Pepsi's bottled water, has a picture of mountains and snow on the label. In reality, it is bottled at Pepsi plants using processed municipal water. In 2004 Coca-Cola's new brand of 'pure' bottled water, Dasani, was revealed to be tap water taken from the Thames Water mains supply at their factory in Sidcup, Kent. After a £7m marketing campaign the entire UK supply of Dasani was pulled off the shelves when it was found to contain twice the legal limit for bromate, a cancer-causing chemical.

JUICE Fruit and vegetable juices are about 80% water by weight. In 2000, about 44% of all fruits in the US were consumed as juice, and the figure continues to climb, as consumption of whole fruit drops. A glass of fruit and/or vegetable juice (150ml (5fl oz)) counts as a portion of fruit or veg, but juice can't make up more than one portion a day because you don't get the same nutritional benefits. When juice is extracted from a fruit or vegetable, it reduces the fibre content and releases a type of sugar that can cause as much tooth decay as processed sugars, especially if you drink it frequently. Make sure you only drink fresh juice. Avoid concentrates and don't be fooled by deceptive labelling. Anything branded as 'fruit drink' or 'fruit flavoured' drink is not the real thing. Although fresh versions are rich in vitamin C, minerals and phytochemicals, they can be deceptively high in calories. Fresh juices can range between 70 and 200 calories for a 200ml (7fl oz) carton and they can be high on the glycaemic index so watch for the sugar rush, sugar crash syndrome. Fresh juice should have only one ingredient.

Drinking tap water is out of the question in Tokyo because there is too much chlorine. But I have no space to put a water purifier in my tiny kitchen so I put some wood charcoal in water and leave the pitcher in the fridge. Charcoal is said to absorb some harmful substances and make water more tasty.
Yoko, 33, Japan

I live in a very hot climate so I drink approximately 3 litres of still mineral water a day! I drink sparkling mineral water with meals but I find still is more thirst quenching.
Carra, 31, La Réunion

My husband seems to think that because a pint of beer is 75% water that is enough to keep him hydrated.
Tara, 29, UK

Paying for brand name waters is a classic example of manufac-turers selling sand to the Arabs. The stuff is about the only thing on the planet that is still free yet we insist on buying it in plastic bottles with plastic caps and fancy labels. SO dumb!!!!!!!!!!!!!!!!
Geraldine, 28, US

GREEN TEA Regular tea contains caffeine but not in great quantities so you can have up to seven cups of tea a day without going over your caffeine limit. Green tea is a better option because it is thought to protect against cancer and it also contains polyphenols, chemicals that have antioxidant properties that slow ageing which is why it is now the hippest ingredient in beauty products. It also contains the amino acid theonine, which promotes a sense of calm and improves mood. A Swiss study found that people who took extract of green tea burned significantly more calories than people who didn't. It seems that 'phytochemical flavonoids' contained in green tea effect the energy hormone noradrenaline (norepinephrine), which then speeds up the process of fat oxidation.

COFFEE Caffeine is a stimulant that arouses the nervous system and stimulates the production of adrenaline (epinephrine), increasing heart rate and generally making you more alert. Caffeine directly raises blood cortisol (three cups of coffee will increase cortisol for two to three hours), which encourages the body to store fat and speeds up the ageing process. To minimize the effect, you should avoid eating carbohydrates with your coffee. Coffee is acidic and it is thought that drinking several cups of coffee per day increases the risk of postmenopausal bone loss, arthritis and high blood pressure. Research from scientists at Harvard Medical School suggests that consuming more than two cups of coffee each day could boost oestrogen levels in women and exacerbate conditions like endometriosis and breast pain. According to their study, women who consumed at least 500mg of caffeine each day (four to five cups of coffee) had close to 70% more oestrogen during the follicular phase (days one to five of their menstrual cycle) than women who had no more than 100mg of caffeine (one average mug of instant or brewed coffee). For most people, moderate coffee drinking has minimal side effects but the maximum recommended intake of coffee daily is 300mg. Though coffee doesn't contain any calories on its own, add regular milk and a sprinkle of chocolate and a medium cappuccino (400ml (14fl oz)) turns into 110 calories and 6g of fat, a medium caffè latte with whole milk contains 180 calories and 10g of fat, and a medium mocha coffee contains a whopping great 290 calories and 18g of fat.

SOFT DRINKS In 2003 the WHO launched a tough assault on the food industry with a scientific report blaming sugar in soft drinks for the rise in childhood obesity. In 2003, the average person in the UK consumed 111 litres of soft drinks. That's a lot of sugar. A can of coke has about 7 tsps or 13 lumps of sugar per can, and sugar and corn syrup from soft drinks now supply more than 10% of our total calories. Recent research has linked increased fizzy drink consumption with an escalation in the incidence of cancer of the oesophagus. Cases of this unusual cancer have risen by 570% in white American men in the last 25 years and the

My husband and I like to have a cup of green tea every night before we go to bed. I don't know if it is really any good for us but since we like to have a cup of tea anyway we decided to try it out. We have become accustomed to the taste now and we both believe that it makes us feel more restful.
Donna, 65, Gibraltar

I quit drinking Nescafé because their behaviour in Africa is so dreadful. I now drink Fairtrade coffee because profit goes to the local grower rather than some greedy multinational.
Primrose, 21, UK

Some mornings I will have about four diet cokes between 9.30am and lunch time. If I have a hangover or I am feeling really tired, I will have real coke because I need the energy but most of the time diet does the trick. I know I am probably taking in too much caffeine because I also drink coffee but I work from 8am to midnight four days a week and I don't know how I would stay awake otherwise. Other girls use herbal supplements like guaranna, which they say work better but coke does the trick for me.
Dana, 24, US

disease now hits more than 7,200 people in the UK every year, a rise of 655% in 30 years. At least 40% of fizzy drinks are consumed by children but heavy soft drinkers are almost four times more likely to drink less than one glass of milk a day so they are more likely to have lower calcium intakes, a fact that is particularly pertinent to growing girls. The risk of osteoporosis depends in part on how much bone mass is built early in life. Girls build 92% of their bone mass by age 18 but if they don't consume enough calcium in their teenage years they cannot 'catch up' later. While osteoporosis takes decades to develop, preliminary research suggests that drinking soft drinks instead of milk is already contributing to an increase in broken bones among children. The caffeine in soft drinks adds to the problem because it increases the excretion of calcium in urine. Drinking 350ml (12fl oz) of caffeine-containing soft drinks causes the loss of about 20mg of calcium, or 2% of the US RDA (or Recommended Daily Allowance). That loss, compounded by the relatively low calcium intake in young girls, who are heavy consumers of soft drinks, may substantially increase the risk of osteoporosis in the long term. Caffeine also causes nervousness, irritability, sleeplessness, rapid heart beat and headache. Several additives used in soft drinks cause occasional allergic reactions. Yellow and red dye can cause asthma, hives, runny nose and hyperactivity in sensitive children.

DIET SODA Diet drinks account for less than a quarter of the soda market but they are not as bad for us as was previously thought. There's nothing natural about a product that lists its 'nutritional information per 100ml' as 'carbohydrates 0g; protein 0g, fat 0g energy, 0.4 cal'. but previous reports of aspartame, the artificial sweetener used in many diet drinks being responsible for causing epilepsy, multiple sclerosis and brain tumours have now been rubbished. Diet drinks are still a caffeine fuelled chemical cocktail, but studies from the Scientific Committee on Food in Brussels, the Food and Drug Administration, the American Medical Association in the US and the FSA in the UK say that there is no reliable scientific evidence to back up claims that aspartame causes any of the serious disorders with which it has been linked. Experts say that an adult should consume no more than 40mg of aspartame per kg of body weight per day. To exeed that level a woman of average weight would have to drink more than 14 cans of diet drinks a day! Saccharin, on the other hand, does cause some concern because it has caused bladder cancer in laboratory rats.

ALCOHOL: THE BAD NEWS In excess, alcohol has a toxic effect on the brain, heart, bone marrow, gastrointestinal tract and liver. It can lead to the development of fatty liver, alcoholic hepatitis, fibrosis and cirrhosis. Long-term heavy drinking increases the risk of high blood pressure, heart disease, stroke, certain forms of cancer and death. Women can be at a slightly greater risk of developing breast cancer if they consume two or more alcoholic drinks per day. Women are meant to drink less alcohol than men because they generally have smaller livers and less of the alcohol processing enzyme ADH in their stomach. Women who are pregnant or trying to get pregnant should drink two units or less a week though many doctors advise them to eliminate alcohol completely. Short and overweight women tend to be less well able to tolerate alcohol. Alcohol with fizz is absorbed into the bloodstream quicker and if you are tired, stressed, premenstrual or haven't eaten, you may find that your tolerance is affected. Alcohol can get you drunk but it can also make you fat. At seven calories/g, alcohol adds about three calories/g more than protein or carbohydrate. 125ml (4fl oz) of wine: 100 calories; sherry or port: 200; 350ml (12fl oz) of beer:169; 50ml (1½fl oz) of gin, rum, vodka, or whiskey:110 calories. The addition of a mixer other than water or soda drives the calories even higher. For every 125ml (4fl oz), juices add from 25 calories for tomato juice to 80 calories for cranberry juice; soft drinks range from 30 calories for ginger ale to 50 for cola. Over the course of a year, two cans of beer a day in excess of your normal caloric needs could result in a 15kg (33lb) weight gain. A daily glass of wine with dinner could add 4.5kg (10lb) a year.

ALCOHOL: THE GOOD NEWS Guidelines suggest that women who drink less than two to three units of alcohol a day do not face significant health risks. A unit = 300ml (½ pint) of beer or cider, 1 measure of spirits, port or sherry. However most wine is now 12% alcohol by volume which means that one small 125ml (4floz) glass of wine counts as 1.5 units, as does one glass of champagne. And splitting a bottle of wine puts your consumption at closer to five units, well above your daily allowance. If you keep within the limits, there is mounting evidence that moderate (as opposed to heavy) drinkers have lower levels of coronary heart disease and live longer than those who don't drink at all. These benefits appear to be linked to polyphenoloic phytochemicals, flavonoids such as reservatol in red wine and antioxidants in dark beers. Research suggests that the ethanol in all alcohol probably helps because it reduces levels of bad cholesterol, increases good cholesterol, thins the blood and reduces levels of fibrinogen, which clots the blood. However, red wine is universally considered to be the healthiest alcoholic drink because it contains iron and certain polyphenols in the skin of the grape and a glass of red with your meal is now thought to favourably influence lipid profiles. Research carried out at the University of California to determine which red wines have the highest concentrations of flavonoids concluded that the flavonoid favourite is Cabernet Sauvignon, followed closely by Petit Syrah and Pinot Noir. Merlots and red Zinfandels have fewer flavonoids and white wine had significantly smaller amounts than any reds. The sweeter the wine, the fewer the flavonoids, so if you are drinking, opt for dryer red.

Every woman I know drinks more alcohol than she should. Most of the women I know, including myself, use it as a way of alleviating stress. It works quickly, it is cheaper than a massage. I know it's bad for you but, come on, we live in a totally toxic and polluted city, we are surrounded by fumes and smoke and the food we eat is loaded with additives and preservatives. At what point do we stop denying ourselves simple pleasures like a few glasses of wine every night?
Esther, 37, US

I drink two to three glasses of wine about three to four times a week, sometimes more. I'm aware that the limit is about 14 units a week and that I am often over that but few people of my age group stick to that. It's part of unwinding for us now, a hard habit to break.
Hanna, 25, UK

I craved red wine before my periods. It was the only alcoholic beverage I wanted to drink. I realize now that it contains iron and is rather good for you so I guess my body was just craving it.
Louise, 43, UK

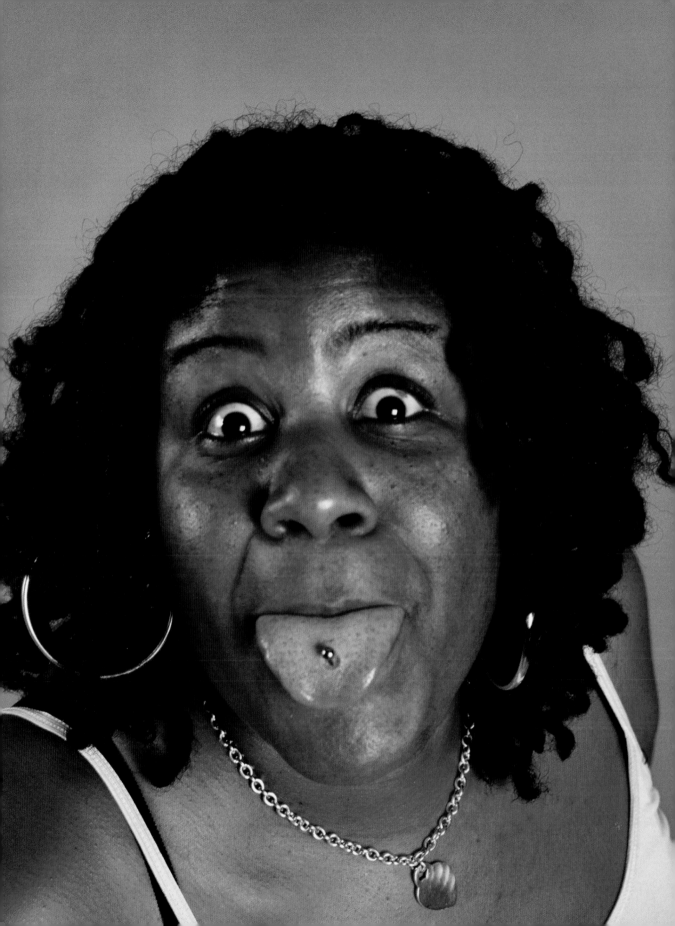

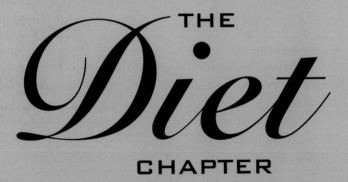

THE

Diet

CHAPTER

From eating to live to living to eat

Fossil records show that bacteria, life's most common design, have been around for 3.5 billion years. Given that it takes a thousand million years to make a billion, having only been here for half a million years or so, humans are relative newcomers to the planet. However, despite the enormous impact we have had in that time, human genetic make up hasn't actually changed that much and many experts now believe that over the last 10,000 years, a conflict between our genes and our environment has resuted in a predisposition to plumpness that has triggered the current epidemic of obesity.

In the Stone Age, our ancestors were hunter-gatherers. Their lifestyle was a pattern of feast and famine, and survival was largely dependent on their ability to pack away enough food to create stores of body fat to see them through leaner times. In 1962, geneticist James Neel proposed that that this advantageous tendency to store fat had evolved into a 'thrifty gene'. He believed that depite the dramatic evolution of the human brain, the 'thrifty genes' in our bodies are still operating on a feast or famine basis and have not yet adapted to an age where food is plentiful. According to Neel, the mismatch between our genes which are still trying to store fat and our diet which contains more fat than we need is the root cause of obesity and many, if not all, of our degenerative vascular diseases. Since Neel is now dead and none of us will be around in 10,000 years to find out whether it is true or not, it is a difficult theory to prove, or disprove, but since its proposal, many experts have agreed that because mankind evolved to resist famine and there is now far too much food around, we are all putting on weight at an alarming rate.

The fact that our diet has changed dramatically (not for the better) hasn't helped. Until the invention of agriculture about 10,000 years ago, humans existed on a diet of meat, fish, fruits and vegetables, but since then, humans have become increasingly dependent upon cereals, grains and potatoes. Today, approximately 17 plant species provide 90% of the world's food supply. The top ten crops are wheat, maize, rice, barley, soybean, cane sugar, sorghum, potato, oats and cassava and it is virtually impossible to avoid bumping into at least one of them at every meal. Without these plants there is no way that the world could support its existing population of 6 billion people and the anticipated 12–15 billion people expected during the next century but the more grain products people eat, the less they eat of important nutrients such as vegetables, fish and fruits. And since grains and cereals are not as filling as fats and proteins, people tend to eat more of them than they should.

In half the world, bread provides more than 50% of the total caloric intake, and in some countries in southern Asia, Central America, the Far East and Africa, cereal products comprise up to 80% or more of the total caloric intake. Developed countries are experiencing a well publicized obesity epidemic but, in the past 20 years, rates of obesity have been increasing just as dramatically in developing countries too. Médecins Sans Frontières believes this is because the poor are largely fed on a diet of cheap, filling starches like bread and potatoes, which makes them overweight but leaves them suffering from malnutrition.

The suggestion that a diet based on cereals, grains and potatoes is related to obesity is not new. Back in the 18th century French gastronome Jean Anthelme Brillat-Savarin identified 'floury and feculent (bread, rice, potatoes and sugar) substances to be the primary culprits in corpulence' and in the 1970s, the accepted wisdom was that fat and protein protected against overeating by making you feel full, while carbohydrates made you fat. It was thought that the ideal diet was one that prevented snacking and excessive sugar consumption, so people were encouraged to eat plenty of eggs, beef, lamb, chicken, butter and well-cooked vegetables. However this thinking goes against the advice of the US food pyramid and the UK balance of good health guide, both of which promote a diet that is high in grains and cereals and low in fat (p.39).

As long as you get a broad enough nutritional range and don't eat too much of any single food, it doesn't matter what you eat. However the more pre-packaged or processed foods you consume, the more difficult it becomes to have any idea of exactly how many calories foods contain. Food manufacturers rely on added sugar and fat to make their products tasty, but an extra 50 calories a day over and above what you normally eat leads to a 2.2kg (5lb) weight gain in a year. And it is very difficult to lose that weight. One 450g (1lb) of fat on your body is the calorific equivalent to 3500 calories. What that means is that to lose 450g (1lb) of fat a week you need to decrease your calorie intake by about 500 calories (the equivalent of five slices of bread) every day.

At the end of the day, scientific theories about why the global waistband has expanded all boil down to the same thing: people eat too much and do too little exercise. And although there are a million diets on the market, the basic principle is the same for all of them – eat fewer calories than you use up. How this idea is dressed up differs from one guru to another, but whether you are doing Atkins, Pritikin, Weight Watchers or the Zone, you are simply cutting the number of calories you consume. The truth is that all diets work, but only if, and while, you stick to them and the minute you resume your normal eating pattern you pile the pounds back on again. So, this chapter explores the practical and emotional reasons behind why so many women repeatedly lose the same 10lbs and it promotes diet plans that offer sustainable long-term change rather than short-term results.

I have been a fish-eating vegetarian for 15 years now. I felt, emotionally, that eating meat wasn't right for me. I then looked for intellectual reasons that might support this feeling and realized there were many: better health; less risk of eating genetically engineered meat; cheaper; environmentally more sound and a sound conscience that I wasn't killing anything just 'because it tastes good'. I think, like many other people, my diet is still dominated by simple carbohydrates but I try to avoid bread as the wheat can make you feel bloated and there isn't much nutritional goodness in it. I try to choose more complex carbohydrates and opt for rice and rye when possible. The key to a healthy diet is eating lots of fruit, veg, fish, nuts and seeds whilst avoiding most things in packets! My diet affects what I buy but I don't let it rule my life if I am a guest at someone else's house or cannot eat as I might prefer for some reason. I think you can be committed without taking yourself too seriously.
Charlotte, 28, UK

Appetite and the brain

Appetite is controlled by neuronal circuits in the hypothalamus, a part of the brain that controls the pituitary gland. The pituitary gland is the master gland in the endocrine system, and as such maintains the body's hormonal balance. When you get hungry, a complex interaction between the brain, hormones and enzymes in the gut tells you that your body needs food. Similarly, when you feel full, your stomach secretes a hormone which tells your brain that you don't need to have a second helping because you are not hungry anymore.

In 2002, Professor Steve Bloom at the Hammersmith Hospital discovered that people who are obese have a deficiency of PYY_{3-36}, a stomach hormone which helps to regulate appetite by telling people that they are full (p.100). This deficiency means that obese people eat more than they need to, and naturally their weight escalates. There are two possible reasons for this. One is that obese people are born with the deficiency. The other is that being overweight somehow turns the hormone off, creating a vicious circle whereby, once you get to be fat, you can't get thin again because there is nothing to tell you to stop eating. Though it's impossible to say for sure as yet, the latter theory is more likely to be true because when obese people do lose weight, their hormone levels returns to normal.

Now that it is understood that people who are obese are unable to regulate their appetite, research into obesity is concentrating on finding ways of tricking the brain into believing that it is either not hungry, or already full. Several prescription appetite suppressants are already available (p.92) but none are effective enough and many have side effects. However, several scientists now feel that they are close to unravelling the complex relationship between appetite and the brain and they hope to find an effective phamacological solution in the next few years. (p.101).

Though the fact that overweight people are unable to 'diet' shatters the myth that people who are overweight don't overeat or have 'slow metabolisms', it does suggest that by the time a person becomes obese they cannot stop eating because their brain fails to tell them that they are full. As Professor Bloom says, "no one chooses to be obese. There's twice the suicide rate in the overweight, they get divorced more frequently, they get married less frequently, they have two-thirds of the average wage of the thin person and their lives are actually fairly unhappy." There are over a thousand obesity related deaths in the UK every week so a pharmaceutical solution would be welcomed by the medical profession and the seriously overweight. However it probably wouldn't be welcomed by the billion dollar diet industry. If scientists prove that appetite cannot be controlled without medical help, then behavioural modification, weight-reduction programmes, and will power, will be a thing of the past.

The diet trap

MONEY FOR NOTHING Americans now spend an estimated $30 billion a year on diet programmes, diet foods and diet drinks. Comparatively, the UK spends even more – £10.3 billion. Yet the majority of diet claims are misleading, unproven or just plain false. In reality, all diets work because all diets decrease the number of calories that a person consumes, but most are impossible to sustain long term and the majority of people who do manage to lose weight end up putting it all on again as soon as they revert to their normal eating patterns. What this says is that it is normal eating patterns that have to change, not diets. But that's not what women want to hear.

DIETING IS BAD FOR YOU Women who diet rarely do it because of the long-term health benefits (unless they have been ordered to do so by a doctor). The majority are looking for a fast track to skinny and they are not particularly concerned about the health implications of diet pills, supplements, quack diets or diet foods. But crash diet programmes and pills often do more harm than good. They send your metabolism into a cycle of rapid weight loss, followed by a rapid 'rebound' weight gain once normal eating resumes.

Our bodies do not respond well to extremely low calorie diets. In an experiment at the University of Minnesota, a group of 36 young, healthy, emotionally stable men were put on a balanced diet for six months. The men ate about half the number of calories that they would have done ordinarily and followed a programme comparable to many commercial diets. After losing about 25% of their body weight, which is the point at which an average woman would weigh about the same as a supermodel, the men became irritable, tense and developed obsessional fixations with food. They also showed signs of depression, hysteria and lethargy and completely lost interest in sex. Most obesity researchers now believe that stringent dieting (unless carefully monitored and combined with counselling), can actually be a major trigger for binge eating.

THE BIG CON Nearly 50% of women say that the one thing that would make them happy is to be the right weight and more than 50% of women are on a diet right now. Most will fail in their efforts to lose weight, but dieting is a repeat business. Instead of addressing the futility of the method, women simply blame themselves for not succeeding. And try again. Sales of diet foods, pills, drinks, scales, creams, shakes, clubs etc continue to grow but cosmetic surgeons now have their eye on a share of the slimming pie. Liposuction is now the leading form of cosmetic surgery in the US with 400,000 operations carried out every year. It certainly works but unfortunately, while liposuction might get you back in to your trousers again, it has absolutely no effect on clogged arteries or out-of-control eating habits.

From the age of about four I realized I was a plump girl in a very slim family. Looking at photos now I realize I wasn't nearly as fat as I felt but I've always had that feeling – it is very much part of my self-image. I behave plump. I am sensible, caring and maternal towards others and bad at flirting and expressing a sexual side.
Jane, 38, UK

I sometimes comfort eat at the time of the month. I don't know if it is psychological or hormonal but I have put on a bit of weight around the tummy. I think that is due to a new contraceptive pill I am on, which I think I will be changing in the near future to see if it makes a difference.
Nicole, 22, UK

When I diet, as I do most of the time, I feel my mood changing. I start out full of enthusiasm but as I get hungry and I try and persuade my body to accept apples instead of the thick slices of buttered white bread that it is really craving, I begin to feel a bit like an apple, cold, hard and very acidic.
Stacey, 24, Canada

The discomfort zone

EAT UP The majority of women are aware that food that doesn't make it into their mouth, doesn't make it onto their hips. But if eating was just about satisfying hunger, life would be very simple. Women have a complex relationship with food. Feelings that are established in childhood are compounded when women have their own children. Feeding a child is one of the primary care-giving roles for mothers. And for infants, it is one of the first areas in which they can exert a degree of independence. When a child learns how to feed itself and realizes that it can refuse some foods, or demand more of others, it begins to establish a degree of autonomy. Mothers often find this period quite difficult. Nutritional concerns coupled with the frustration of a demanding infant can turn mealtimes into a battle. If feeding becomes an 'issue' , as children get older food can become a method of controlling, appeasing, bribing and rewarding.

NOT FOR ME THANKS A mother's anxieties about her child's diet often sit very uncomfortably with her own feelings about eating. She wants her child to eat, but at the same time, she may be trying to control what she allows herself to eat. This sends very mixed messages to daughters in particular. Many women don't realize how much they moan about their weight, but they do. A lot. And when anxieties about weight are transmitted to children who have not yet established their own relationship with food, a switch of consciousness takes place and the child becomes aware that diet, and thinness in particular, have a powerful relationship with confidence and control. Food is a pleasure, a comfort, a social connection, an inter-familial experience. But it is also a source of anxiety and, as such, it becomes easy, inevitable even, for girls to develop a confused and masochistic relationship with food.

THE YO-YO SYNDROME Psychologists believe that women who focus on appearance as their main reason for losing weight are less likely to succeed because their motivation is so deeply grounded in negative body image, feelings of guilt, failure and lack of control. They explain the predictable cycle to the patterns of behaviour that drive women into overeating and yo-yo dieting in the following terms. A woman who feels bad about her body decides she must become 'thinner' and in order to do that, she has to deny herself certain foods. If she becomes 'thin', she believes she will be happy and confident, and she will like herself more. So she goes on a 'diet'. But she is ill-prepared for the experience. She doesn't address her lifestyle or her emotional state, or question the possibility that she might still disap-prove of herself, even if she becomes thinner. If she is substantially overweight, she is likely to lose quite a lot of weight relatively quickly. But then her metabolism slows down (p.18) and she hits a plateau. At this point her resolve weakens. She feels good because she realizes that she can lose weight if she wants to, but hunger has left her tired, ratty, and fed up with dieting. She may be slimmer but she doesn't feel any happier, which depresses her and since she is used to using food as a way of cheering herself up, she breaks her diet. A quick fix of chocolate boosts her glucose levels and makes her feel better temporarily, but once the diet is broken, she feels guilty and thinks she has failed. Her eating becomes a little chaotic and she gains weight. She feels bad about it, but part of her feels that since she has broken the diet, it doesn't really matter what she does. Gradually she returns to the weight she was before, or she may find herself even heavier. Feeling guilty and overweight, she goes back on the diet, yet again having failed to address what she is really hoping to achieve or how realistic her goals are.

THE INVISIBLE WOMAN Although being thin is assumed to be every woman's ideal, there are many women who find it easier not to be. That may be hard to believe considering the amount of discrimination overweight people have to put up with, but in a culture of thin, being overweight can be a means of protection. Creating a barrier of fat shields an overweight woman from the rest of the world. A large woman may take up more physical space, but overweight women often describe themselves as feeling 'invisible' because society ignores people who don't conform to certain physical stereotypes. It can make a woman feel less, rather than more vulnerable because she is less likely to be the target of unwanted sexual attention, or indeed any attention at all, and for someone who has low self-esteem, has suffered abuse, is shy or lacking in confidence, hiding behind an extra 36kg (80lb) appears to make life easier rather than harder. Which is not to say it is a good idea, because carrying extra weight has huge negative health implications.

THE SHRINK DIET Losing weight successfully requires a massive cognitive reshuffle. It involves enormous commitment and a permanent and wholescale change of attitude to both eating habits and levels of fitness. So, before you go on a diet it is important to analyse whether there are any underlying issues that might be triggering the eating pattern that has lead to your weight gain. If you have dieted before and failed, you need to consider what went wrong during your previous attempts and examine whether you are likely to be any more successful if you try again. If, for example, you suspect that your weight is a response to unhappiness, or lonliness or frustration, you may actually be better off seeing a counsellor or getting psychological help before you attempt to lose weight. There is no point dieting if you really ought to be trying to fix some aspect of your emotional wellbeing, because although a diet will make you thinner temporarily, it won't sort out the behavioural and psychological triggers that influence your eating. If these aren't addressed, you will never be able to be 'off the diet' without gaining back all the weight that you have tried so hard to lose.

When I was little I had hepatitis and was not allowed to have foods high in animal fat for four years. If I get depressed, I live on a diet of ice cream, butter, cakes, cream, you name it. It has everything to do with the fact that I wasn't allowed to have it when I was little. As a grown-up, I can have it as much as I like.
Karen, 48, UK

My obsession with not being overweight has probably had the opposite effect on my daughters who are both very heavy. My son does not have the same problem.
Rosalyn, 56, Scotland

In my late 30s I went out with a man who had an inconsistent, demanding personality. He was a control freak who tried to dominate me. I stopped eating to exert control over my own life. I went from a size 12 to a size 8 in two months. He loved skinny women but wouldn't have sex with me. I thought if I was skinnier, he'd want to have sex with me. In the end, I left him. I'm back to a size 12. I don't know if I was anorexic, but it was dramatic weight loss brought on by control and lack of love from him.
Ellen, 37, UK

Monitoring what you eat

Keeping a food diary for a week or more is the easiest way to establish how your lifestyle and your emotions interfere with your efforts to lose weight. Once you have identified the triggers that make you overeat you can begin to eliminate them. While keeping your diary you shouldn't change your routine, the amount you eat or when you eat, in any way. Keep a notebook with you and record everything you consume, when, where, how hungry you were and how you felt at the time.

KEEPING A FOOD DIARY Tina is a 35-year-old working mum who feels she could lose a couple of pounds. She has quite a healthy diet and understands the basics of nutrition, but her weight has been creeping up since she had kids. She kept a food diary for a week and began to understand a few of the key issues that were causing her problems. Below is a sample day from her diary with the calorific values of the food and drink she consumed in brackets.

Time: 8.05am. *Food and drink:* Coffee. (0) Bagel with full-fat cream cheese (400). *Where:* At home, standing up, trying to get the kids to school and find my papers for work. *Feeling:* Rushed. *Hungry:* Not really hungry.

Time: 9.40am. *Food and drink:* Black coffee, glass of water (0). *Where:* At the office. *Feeling:* Trying to gear up to do some work. *Hungry:* Not really.

Time: 11am. *Food and drink:* Caffè latte (132) with three chocolate biscuits (150). *Where:* At my desk. *Feeling:* A bit tired. Need to perk up. *Hungry:* Yes.

Time: 1pm. *Food and drink:* Box of sushi (500), fruit juice (100), apple (85), caffè latte (132). *Where:* At my desk. *Feeling:* A bit guilty about the biscuits so I am having a healthy lunch. *Hungry:* Yes and I don't feel full either.

Time: 3.45pm. *Food and drink:* Coke (129). *Where:* Desk. *Feeling:* Bored, still hungry.

Time: 5.30pm. *Food and drink:* Two glasses of white wine (240), and a packet of crisps (150). *Where:* At the pub after work. *Feeling:* In a good mood. *Hungry:* Yes.

Time: 7.30pm. *Food and drink:* Cook for the kids, then finish their fish fingers and chips (162). *Where:* Home. *Feeling:* Hate waste. *Hungry:* Absolutely starving.

Time: 9.30pm. *Food and drink:* Chicken salad and pitta bread (500), glass of red wine (120). *Where:* In front of the TV with partner. *Feeling:* The kids are finally in bed and I am exhausted. *Hungry:* Less so but my partner wanted supper so I felt obliged to eat with him.

TRIGGERS Tina's food diary helped her to recognize the fact that she eats when she is stressed, rushed and bored. She doesn't need to go on a diet, but she does need to pay more attention to how, and when she eats. Eating on the run, snacking to alleviate boredom and eating because she feels she has to are all contributory factors to her gradual weight gain. As a busy working mother, Tina doesn't have much time to pay attention to her own diet, so she tends to eat when she is not hungry or waits till she is so famished that she will eat anything in sight. Simplifying things would help. Ideally, Tina and her partner should eat their main meal earlier so that she doesn't snack. And she should avoid eating in front of the TV because people eat more when they are visually distracted.

BEHAVIOUR PATTERNS In the rest of her food diary, Tina makes some classic mistakes. She goes to the supermarket after work when she is starving and ends up polishing off half a box of Pringles while she is shopping. It takes 15–20 minutes for your brain to feel that you have eaten enough but Tina doesn't wait for her food to digest before deciding that she is still hungry and having a pudding. She doesn't like waste but she often cooks more food than either she, the kids or her partner needs, which she then feels obliged to finish rather than throw away. In thinking about this, Tina suspects that she may actually do this subconsciously because she wants to eat more than she allows herself on her plate.

SERVING SIZES By following recipes and using serving guides, Tina should be able to cook more exact portions and, if she feels she is not getting enough to eat, she can increase the volume of vegetables in her diet to bulk up the mass. Tina should snack on crudités with yogurt dip or a small amount of reduced fat hummus and keep packets of chopped vegetables in the fridge so that she can whisk up dishes such as stir-fried vegetables with ginger, chilli oil and a portion of straight-to-wok noodles when she gets home from work. It takes minutes to make and is delicious, filling and very low in calories.

CALORIES Though Tina's food diary has lots of positive elements, her total calorie intake for the day is 2305 calories, 365 calories over the recommended daily allowance for a 35-year-old woman. What is interesting is that 753 of those calories come from drinks. She should cut back on alcohol, but simply swapping lattès, juice and coke for water and the occasional diet soda would take her down to well within the weight maintenance range. To lose weight Tina needs to make some basic changes. Swapping her morning bagel for a bowl of cereal, cutting out crisps, choco- late biscuits and her habit of finishing the kids' dinners would be a good place to start. If Tina could cut back by about 500 calories a day she would see a gradual and sustainable weight loss without actually feeling like she was dieting.

When I keep a food diary I realize that I consciously eat less because I am more aware of numbers of calories and the amount of junk I am consuming.
Gabrielle, 23, Canada

I don't really think about what I eat but I don't like eating a lot of sweet stuff because it makes me feel sick.. Sometimes I eat when I am not particularly hungry, especially if I have something delicious in front of me. I hate people feeling as if they have to eat and I hate people being forced to eat. I think we should just be allowed to eat what we want and leave the rest but my mother often threatens me with stories of starving children in Africa. I tell her to pack it up and send it to them if it makes her so upset.
Scarlet, 13, UK

My diet is fine if I am eating in front of anyone. My problem is that whenever I get stressed out or tired I turn to the cookie jar and once I start I can not stop. I can get through a batch of chocolate chip in ten minutes without even noticing. I will also eat ice cream, maybe a litre, on my own if I am unhappy.

Calories, servings and portions

I was called Boney M at school because I was so skinny, but in my early 20s I started to fill out a bit. I am only 5' 7" and I had always been about 8½st [54kg] but I used to smoke a lot. I stopped smoking on New Year's Day 1998 and four years later, in 2002, I was 11½st [73kg]. At that point I realised I needed to go on a diet. I have tried Weight Watchers and Slimming World and I thought they were good, but unless you keep it up you don't lose the weight. I decided to do calorie counting so I know the calories in everything. I ate 1000 calories a day, though if I was going out I would eat more. Between August and Christmas I lost a stone and I feel much more confident and happier about myself. People told me I looked great when I lost weight but after a while they stopped commenting. Now they don't say anything. I suppose they are just used to it but it makes me wonder whether I should try and lose more weight. I suppose I just crave appreciation. I felt invisible when I was fatter. I think it is probably different if you were always heavy, but if you gain weight you don't feel good.
Marion, 44, UK
(Pictured right)

All diets revolve around a simple equation: in order to lose weight, energy expended must be greater than energy consumed. Energy in dietary terms is defined in calorie units. If you eat less than the number of calories your body requires you will lose weight. Whether you do it by confining yourself to mangoes, muffins or martinis is irrelevant. As long as you take in less than you use up, you will get thinner. However, although in theory a diet of six Mars bars a day (1380 calories) would induce a weight loss of 900g–1.3kg (2–3lb) a week, in reality you would feel sick, and wouldn't be meeting any of your nutritional needs.

CALORIES The average woman needs about 1,940 calories a day. Any less than that and she will lose weight. Any more than that and she will gain weight. 1940 calories sounds like quite a lot, but when you consider that a McDonald's Big Mac and large fries contains 1130 calories you can see how easy it is to get through twice that amount in a day without even feeling full. Any woman who eats between 1400 and 1600 calories a day will lose about 450g (1lb) a week. To do this you need to be aware of the numbers of calories in the foods you are eating. You can buy pocket books that list the calorie content of most foods or you can buy a calorie counter that weighs and estimates quantities of foods before you eat them.

SERVINGS Both the US food pyramid and the UK balance of good health plate guide operate on the basis of 'servings' (eyeball guide p.38) but most women have no visual concept of what a serving looks like so they hugely underestimate how much they are eating. One would automatically assume a small bagel or an English muffin to be a single serving of carbohydrate. In fact, both items count as two servings. A breast of chicken might be considered a serving of protein but a serving, according to medical guidelines, is no more than a thin 25g (1oz) 'sandwich slice' of chicken. On packaged foods, look at the 'serving size' measurement on the nutrition label of the food's package. On a packet of brown rice, the serving size is 50g (2oz) of uncooked rice per person which looks about the size of a small scoop of ice cream and creates about 110g (4oz) of cooked rice. When following a recipe, look for how many 'servings' the recipe makes. If the recipe says 'serves four', that means that one portion is one fourth of the total amount of the food you prepare by following the ingredients and measurements in the recipe.

PORTIONS 'Servings' as recognized by nutritionists and dieticians bear little relationship to the portions served by restaurants. But studies show that people eat what is put in front of them, regardless of how hungry they feel, so today's oversized portions get eaten even though they are neither wanted nor needed. Remember, your unfed stomach is about the size of your clenched fist and if you are trying to lose weight, no portion of food that you eat should ever be any larger than that.

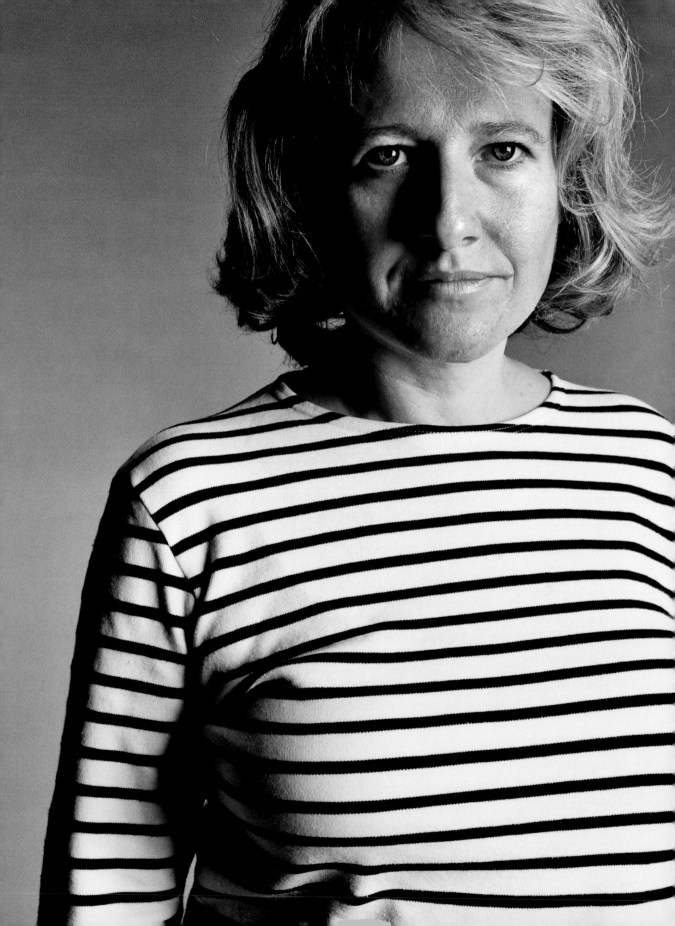

Dieting

How many calories do you need to consume every day?

Girls aged 12–14:
1845 calories

Girls aged 15–18:
2110 calories

Adult women:
1940 calories

Women aged 64+:
1900 calories

Women aged 75+:
1810 calories

Dieting actually makes me feel more energetic and alive than I do normally. I feel more physically sensitive to the environment around me and I love the feeling of my emerging hip bones.
Kay, 27, US

I haven't weighed myself for a couple of years because I'm too scared to. I'm always trying to lose a bit because I eat too much but it tends to be a push pull situation. I tend to eat a lot all the time and the way I try and make myself feel better about it is by trying to eat healthy food. I did a food diary once and my consumption is huge. I tried the Mayo clinic diet and I did lose weight around my stomach but I came out in hives also. Nothing works for me.
Lily, 30, Australia

THE FIRST STEP Eating is pleasurable. Exercise is hard work. Dieting is both boring and hard work, and because there really is no way around that, most women give up trying very quickly. Losing weight and keeping it off is a big commitment and unless you are willing to take the process seriously there is no point even thinking about it. If you feel you need to lose weight, your first step should be to see your GP. Tell your doctor that you plan to go on a diet. Get yourself weighed at the surgery and discuss how much weight you should be aiming to lose. Then make another appointment to be weighed in about three months' time. Be realistic about how much weight you should try and lose and plan out a monthly weight-loss target. Weigh yourself just once a week, preferably on Wednesday morning.

Your first week should be spent monitoring your normal eating habits (p.72). If you see a pattern emerging, you may want to change the times that you eat your main meals to coincide with when you get hungry and end up snacking.

Choose a diet that features food you enjoy, e.g. a high carb, low fat diet if you enjoy carbs, or a protein diet if you enjoy meat. Learn to calorie count and monitor serving sizes. Most people simply don't realize how much they eat (p.74)

Don't tell anyone that you are going on a diet so you won't have to deal with continual enquiries about your progress. However, if you have a partner or friend who needs to lose weight, consider doing it together so that you can monitor each other's progress or join a slimming club so that you have some support.

Exercise every day and do it when other people are eating. Gyms tend to be quieter at around 8pm and you will be less tempted to break your diet if you keep busy. Eat a light supper before you work out, and have a small snack afterwards when your metabolic rate is faster than normal. If you break your diet, don't give up, just exercise the next day.

Though diets such as Atkins do encourage rapid weight loss research shows that when women who have been on rigid diets go back to eating normally, they put the weight they have lost back on again within a year.

Medical experts believe yo-yo dieting where a woman repeatedly loses the same 4.5kg (10lb) is bad for health and may increase the risk of heart disease. They encourage a sensible approach to dieting, i.e. committing to a long-term weight-loss plan, developing better eating habits and taking exercise. As such, the diets in the section listed as Diets that work (p.78) are ones that are sustainable and more likely to be adopted as a way of life rather than a diet.

Losing it

KETOSIS When your body is deprived of food for a couple of days, it begins to run out of its reserves of glycogen (energy) and has to draw on its stores of body fat as an alternative energy source. This process is called ketosis and it occurs on all 'starvation diets'. However the process is accelerated if you cut carbohydrates (energy foods) completely. Ketosis is a sign that you are losing weight, but your body doesn't give up fat without a fight so there are some interesting side effects.

SMELLITOSIS During the first day or two of a starvation diet you will begin to feel very hungry and light headed. Your blood sugar levels will dip and you will lose several pounds in weight, most of which will be water. After about three days you can tell that your body is beginning to burn its own fat as fuel (ketosis) because your breath will begin to smell quite strange. The smell is sometimes described as being like pear drops or a cross between apples and nail polish remover. The smell is due to the production of ketones in your liver. Ketones are an acid by-product, which are normally excreted in urine but, during extreme weight loss, volatile ketones such as acetone are expelled as gas from the lungs, which cause the distinctive odour.

RAPID WEIGHT LOSS Weight loss is very rapid with ketosis because your kidneys go into overdrive, excreting urine in an effort to balance the salt levels in your body. Since sodium, potassium and phosphorus are also excreted in urine, if it goes on for too long, it can create a serious chemical imbalance in the body.

SLOW RESPONSE TIMES With little or no glucose available, fat cells release fats into the blood as an alternative fuel source. But the brain needs a certain amount of carbohydrate to function properly – about 150g (5oz) a day. If you eat a very low carbohydrate diet for a while, or if you starve yourself, your brain stops working as well and your thinking and reaction times tend to slow down. You tend not to notice these changes when you are on a diet, because the changes in your brain make you slower to react to stimuli and you become less self-aware. This can make a difference if you are doing anything such as driving, which can require quick thinking and reflexes, though in evolutionary terms it would have been an advantage, because the brain would have been less sensitive to feelings of hunger.

Sometimes ketogenic diets are used specifically because they slow down reaction times. People with epilepsy are sometimes put on them to make their brains less likely to react to triggers that make them fit. Furthermore, on a low to no carbohydrate diet, the protein you eat – and protein from muscles – is converted to glucose to supply the brain's needs. So if you go on this diet, you may feel tired because you have lost muscle mass as well.

When I am totally stressed I can feel my body changing. I don't really realize it but I stop eating enough and then everything just seems to speed up. I feel the adrenaline pumping and my heartbeat is elevated and I get a tinny taste in my mouth. I suffer from anxiety and it is all related. It's not a healthy or natural state.
Helen, 39, UK

I lost about 2st [13kg] in weight through exercise in about eight months. I stopped eating rubbish and I made more time for myself. I hired a personal trainer who went through nutrition and planned my training. She looked at my lifestyle and told me how to look at my food intake and find out where I was going wrong. I wasn't eating pie and chips but I was taking in too many calories and my lifestyle was too sedentary. I now try and walk more and I am a lot more active than I used to be. I am not anal about food but I am conscious of what I am taking in because before I just didn't think about it. Now if I have a huge meal, I will keep myself in check for a few days. Before I would just keep piling into the food.
Ant, 34, UK

Diets that work if you stick to them

WEIGHT WATCHERS Established in the US in 1963, over the years Weight Watchers has helped millions of people to lose weight and is a much copied formula. Weight Watchers combines weekly meetings and weigh-ins with a personalized diet plan, which is essentially based on calorie counting. Dieters pay a joining fee and when they come to weekly meetings they pay a small attendance fee. The meetings motivate dieters to stick to the programmes and the Points Plan (a system whereby food and drink is allocated a number of points depending on their calorie content) makes working out how much you are consuming relatively easy. The eat-what-you-want approach directs members towards an all-things-in-moderation way of living, rather than a diet mentality, which is essentially what any good diet programme should hope to do.

During the week, you record the number of points you eat at each meal on a pre-printed food journal and you plan your evening meal around your remaining points. You are also required to check off the dairy products, veggies and fruit you eat, as well as the water you drink, to ensure you are getting a good nutritional balance. Vegetables are allowed in unlimited quantities so you won't go hungry. You can eat anything you want on Weight Watchers. The key is deciding what foods you want to allot your points for the day to. You can also do what is called 'banking' points. If you have a special event coming up, you can reserve some of your points from one day and use them another. As you begin to lose weight, the number of points you are allocated is reduced so that weight loss doesn't plateau and it can be difficult to accustom yourself to increasingly smaller portions of food.

Generally, most women find the weekly weigh-ins and group support very helpful as the diet becomes more difficult and the programme is good for women who want to track their long-term progress. If the programme is followed accurately, you will probably lose about 450–900g (1–2lb) a week after your first week and weight loss at this rate is more likely to be permanent. Weight Watchers also encourages participants to exercise and you can earn points by working out. It does prove costly, especially if you have a lot of weight to lose – and you have to pay the attendance fee even if you miss a meeting. Weight Watchers have now introduced an online plan, though the group support provided by the meetings appears to be the secret to Weight Watchers' success. Weight Watchers sell ready meals, snacks and desserts at most supermarkets and the Lean Cuisine range of ready meals also provides the Weight Watchers points plan on their packaging.

There are several variations on the Weight Watchers theme. Slimmers World is one of the biggest with over 5,500 groups nationwide. Less widely available is Curves, a promising US initiative which combinines group exercise with a low carb diet.

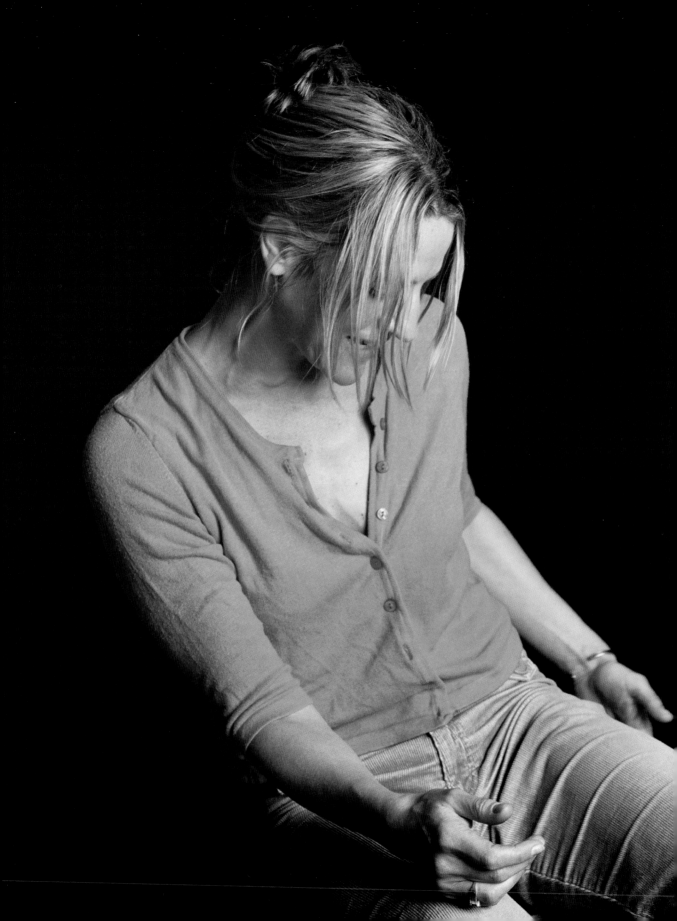

I don't think diets are healthy. For a short-term period you are changing your diet and denying your body stuff that it wants and needs (Atkins is a perfect example), but is it realistic to believe that you will spend the rest of your life eating no starches or all cantaloupes? NO! You are just setting yourself up for long-term failure. Eat good food is my long-term diet plan. You can find an apple in almost any store you go into. Eat that instead of the Snickers bar. Or eat ½ the Snickers bar and save the rest for later. Moderation is best, Aristotle said it. 'Everyone feasts but no one is full.'
Bobby, 31, US

Since sushi is my favourite food I have no trouble getting enough good fat in my diet. I like all Japanese food really and my favourite restaurant in London is Nobu because they make the best oriental food. Better than Japan even. You have to be careful buying raw fish because it needs to be good quality, especially if you are buying it pre packed. I can say that Marks and Spencer do absolutely the worst sushi in london. Yeuch.
Star, 24, UK

JAPANESE DIET According to the WHO, Japanese people have the best life expectancy in the world. Their traditional low fat diet has always been a major factor in the low rates of heart disease and lung cancer (though Japanese women who adopt a Western-style diet are now suffering from increased rates of breast cancer, coronary heart disease and diabetes). The negative aspects of the traditional Japanese diet are few, though salt intake is very high. Soy sauce, for example, contains 16% salt and stomach cancer, the biggest cause of death in Japan, is thought to be directly related to that. It may also be related to a high intake of pickled foods, which contain cancer-causing chemicals called nitrosamines.

Research shows that the greater the variety of foods a person eats, the lower the risk of many diseases. A survey of the diets of 200 elderly Japanese women revealed that they consumed a variety of over 100 biologically different foods per week. By contrast, in most Western countries, the recommended minimum is only 30, and most of us don't even manage that. Westerners, on average, eat 47 times more meat than fish. By contrast, the Japanese consume three times more fish than meat and this healthy combination of fish and a variety of plant foods provides a great nutritional base. White rice is the main dietary staple balanced with lots of oily fish such as tuna, mackerel and, more recently, salmon, which contains good fats like omega-3 fatty acids, which lower cholesterol. Red meat is minimal though nothing is excluded and the general approach is a little of everything. Vegetables, such as bamboo shoots, eggplant, mushrooms, sweet potato and Chinese cabbage play an important role and natural flavourings such as herbs, spices and condiments such as ginger, lemon, sesame seed, wasabi horseradish, shiso oba leaves and mustard add other essential nutrients. And fresh fruit is served at the end of every meal.

Japanese women also consume approximately 40 times more soy products than Western women. Soy contains naturally occurring plant oestrogens (phyto-oestrogens) and scientists believe that this may explain the absence of negative menopausal symptoms amongst Japanese women, though some experts argue that Japanese women just don't whinge as much. Phyto-oestrogens are also thought to protect against breast cancer and osteoporosis. Japanese women who stick to a traditional diet generally don't have to worry about their weight or their health and they have great skin because they drink tons of green tea, which is particularly rich in antioxidants. Our own black tea is also antioxidant-rich, but the effect is destroyed with the addition of milk, which prevents their absorption.

Although making Japanese food requires an enormous amount of planning and preparation, so many restaurants and delis now sell pre-prepared Japanese food that this diet is actually a very easy option for women who are working or haven't got much time to cook. And because packaged foods give a complete breakdown of their ingredients, it is relatively easy to construct a plan that is nutritionally sound and stays within your calorie-controlled diet. The secret is to try and vary the range of fish, vegetables, salads, seeds, nuts and fruits that you consume.

A one-day menu might include: *Breakfast*: a small bowl of muesli with chopped fruit and skimmed milk or a soft boiled egg, with one slice of soy and linseed toast and a cup of green tea. *Lunch*: might be a miso soup with either a sashimi platter or a sushi selection box with a large mixed chopped salad, a small fresh fruit salad and a cup of green tea. *Dinner*: might be a stir-fry of chopped vegetables, cashews and beansprouts with noodles flavoured with lemon, garlic and sesame oil, or a large bowl of broth with chopped vegetables, tofu or chicken and noodles with a large salad of chopped veg with sunflower and pumpkin seeds followed by a raspberry and kiwi fruit salad. The daily calorie total is less than 1400 but it includes a broad range of nutritious foods, is high in omega-3 and omega-6 fatty acids. Weight loss should be about 450g (1lb) a week.

LOW FAT DIET In many ways, the term low fat diet is a misnomer because, in an ideal world, these eating plans would not actually be considered diets, but healthy eating programmes, that should be adhered to all the time. Low fat diets enjoy continued support from the medical establishment who believe that reducing the amount of saturated fat we eat lowers cholesterol and decreases our chances of developing coronary heart disease. Low fat plans encourage people to fill about 60% of a moderated calorie intake with complex carbohydrates, such as unrefined cereals, wholemeal bread, brown rice, fruits, vegetables, beans and legumes, with the other 40% being made up of protein and fat.

Unrefined carbohydrates burn about 25% of their own calories in converting themselves into energy – whereas fat is seven times more easily converted to bulge. But very few of us have any idea about how much fat is in the foods we eat. As a guideline, any food that is labelled as containing 20g+ fat per 100g with 5g+ as saturates is a high fat food. Any food that contains 3g fat per 100g with 1g as saturates is a low fat food. We also have several misconceptions about the fat content of meat. Often demonized as fatty, a sirloin steak with the visible fat removed is actually quite low in fat at 4–8g per 100g (minced meat has a higher fat content) while skinless chicken only contains about 1–3g fat per 100g, though the darker meat contains more fat than the white meat.

There are several different low fat diets on the market, the most famous ones being the *Hip and Thigh Diet* by Rosemary Conley, *The Diet* by Dr Dean Ornish and *The*

I was so much healthier when I lived in Japan because I ate a lot of tofu and fish and girls don't really drink beer there. Since I moved to the UK I drink a lot of beer and it is hard to find fresh food so I have become more unhealthy.
Kana, 25, Japan

Japanese food is the perfect combination for me. The oily fish and rice is filling but healthy and low in calories. I try and eat sushi as often as I can though I am now concerned about the health warnings on salmon so I tend to choose tuna sashimi and prawn or squid sushi. I also believe that green tea is very good for my skin.
Angie, 36, US

My lunch used to be a hit and miss affair. I'd grab a sandwich and chips and maybe a latte and cake but my weight shot up so now, before I go to lunch I check the website of my local sandwich chain and make a calorie controlled choice. Sushi 500 calories or humous and vegetable wrap 300 calories plus a fruit salad. I haven't lost weight yet but I haven't gained any weight either.
Kerry, 25, US

Pritikin Weight Loss Breakthrough by Robert Pritikin. All three programmes restrict calorie intake to around 1300 calories a day and provide lists of foods that can be eaten freely, so there is no need to count calories. The list of banned foods is extensive – all fats, oils, nuts, seeds, avocados and refined carbohydrates such as white flour, white rice and sugars. Though the Rosemary Conley Hip and Thigh Diet won't target fat on the hips and thighs as the title implies, it does contain a decent exercise programme, which puts it streets ahead of other diet plans. Because these diets are both very low in calories and very low in fats, there is some concern that good HDL cholesterol levels might be negatively affected, so adding a fish oil supplement would probably be a good idea.

The problem with low fat diets is that because they are balanced and not too stringent, they can take months to deliver a noticeable result and most women are just too impatient to stick to them. Many women also go wrong on low fat diets because of the misconception that anything labelled 'low fat' is actually low calorie. You can't eat low fat yogurts on a low fat diet without factoring in the fact that each one adds up to 100 calories to your daily total. A packet of salt and vinegar lite crisps (33% less fat) implies fewer calories. In fact, they contain 465 calories per 100g, just 60 calories less than the full fat version. It still counts as a saving, but studies show that because people who choose low fat products believe they are eating something healthy, they tend to eat more of the food than they would if they had opted for the full fat version in the first place. Subconsciously, the loss of fat appears to register as deprivation, so dieters console themselves with greater quantities.

A one-day menu might include: *Breakfast*: a small bowl of bran or muesli topped with fresh strawberries and a slice of wholegrain toast with low fat spread. *Lunch*: a large mixed salad with some tuna and an oil and vinegar dressing and an apple for pudding. *Dinner*: a small grilled chicken breast with roasted vegetables and a small salad. You can enjoy a glass of wine and a banana for pudding and you can drink water, tea, coffee or diet sodas throughout the day. The calorie count per day is about 1500, which should lead to a weight loss of about 450g (1lb) a week, though obviously if you eat less that ratio will increase.

EAT RIGHT 4 YOUR TYPE Written by Dr Peter D'Adamo, a naturopathic specialist, this diet is based on the premise that our blood type controls whether we view certain things in our diet as foreign or friendly. Though sceptics have called his theories 'pure horse manure' and there is no scientific backing or even approval for this diet, the book has sold 2 million copies, so it is unlikely that D'Adamo actually cares that much. D'Adamo's ideas are based on evidence that the most common blood type, 'O', goes back to the pre-historic age of hunter-gatherers. His theory suggests that people with type-O blood do best eating foods rich in fat and protein, such as meat or fish, skimping on carbohydrates and dairy and avoiding foods like lentils, brazil nuts, avocados and oranges altogether. Type-A blood appeared later in farming cultures, making modern-day 'A' and 'A–B' blood types better off with diets heavy on grains, carbohydrates, fish and plant foods, skimping on dairy and avoiding red meat altogether. Blood type-B evolved after 'O' and 'A' and is a balance of both.

An overview of the type-O diet suggests that this is basically a calorie controlled high protein, low carbohydrate diet, but because the diet is based on natural foods and plenty of fruit and veg with a ban on refined foods, it is more nutritionally sound than diets like Atkins. However, it requires the kind of forward planning and shopping that most women find to be a real pain in the ass. D'Adamo also suggests that exercise should be tailored to your blood group which is frankly stretching it a bit. Type 'O' should engage in vigorous exercise, while type 'A' should do light activities like yoga and golf.

A typical diet day for someone with blood group 'O' would be: *Breakfast*: rye bread, plums, walnuts and pineapple juice. *Lunch*: mackerel fillet, spinach, red pepper and onion salad, with fresh figs. *Dinner*: lamb chops with broccoli, parsnips and an apple. The calorie intake is about 1400 a day. Although the programme is aimed at health rather than weight loss, and D'Adamo claims the diet has successfully helped treat unexplained symptoms such as rashes or itching in patients, the drop in daily calories should lead to losses of about 450–900g (1–2lb) a week.

FOOD COMBINING Food combining was first introduced in 1911 by Dr William Howard Hay who believed that eating certain foods together caused a chemical imbalance in the digestive system. The diet wasn't originally devised as a weight loss plan and there is no scientific evidence to support Hay's theories because the body is perfectly capable of digesting pretty much anything put into it. However, the diet is nutritionally sound because it allows you to eat from all the food groups, albeit at different times. Consuming only one major calorie source per meal, i.e. protein or carbohydrate, automatically limits the number of calories you consume, so, assuming you don't overeat, you can expect to lose weight this way.

The basic rules of the diet are relatively simple once you get the hang of it. Hay suggests that protein (meat, fish, chicken, dairy, tofu) and allowed carbohydrates (wholegrain rice, wholegrain bread, potatoes, pulses) should never be eaten together at the same meal, because starches are broken down by alkaline saliva and proteins require gastric acid. Vegetables can be eaten with both. Hay believed that

I used to be incredibly strict with myself about everything I ate. I knew the calorie content and nutritional value of absolutely everything. Now I take a more relaxed approach and although I have gained some weight I do feel healthier.
Fiona, 37, UK

Sometimes I feel very good about my diet and then at other times I feel like I get sucked down into a food vortex. If I'm not eating properly my naval piercing starts acting up. That's when I know I've gone too far. At that point I'm uncomfortable with my body.
Tara, 24, Canada

I think I've been on a diet since I was about seven. I have always seen myself as fat. I never ate like a normal child and was very body conscious, especially in the changing rooms at school.
Sam, 24, UK

I felt so hungry on a low fat diet that I gave up very quickly. I need to eat some protein and carb to feel full. Rabbit food just leaves me too hungry. I think that as long as you cut down on sugar and alcohol you should be able to find a balance.
Julie, 29, Scotland

fruits should always be eaten on their own because they digest very rapidly, a process that is held up if they are eaten with foods that take longer to digest in the stomach. Only a single protein or a single carbohydrate can be eaten at a time and all refined starches such as white bread, white rice, pasta, biscuits, cakes and sweets, have to be avoided completely. Milk should be taken in minimal quantities and 70% of the diet should be high water content foods such as fruit, salads and vegetables. There should be no less than four hours between starch and protein meals.

A typical Hay Day would consist of: *Breakfast*: a fresh fruit salad or boiled eggs with slices of cucumber. *Lunch*: might be a salad sandwich on wholemeal bread with mayo. *Dinner*: you might have grilled fish or chicken with veg. The calorie count should come in at about 1000–1500, depending on serving sizes and generally it is easy enough to follow because there is no weighing and measuring. You can vary meals quite a lot and if you eat out, just ditch the side order of potatoes and stick to meat, chicken or fish with salad.

THE VEGETARIAN DIET Becoming a vegetarian is often a matter of principle but many women, particularly teenage girls, decide to adopt a vegetarian diet because they presume it will make them thinner. Sadly not. Non-meat simply doesn't mean non-fat. In fact, convenience vegetarian foods such as veggie burgers often contain more fat than meat; check the label! Much of the nutrition that is supplied by meat can be found in non-meat foods like dairy products, cheese and eggs. However, cheese contains more fat than many meat products and egg yolks are high in cholesterol. Your total daily cholesterol intake should be no more than 300mg; an egg yolk contains 213mg.

You can lose weight by cutting out meat, chicken and fish, but you need to know how to get the right protein balance and should have a sound understanding of nutrition. You will need to switch to low fat dairy and eat plenty of pulses, tofu and dark green leafy vegetables to maintain an adequate nutritional and calcium intake. Weight loss means light eating, even if you are a vegetarian.

To keep your diet as non-fattening as possible, go easy on dairy, egg yolks and mayonnaise and aim to buy low fat dairy products and skimmed or fat free milk. Check the sugar content in any low fat foods that you buy and avoid the usual suspects, sweet stuff such as biscuits, cakes and sweets and fizzy drinks – and although you should drink juice, eating fresh fruit or juicing it yourself is preferable. Vegans should include vitamin B12 in their diets (fortified cereal and fortified soy milk) along with vitamin D (soy milk, margarine and fortified cereals), particularly if exposure to sunshine is limited.

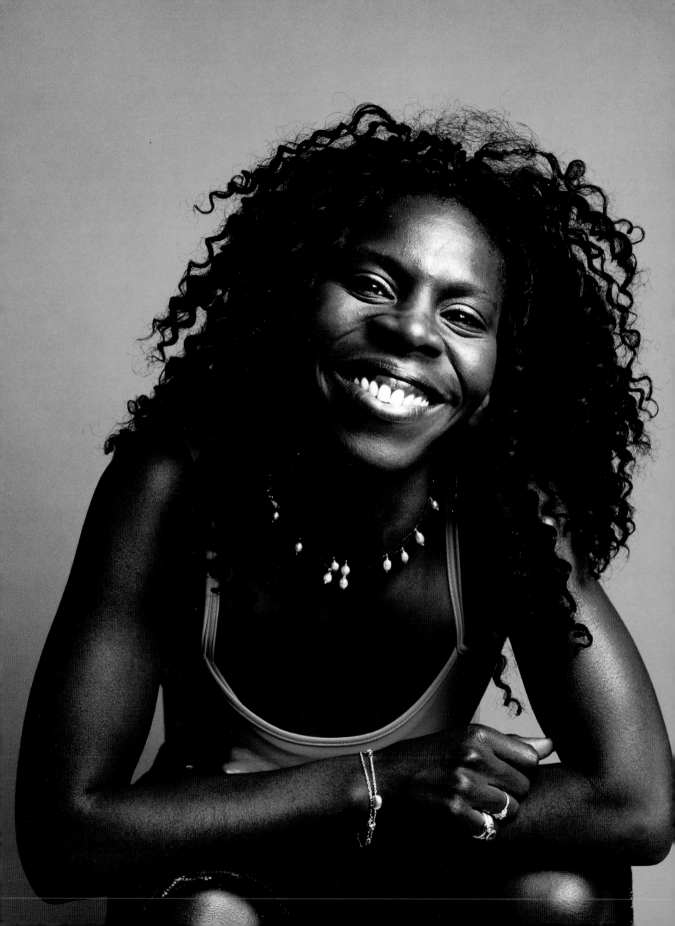

Lighter life, detox diets and fasting

LIGHTER LIFE Developed by experts in the UK and delivered by trained counsellors, this programme is a GP monitored plan which aims to assist controlled weight loss, whilst at the same time promoting greater understanding of food issues. It has only been operating for six years so it is not completely nationwide but details are available at www.lighterlife.com. This is not a cosmetic diet programme and is only aimed at the seriously overweight. It involves consuming mainly liquids and nutritionally balanced powders for three months to get the body into a constant state of ketosis, and encourage rapid weight loss. Removing normal food from the programme gives dieters time and space to understand what triggers their overeating and bi-weekly sessions with a counsellor help dieters to examine issues such as lifestyle, stress, boredom, addictive cravings and emotional eating. The people behind the Lighter Life programme believe that normal diets treat the symptoms of obesity, without treating the cause. This programme attempts to help dieters question why they feel they need to 'use' food. They believe that losing weight, without understanding why you put it on in the first place is a lost cause, because the weight will go back on again as soon as you stop dieting since you haven't developed an alternative coping mechanism for dealing with your triggers. It is very tought but the focus on counselling means it has a better success rate. Dieters should become more aware of their eating habits and their nutritional needs and weighing 19–31kg (3–5st) lighter but maintaining that weight loss once you go back to eating solids can be difficult unless you adhere to a strict maintenance programme The programme costs £45 per week and for that you get all the food you are allowed to eat (not much) and two sessions of counselling.

DETOX LIQUIDS Detox liquids contain natural ingredients (cloves, liquorice, kelp, juniper, fruit juice) which are supposed to 'eliminate toxins' but essentially they have a diuretic effect. The liquid is diluted in a litre of water and drunk throughout the day for three days. You can have three small meals: *Breakfast*: any wholewheat cereal. *Dinner and lunch*: a protein, a carb and veg. Prohibited foods include bread (not rye bread), salt, meat, cakes, biscuits, processed foods, coffee and alcohol. If you can stick to it, you will lose water weight so it is a good short-term plan if you are desperate to get into a little black dress – or even a big white one.

FASTING Most people who fast swear they feel re-energized and since none of us suffer from starvation there is no harm in doing it for one day each week, as long as you drink lots of water, unsweetened fruit juice and clear broth to keep yourself hydrated. Not eating allows your insulin levels to drop and boosts your adrenaline. Don't do it for longer than 24 hours and, if your aim is temporary weight loss, make sure you eat a good breakfast the following morning so you are not light headed during the day. Avoid caffeine and alcohol.

Diets that you can't or shouldn't stick to

ATKINS Yes, yes, yes, the Atkins diet does help people lose weight and it shows rapid results, *but* the only diets that can really be said to work are those that are both sustainable and don't do harm. And the jury is still out on Atkins in this respect. The original Dr Atkins Diet Revolution was first published in the 1970s. It is based on the premise that starches (rice and potatoes), refined carbohydrates (bread, bagels, pasta) and sugars (anything sweet, even fruit juice) are the primary cause of obesity (and even heart disease), and that, contrary to medical opinion, fat is harmless, filling and does not incur the increased insulin production and blood sugar swings associated with a diet high in carbohydrates and sugars. Atkins believed that a high protein, high fat, low carbohydrate diet induces ketosis (p.77), which forces the muscles and tissues to burn body fat for energy, creating more efficient weight loss with minimal hunger and increased energy levels.

The diet received its most powerful scientific support in May 2003 when two studies published in the *New England Journal of Medicine* demonstrated that the diet helps people lose weight faster without raising their cholesterol. The research found that people on the Atkins diet lost twice as much weight over six months as those on a standard low fat diet. And Atkins dieters generally had better levels of 'good' cholesterol and triglycerides, or fats, in the blood than those on a low fat diet – though some experts believe that this is because the Atkins dieters were given daily fish oil supplements and those on a low fat diet were not. However, as with most stringent diets, the Atkins control group managed to put on all the weight they had lost within a year of coming off the diet.

15 million followers believe in Atkins but the WHO, the UK and US Departments of Health, the American Medical Association and the American Dietetic Association don't. They are concerned about the links between a high fat, high protein diet and heart disease, high cholesterol and kidney failure, while the American Institute for Cancer Research (AICR) say that inducing ketosis can lead to muscle breakdown, dehydration, headaches, nausea and kidney problems. They believe long-term use of the diet increases the chance of kidney failure and can lead to ketoacidosis, a fatal variant of ketosis. Other studies have shown that low carb diets increase the amount of calcium excreted in urine by up to 130mg which, over several years, would significantly increase the risk of osteoporosis in later life. Recent studies also link the Atkins diet to infertility. The final nail in the coffin comes from Robert Atkins himself. According to details from a leaked coroner's report, at the time of his death in 2003 April he was clinically obese (18st 6lb) and had a history of heart attack, congestive heart failure and hypertension. In January 2004, after mounting pressure and fear of lawsuits, his company was finally forced to issue a warning stating that only 20% of fat on the diet should be saturated.

I am the right weight for my height according to BMI scales but there isn't a day that goes by when I don't think about being lighter at least five times. I measure my weight by whether I fit into my clothes and I try to avoid the scales at all costs. If I don't have enough to do, I eat and eat, constantly visiting the fridge as I aimlessly pad around my apartment. Depression makes me eat more but that only makes me more depressed. I have done all the diets – Slimfast, Cabbage Soup, Grapefruit diet and Atkins. Atkins really works and is not too difficult. On Atkins I lost 10lb [4.5kg] in two weeks and pretty much kept it off.
Sarah, 37, UK

I tried an emergency crash diet before a big date once and I broke down about five hours in. It's foolish really and, to be honest, if you can't go to your ten year reunion the way you are then you are silly. Just be happy with who you are.
Marina, 32, US

The Atkins diet is great for about three days but that is about all anyone can stick.
Kim, 37, UK

The diet is relatively simple to follow. During the 14-day induction phase, only pure proteins are allowed. Pure proteins include meat, fish and shellfish, poultry and eggs, along with pure fats, such as butter, olive oil and mayonnaise. No more than 20g (¾oz) of carbohydrates are allowed during this period. These should be weighed exactly and should come in the form of vegetables such as salad, asparagus, broccoli and kale. No fruit, bread, grains or starchy vegetables such as potatoes are allowed. Because so many foods are omitted on the diet it is advisable that you take a multi-vitamin and a fish oil supplement. A typical menu might include: *Breakfast*: eggs, bacon and decaf coffee. *Lunch*: cheeseburger with no bun, diet soda and a small amount of broccoli. *Dinner*: chicken, romaine lettuce and mayonnaise rolled up together. After 14 days you can increase your carb intake by 5g (¼oz) but you will eventually hit a plateau and have to slack off your carb intake once again. Once you reach your goal weight, you can introduce a few more carbs back into your diet, but if you pile into the bagels, you will soon see your weight shoot up again.

Because you don't have to weigh or portion any foods other than carbohydrates, the diet is relatively easy to stick to but you do need to adhere to the no-carb policy for the diet to work. The typical calorie count for a day's eating is 1400 but the drastic reduction in carbohydrate consumption causes fluid loss, which makes initial weight loss very rapid (1.8–5.4kg (4–12lb) in the first two weeks). Eating protein is comparatively more expensive than filling up on vegetables, but women who want to lose weight quickly believe it is worth the expense. If viewed as a long-term programme, the Atkins diet fails because it doesn't encourage healthy eating habits, but before becoming overly concerned about the negative health implications, it is probably worth bearing in mind that most women who go on diets don't do so long term and often don't stick rigidly to them anyway. Though it would be irresponsible to suggest that a life-long diet of meat and no veg was suitable for anyone other than our prehistoric ancestors (who only lived to 25), it can be a good way to kick start weight loss for women wishing to shift a few pounds quickly.

THE ZONE The success of the Atkins low carb diet has spawned a number of adaptations such as the South Beach Diet but the most famous is the Zone by Dr Barry Sears. The central premise is based on balancing the ratio of carbs, fat and proteins in your diet in order to control your body's insulin production, but although it is generally a more balanced plan than Atkins, it is incredibly complicated to follow and the quantities have to be very precise, which makes it very fiddly and annoying. Some 40% of your daily calorie intake comes from carbohydrates, 30% from protein, and 30% from fat. Sears talks about blocks of food and stresses the importance of portion sizes, which is a good thing. However, the amount of food allowed in the blocks is tiny and the diet only clocks in at 600–800 calories a day, which is a drastic reduction. There is no doubt that anyone who sticks to the Zone diet will lose weight, but the presence of 40% carbohydrate means ketosis does not occur. Dieticians might see that as a plus, but for dieters it is a big minus because ketosis diminishes appetite. Most people end up feeling hungry and light headed and the minute they go off the programme their weight shoots back up. The Zone essentially follows glycaemic index ratings (p.38). High GI foods, such as carrots, parsnips, sweet potatoes, bananas, bread, pasta, rice, noodles, corn, and sugar, are listed as 'unfavourable', though alcohol may be consumed in moderation. Fish and chicken are the plan's staple foods and you can choose side dishes from the 'favourable' carbs list, which include vegetables like beans, kale and spinach. There are lots of expensive ingredients so planning meals and shopping becomes a nightmare.

One of the simpler days might include: *Breakfast*: four egg-white omelette, half a grapefruit, half an English muffin and 25g (1oz) lean Canadian bacon. *Lunch*: might be 75g (3oz) turkey breast, half green bell pepper, and 1½ tbsp guacamole in a mini pitta pocket with a plum. *Afternoon snack*: two hard-boiled eggs, half an apple and three almonds. *Dinner*: 130g (4½oz) poached salmon with 1 small courgette, two tomatoes and a half an apple. *Late night snack*: 25g (1oz) turkey breast with ½ tbsp guacamole and a small bowl of strawberries. You can also eat at fast food restaurants if you fancy eating two meat patties with one bun. Mmm. Sears also sells Zone supplement bars and snacks, which are part of the plan. In Hollywood, most Zone dieters use Zone Gourmet and get all their meals delivered to ensure they stick to the plan but for lesser mortals, the idea of shelling out 50 bucks a day for diet food is a bit hard to stomach.

SLIMFAST Liquid meal replacement plans were started back in the 1960s with the Optifast diet. Very low calorie meal replacement plans are generally medically supervised and only for very obese people who need to lose a lot of weight quickly as the drinks provide only 500–800 calories per day in seven shakes. But commercial versions, such as the Slimfast diet, integrate shakes with solid food. The Slimfast diet involves replacing breakfast and lunch with a nutritionally balanced shake made from skimmed milk powder, fibre, vitamins, minerals and sweeteners.

Each shake contains about 220 calories and you are also allowed two additional pieces of fruit and a Slimfast Bar as needed during the day. In the evening, you can have a calorie controlled meal containing approximately 600 calories, e.g. 110–175g (4–6oz) of poultry, fish, or lean meat; half baked potato; three servings of steamed vegetables (1½ cups of cooked vegetables); a large salad; and fruit for dessert. Slimfast also encourages dieters to drink six to eight cups of water daily.

I have used an enema kit to detox and lose weight. You string it up on the towel rail, lay on the floor, and insert the tube into your rectum, then slowly release about 1–1½ litres [1¾–2½ pints] of water into your anus. The water is luke warm and is usually mixed with linseed extract. As you lie there, the rectum and intestines start to contract quite powerfully, and you feel quite sick. After holding on for about 15 minutes you go to the toilet, and it is very surprising what comes out ... after fasting for a few days, what is flushed out is the very black pebble-like bits that have been there for quite some time. I think that releasing this old toxic fecal matter is extremely beneficial and can help clear up skin problems, sharpen the mind, and give better overall health.
Katie, 31, NZ

I did the Slimfast diet and it is the only diet that ever worked for me. I only found out why recently. It turns out that I am completely allergic to wheat and the Slimfast meant I didn't eat wheat, just an evening meal of meat and veg. As a result, I felt better on it.
Alex, 29, UK

Any diet that restricts the number of calories you consume will make you lose weight and anyone who sticks to a Slimfast programme can expect to lose approximately 900g (2lb) a week. However, once you return to eating normally the weight usually goes right back on. And God is it boring. The shakes themselves taste pretty revolting and with nothing to chew on you just yearn for a hunk of bread or something to get your teeth into. The shakes are nutritionally balanced and their composition is covered by legislation so you won't go short of vitamins and minerals. However, although two different studies have shown that meal replacement dieting is both safe and effective, as a programme it doesn't encourage dieters to address their eating habits and, as a result, they are highly unlikely to deal with the root cause of their weight problem and make the necessary dietary changes to ensure that weight loss is sustainable in the long term.

Liquid meal replacements cater for people who can't be bothered to invest in the necessary planning, shopping and cooking that most diets require. In fact, anyone who eats a bowl of cornflakes with low fat milk and chopped strawberries for breakfast and some steamed fish with a large salad for lunch is actually consuming fewer calories than a person drinking two to three shakes. Essentially, Slimfast drinks are a quick, unimaginative and ultimately unsustainable option for people who are trying to lose weight.

THE HOLLYWOOD 48-HOUR MIRACLE DIET This 'Miracle Juice' has supposedly been scientifically formulated, so that in just 48 hours you will cleanse your body and lose up to 4.5kg (10lb) in weight. Well, you just know that is never going to happen, but you may well lose a lot of water if you drink this $20 diuretic. The diet is a two-day juice fast. Four times a day, you dilute 125ml (4fl oz) of the juice with 125ml (4fl oz) of water, and sip the drink over the next four hours. You also drink eight 225ml (8fl oz) glasses of water each day and you eat no food during this period. Because your body is taking in so much water you will urinate a lot and as you are not taking in any sodium, your body sheds even more water in an effort to keep your salt levels balanced. However, two days without eating any food is actually quite excessive and not many people can stick it through the second day without feeling absolutely dreadful. Anyone who wants to try a juice fast would be better advised to combine a mixture of water, and fresh unsweetened juices. This would provide at least some guaranteed nutrients and it would cost less too.

THE CABBAGE SOUP DIET The New Cabbage Soup Diet by Margaret Danbrot is a barking mad approach to dieting that promises a ten pound weight loss in seven days. Which is probably true, but anyone who is tempted by the thought of unlimited quantities of cabbage soup needs their head examined. To be fair, the author does make it clear the diet is not designed to be a substitution for good nutrition. She says it is designed to run for seven days and then be abandoned for at least another two weeks before it can be used again. The diet works because it is very low in calories and gives you guidelines of certain ingredients to use on specific days. While there are no 'magical' ingredients in the soup, Danbrot says that the working agents, antioxidants, phytochemicals and a combination of the 'superfoods' in the rest of the diet, rid the body of toxins and make the weight disappear. Chances are, you will also burn up a few calories lugging home pounds of cabbage and trying not to fart in front of people.

The soup is roughly made from: 1 head of cabbage, 6 large onions, 2 green peppers, 1 × 800g (28oz) can tomatoes, 1 bunch of celery, 1 packet onion soup mix and lots of water. Each day, dieters can eat as much cabbage soup as they please, plus on: *Day 1*: Any amount of any fruit excluding bananas. *Day 2*: Any amount of any vegetables, including one baked potato with butter. *Day 3*: Unlimited fruit and vegetables. *Day 4*: Eight bananas and up to eight glasses of skimmed milk. *Day 5*: Six tomatoes and 500g (20oz) of beef, chicken or fish. *Day 6*: Unlimited beef, chicken or fish and vegetables. *Day 7*: Unlimited boiled brown rice and unlimited vegetables. The diet is effective for temporarily losing a few pounds, but many dieters complain of nausea, gas and lightheadedness after just a couple of days. Most of the weight you lose is water, but if you have a hot date in a week's time, it may be worth giving it a try but remember to go off it several days beforehand. (It's a gas thing).

THE EGG AND GRAPEFRUIT DIET If the idea of juice or cabbage soup doesn't rock your boat, what about 48 hours on egg and grapefruit? This is about as unpalatable as crash diets get and provides very little nutrition so you should definitely take multi-vitamin and fish oil supplements while you are doing it. Grapefruit is fat free, low in calories and full of vitamin C and pink grapefruits also contain some beta carotene, but although grapefruits have long been associated with weight loss programmes, there is no scientific proof that they contain any particular fat-burning enzymes.

A typical day's menu might be: *Breakfast*: Half a grapefruit, a boiled egg and black coffee. *Lunch*: Half a grapefruit, one egg, some salad, a piece of dry toast and black tea or coffee. *Dinner*: Half a grapefruit, two eggs, half a head of lettuce with tomato and balsamic vinegar and black tea or coffee. Six to eight glasses of water will keep you hydrated and you can drink diet sodas too. The 'diet' is unhealthy, monotonous and adds up to less than 600 calories a day, which is unsustainable and frankly masochistic for anything longer than 48 hours. And two days of egg does nothing for your breath.

My heavy heavy weight continued into my 20s and I suspect at some point I just shrugged it off and just got on with life. Of course I was always aware of food and exercise but during my university years I learned a lot about women, body myths and issues. It really made me realize that I fitted into a story and it gave me a dialogue of how to explain what had happened to me. I still feel that if only I could get my body sorted out, then everything else will just fall into place. And I wonder if I'm doing it all on purpose.
Michaela, 31, NZ

As a teenager I knew I was overweight. I would hear comments from random people on the street and I was teased. I was very fat and very frustrated about it so I began to comfort eat. My stomach, bum and thighs were huge. At 16 I weighed nearly 15st [95kg]. I am now more comfortable with my body, but I do feel that I should lose 2st [2.5kg] to look healthier and fit. Looking good makes you feel good and gives you empowerment. My mum has stopped looking after herself in her 50s, but I hope I don't get lazy like her.
Carrie, 22, UK

Diet pills that work

PRESCRIPTION DIET PILLS Prescription diet pills should only be taken under medical supervision and don't work unless they are used in conjunction with an appropriate calorie-controlled diet and exercise programme. In the UK, medical guidelines state that prescription diet pills should only be given to people who have a body mass index (p.16) of 27 or more, who have tried to diet for three months and who have managed to lose at least 2.2kg (5lb) on their own steam. However, most doctors prescribe more liberally, particularly for people who have weight-related health problems and, besides, it is often impossible for a GP to judge whether a person has been on a diet or lost weight without careful monitoring. Although NHS doctors are more likely to take a responsible line on prescribing diet pills, private slimming clinics will basically dole them out to anyone who is willing to pay, as will any website.

Only two products are licensed in the UK as weight-reducing drugs: orlistat and sibutramine. Trials of both drugs over one to two years indicate that it is possible to lose an average of 10.2% of total body weight if following the treatment procedure correctly. However, it is worth bearing in mind that drug trials are generally performed in very overweight people who tend to lose weight more quickly than those who are less heavy.

ORLISTAT (Xenical® in the US) Orlistat is a prescription drug and dosage should be determined by a doctor. As with any prescription medication it is important to tell your doctor if you have any other medical problems or are taking any other medication or dietry or weight loss supplements. It can be prescribed for those with a BMI higher than 28 who are suffering obesity-related health problems (e.g. type-2 diabetes or high cholesterol) or to those with a BMI greater than 30 if they are not suffering from serious health problems. Weight loss helps to reduce blood pressure and improves cholesterol. In diabetics, it also reduces blood sugar which can result in an improvement in the condition. However these benefits need to be monitored by a doctor as doses of oral diabetes medicine or insulin may need to be adjusted. Orlistat should only be used in conjunction with a caolrie controlled diet and users are advised to increase their levels of physical activity during the course of their prescription.

Orlistat works by causing a 30% decrease in the amount of fat your body absorbs from food. It is designed to be used in conjunction with a low fat diet and any more than 30% fat in your diet will increase the side effects of this medicine. It has to be taken during a meal or within one hour of eating. If you occasionally miss a meal or eat a meal that contains no fat, you should skip the dose of orlistat. Because orlistat may decrease the amount of fat-soluble vitamins you absorb, you will need to take a multi-vitamin supplement once a day at least two hours before or after taking orlistat. Orlistat has some particularly nasty side effects such as excess gas, oily, uncontrollable bowel movements and the one everyone dreads, anal leakage. Spare pants are a must.

SIBUTRAMINE HYDROCHLORIDE (Meridia in the US, Reductil in the UK and Germany) Sibutramine can be prescribed to those with a BMI higher than 27 who are suffering obesity-related health problems (e.g. type-2 diabetes or high cholesterol) or to those with a BMI greater than 30 if they are not suffering from serious health problems. Sibutramine should only be prescribed for people who have already attempted to lose weight by dieting or taking exercise and should only be used in conjunction with a calorie-controlled diet.

Anyone looking for a sibutramine prescription needs to be completely honest with their doctor about all non-prescription and prescription medication they are on, particularly psychiatric medications, because of potential interactions. Deaths of patients on sibutramine led to a review of its safety in 2002 but it was re-approved because the benefits were considered to outweigh the risks. The committee decided that patients taking sibutramine had no more chance of dying than other patients of the same age and weight. Sibutramine usage needs to be carefully monitored and it is not recommended for individuals whose blood pressure is above 145/90mm Hg before the start of therapy since it can elevate blood pressure even higher.

Sibutramine decreases appetite but it also seems to have a small effect on energy expenditure. This helps to mitigate the usual fall in metabolic rate associated with dieting and weight loss (so it 'burns off' energy as well as reducing food intake). It has also been shown to help reduce weight in people suffering from type-2 diabetes who tend to find it harder to lose weight than non-diabetics. The recommended starting dose is 10mg per day; doses above 15mg per day are not approved by the Medicines Control Agency (MCA) in the UK and the Food and Drug Administration (FDA) in the US. In the UK, sibutramine treatment is not recommended for longer than one year because it is thought that its effect decreases with time and there has not been enough testing on the health implications for long-term use.

Side effects include insomnia, dry mouth and constipation. It should not be prescribed for patients with a history of high blood pressure, heart disease, stroke, liver or kidney disease, seizures, eating disorders, glaucoma or gall stones. It is not recommended for use during pregnancy or breastfeeding.

The secret to self-acceptance is not comparing yourself to the rest of the world. It is impossible for a woman who is 5' 8" and big boned to compare her body to that of a very petite, small framed woman. It just doesn't work that way. I also think that by working on your mind and spirit, happiness with your body and self-image will follow. A fabulous pair of shoes on a freshly manicured foot, will make any woman forget (for at least 5 minutes) that her pantyhose are not holding everything in!
Kerry, 25, US

When I was younger I took just about anything I could get my hands on to try and bring my weight down. I wasn't fat but I was working in New York and I guess my diet wasn't so good. Lots of junk, shakes and beer. I took speed, guaranna with ephidrine — which was natural but really speedy and I did a fair bit of coke. None of it had any impact because I was bulimic anyway. To be honest, I think it was all a form of self-abuse. I hated myself and until I did therapy my unstable weight matched my unstable mind.
Reece, 38, US

The trouble with amphetamines...

Tolerance to amphetamines, or amphetamine-style drugs develops very quickly and they have the potential to become addictive. They can cause rapid heart rate, agitation and high blood pressure at high doses, and can lead to disturbances in perception and locomotion, abnormal heart rhythms and hypersensitivity to stimulants. People who have diabetes, high blood pressure, hyperthyroidism or abnormal heart rhythms should avoid phentermine and similar drugs.

PHENTERMINE Phentermine first received approval from the FDA in 1959 for the short-term treatment of obesity and is now the most commonly prescribed prescription appetite suppressant in the US, accounting for 50% of all prescriptions but it is not licensed in the UK. Part of the reason it is so popular is because it's significantly cheaper than the other major FDA-approved diet drugs, sibutramine and orlistat. It certainly works as an appetite suppressant but, as with any weight loss pill, once a patient stops treatment they are likely to regain weight.

FEN-PHEN This cocktail of fenfluramine or pondimin (the 'Fen') and phentermine (the 'Phen') became an overnight sensation in 1992, when Dr Michael Weintraub of the University of Rochester published a study citing the drug combination as a more effective method than dieting or exercise in reducing weight in the chronically obese. Although both drugs had been independently approved by the FDA in the 1960s, no testing had been carried out on using them together and neither drug was approved for use longer than 12 weeks. The Fen-Phen regimen is an example of what is known as 'off-label' use, in which doctors can legally prescribe approved drugs for new uses. Many diet clinics were willing to prescribe the Fen-Phen treatment for the mildly overweight as well as the obese and by 1996, US prescriptions for the fenfluramine-phentermine combination exceeded 18 million. However, in 1997 the Mayo Clinic published a report of 24 patients who had developed heart valve disease after taking Fen-Phen, (along with an FDA letter to the editor describing 100 additional cases) in the *New England Journal of Medicine* and the makers subsequently pulled the drugs off the market. Dexfen-Phen, a cocktail of dexfenfluramine or redux and phentermine was also banned.

PHEN-PRO The newest cocktail involving phentermine is Phen-Pro (the 'Pro' stands for Prozac) though other antidepressants can be used in lieu of Prozac. The use of the antidepressant is unrelated to depression but appears to prolong the effects of phentermine and means lower doses of each drug can be used, which reduces side effects. This is also an 'off-label' use but to date, Phen-Pro does not appear to cause the problems that resulted with Fen-Phen. This combination is considered to be less risky because the cases of heart valve disease associated with Fen-Phen were due to the fenfluramine not the phentermine.

Diet pills that don't work

The majority of over-the-counter diet pills are either useless and/or dangerous. Most have not been demonstrated as safe for anyone long term and none have been shown to be safe for pregnant or breast-feeding women. Prescription weight loss medications undergo a strict review process to evaluate safety and effectiveness, but over-the-counter supplements to promote weight loss do not have to undergo any safety or effectiveness review processes whatsoever. Naturally, to avoid being reviewed as a drug, which is costly and time consuming, many companies choose to market their products as dietary supplements. This creates a ridiculous double standard; rigorous regulation to test the safety and effectiveness of prescription medications and virtually no regulation at all for dietary supplements.

If you look at the hundreds of weight loss products for sale, you will see they carry claims that the product is effective for weight loss or for burning fat, but if you read the product label carefully, you will see a statement saying that the product claims made on the label about weight loss or fat burning or muscle building have not been reviewed. Some products are labelled as 'herbal' or 'natural', which gives consumers a misguided notion of safety. In fact, many prescription drugs are derived from bioactive compounds found in herbs obtained from natural sources and there have been several cases of inconsistency, toxicity and dangerous, even fatal, side effects in herbal preparations. Obviously, when adverse effects are found, or the product is found to be mislabelled, or advertising is very misleading, government and health care agencies can intervene, but by then it is often too late for people who have been damaged by the drugs. Furthermore, as use of over-the-counter diet products continues to grow, it becomes increasingly difficult to monitor chemical interactions with other drugs. A US telephone survey carried out between 1996 and 1997 estimated that more than 17 million Americans took over-the-counter weight-loss products. Their results showed that more than 25% of young obese women and 8% of normal weight women used non-prescription weight-loss pills. The internet has dramatically increases the sales of products for weight loss. For example, Americans consume 225,000 capsules of herbal fen-phen, (an ephidrine-based approximation of the banned drug described, see left) every hour with annual retail revenues of approximately $900 million.

The consequences of widespread obesity are certainly serious but so is the use of unregulated diet pills. Easy internet access and the glut of over-the-counter products has normalized self-medication, but as a result, ill health caused by the side effects of drugs is now one of the most common causes of death. If you are struggling with your weight, diet pills may look like the ultimate quick fix, but many products are both addictive and potentially dangerous and they won't encourage you to address the root cause of your weight problem or to adopt a healthier lifestyle.

The diet pill phenomenon fascinates me. The thought of thousands, millions of people, shelling out money for something that so clearly doesn't, couldn't work, is amazing. Obviously if there was a diet pill that worked we would all know about it. The supplements that you can buy without a prescription are no better than vitamins.
Esther, 48, UK

I weigh myself to find out whether I'm putting on or losing weight, but generally I go by how I feel in my clothes. When I'm having to undo the top button on my jeans when I sit down, it's time to eat salad!
Nina, 34, Ireland

My weight dominates my day!! I'm short. I can't change anything about that, so the only thing I can have any power and control over is my weight! In my head I really believe keeping my weight down WILL take the attention away from me being short! - Crazy I know!!!
Aman, 32, UK

Liposuction is the new diet pill. One look at any Hollywood star and you can see that it is not diet but careful fat sucking that creates their shape.
Kim, 54, UK

APPETITE BLOCKERS (Fibre, Psyllium, Plantago, Guar Fibre) Because fibre absorbs liquid and swells or bulks up in the stomach, it supposedly makes you feel fuller and reduces your appetite. Manufacturers also suggest that it 'binds' fat in the gastro-intestinal tract, preventing it from being absorbed. Some studies support the use of fibre to promote weight loss, others don't. In the long term, bulking up with fibre may just stretch the stomach and make it want even more food. Large amounts of fibre can cause gastro-intestinal distress and some fillers, such as guar gum, a complex sugar found in small quantities in foods like cheese and ice cream, can cause obstructions in the gastro-intestinal tract. For this reason, guar gum is banned by the FDA for use in weight-loss drug products.

CAFFEINE Caffeine is often added to weight-loss products because it allegedly helps the body burn up more energy, but it is usually combined with ephidrine so it is difficult to separate the independent effect of caffeine. In 1991, the FDA banned caffeine as an additive to non-prescription weight-loss products because it had not been proven effective. In large doses it can cause insomnia and nervousness. Because it activates the sympathetic nervous system, patients with cardiovascular problems should not take caffeine supplements.

CAPSAICIN There is limited support for capsaicin as a weight-loss aid when consumed in foods such as cayenne pepper or chilli. Capsaicin apparently stimulates saliva, stimulates digestion and accelerates your metabolism at a safer level but the evidence is not very convincing. Capsaicin may increase metabolic rate and body temperature in rats but there is no proof that it does in humans.

CHITOSAN Often labelled as a fat blocker or a fat absorber, chitosan is a polymer of glucosamine produced from the shells of crabs, shrimp and lobster, which purports to bind to fat, blocking absorption in the gut. Limited research has been done but a double-blind study in humans showed no difference in BMI between chitosan and placebo. Minimal safety assessment has been done and its long-term effect on fat-soluble vitamins is unknown. There is concern that people with shellfish allergies may not be aware that the product is both ineffective and has the potential to aggravate allergic reactions.

CHROMIUM PICOLINATE (and other chromium supplements) This a trace mineral found in broccoli, brewer's yeast, wheatgerm, egg yolk, nuts, liver, prunes, apples and cheese, which is promoted as helping the body to burn fat and build muscle. There is a small amount of evidence that chromium supplements can help diabetics bring down high blood sugar levels, but studies show it has no effect on people with normal blood sugar levels and no effect on the body composition of healthy individuals, even when taken in combination with an exercise training programme. Another trial showed that overweight people who took chromium supplements actually put on weight. More recently it has been associated with scare stories about damage to DNA. There is evidence that, as with any supplement, chromium levels in the body become dangerous if allowed to accumulate. There have been reports of severe muscle injury (rhabdomylosis) and kidney damage from a very large dose over 48 hours (rather than a cumulative effect over a longer term).

CONJUGATED LINOLEIC ACID (CLA) CLA is a compound that is naturally obtained from the fat in meat and dairy products. Trials of CLA supplements on 20 men and women in Norway showed a 3kg (7lb) reduction in body fat over three months, while the control group didn't lose any weight. However, this is a result that one would easily hope to achieve with a calorie-controlled diet and moderate exercise. Another 60-person trial in Norway showed weight loss of 2.7kg (6lb) in the same time frame. These are not massive drops so the jury is still out as to whether it has any effect. To get any benefit, 3–4g a day is required. However, supplements can contain as little as 500mg, which means you would need to take seven pills a day. They are expensive and the minute you stop taking them you will gain weight again. There have been no studies done into safety or long-term effects.

DEHYDROEPIANDROSTERONE (DHEA) DHEA is a naturally occurring hormone produced by the adrenal gland. Sometimes referred to as the "mother of all steroid hormones" it is converted in the body into several different hormones, including oestrogen and testosterone. DHEA levels rise during puberty, reach a peak at about age 30, and then drop off dramatically in both men and women as they age. By age 80, people are producing only about 5% of the DHEA they produced at age 30. It is similar to testosterone and limited research suggests a positive effect on increasing lean muscle mass and decreasing fat, with a decrease or no change in body weight. However in 1985, The FDA removed DHEA from the over-the-counter market because there was no support for the health claims that were made for it and it is thought to increase the risk of cancer, especially cancers that are sensitive to oestrogens such as prostate and breast cancer. It can still be obtained on prescription but most of it is bought online.

DHEA is popular with women because it increases lean muscle mass, but increased testosterone is also though to boost libido and that makes it even more attractive. There is growing concern that DHEA is now being abused by young women who have heard about the benefits but don't understand the side effects. Long-term

When I hit 40, a thyroid condition caused my weight to blossom from a size 8 to what seemed a huge 14 – over two months. As I had always eaten masses and NEVER put on an ounce, weight gain like this was weird. My family, who had been telling me to mind my eating or 'one day you'll wake up huge', or 'middle-age spread will get you one day' smugly reacted to their predictions come true. It was literally my 'just desserts' for a life of unbridled gluttony. Only when I collapsed with exhaustion and my throat swelled with a goiter did I realize it was a medical problem. My family did make me feel like I deserved to be fat. ... and I must have believed them, otherwise I would have asked for medical help for such an unusual and rapid change.
Caroline, 40, Austria

I abused laxatives regularly from about the age of 17–23. Even now, if I'm having a 'bad' weight week, I reach for a packet rather than waiting for longer-term solutions to work (i.e. dieting).
Vicky, 31, UK

usage leads to the development of more masculine characteristics; a deeper voice, excessive body hair, acne etc. In adolescents, it can terminate the adolescent growth spurt prematurely, leaving abusers shorter than they would have been without the drugs. And in all age groups, DHEA can cause potentially fatal liver cysts and liver cancer; blood clotting, cholesterol changes, hypertension, heart attack and stroke.

GHB, BD AND GBL Gamma hydroxybutyrate (GHB), butanediol (BD) and gamma butyrolactone (GBL) are synthetic substances believed to have anabolic effects by stimulating the release of growth hormone in the body. All three are considered to be unsafe and also have addictive properties. GHB was investigated as a potential anaesthetic in the 1960s but it caused seizures. It was also heavily used as a recreational drug in the 1980s and was banned by the FDA in 1990. Many manufacturers then switched to GBL and 1,4-butanediol (BD), precursors of GHB, which are broken down by enzymes to form GHB when ingested. However, the FDA determined that dietary supplements containing these chemicals are really unapproved drugs because of the effect they have on the body. It is illegal to sell anything for human consumption that contains GHB, GBL or BD. They can cause breathing problems, coma, vomiting, seizures and death.

GLUCOMANNAN A form of dietary fibre derived from underground tubers of a plant called 'konjac'. There is little evidence that it works but it may provide temporarily feelings of fullness as the fibre bulks up. It has a mainly laxative effect. Like guar gum, it has been linked to cases of oesophageal blocking.

HUMAN GROWTH HORMONE (HGH) HGH claims to help you build muscle and lose weight. It is used medically to stimulate growth in patients with growth hormone deficiencies. It will only work if it is injected or implanted. If eaten, it is simply broken down like any other protein. It can and is injected but it has no real effects when given to normal patients (i.e. not deficient in growth hormone) though there is some evidence it may help the elderly preserve muscle.

HYDROXYCITRIC ACID (HCA) (*Arcinia cambogia*, brindle berry rind) Thought to suppress appetite and inhibit enzymes involved in fat production. There is no convincing evidence it works, because all positive trials had experimental flaws, and at least one study showed negative results. No one has done long-term research. Studies combining HCA with other agents such as chromium, caffeine, L-carnitine, chitosan and/or fibre found greater reductions in body fat compared to placebo, but it is impossible to separate the effects of HCA from the other agents. HCA treatment was not found to increase fat burning during rest or moderately intense exercise. No significant safety concerns have been reported.

LAXATIVES AND DIURETICS Laxatives such as cassia, senna or cascara help to eliminate bodily waste. They are sometimes necessary, but should only be used when medically needed and should never be used as a weight loss tool. Elimination of waste or water is not true weight loss. It will not help you lose fat and extended use causes mineral loss and dehydration. Laxative abuse upsets the salt and water balance that is required for healthy heart function. Abuse can lead to serious electrolyte imbalance causing seizures, permanent heart damage and death. Diuretics cause temporary weight loss as fluid but can lead to dehydration and a loss of potassium and other salts that cause heart irregularities, muscle fatigue, dizziness and fainting. Both laxatives and diuretics (whether they are natural or not) can be extremely dangerous. These products, like all herbal and non-herbal medicines, should be treated with caution and respect.

L-TRYPTOPHAN & 5-HYDROXYTRYPTOPHAN (5-HTP) L-tryptophan is a natural amino acid found in foods like turkey and dietary proteins. It helps the body produce the B-vitamin niacin, which helps the brain release serotonin. Serotonin acts as a calming agent in the brain and there is evidence that it also reduces appetite. In the 1980s, tryptophan became popular as a cure for insomnia, depression and weight loss, but it was banned by the FDA after an outbreak of eosinophilia-myalgia syndrome (EMS) killed 37 people and left 1500 permanently disabled. Though the problem was thought to be due to bacterial contamination in a certain batch, the banning led to the development of a chemical cousin called 5-HTP (short for 5-hydroxytryptophan) as a supplement. The body makes 5-HTP in the brain from tryptophan, but the 5-HTP used in supplements comes from the seeds of an African plant (*Griffonia simplicifolia*). Manufacturers say this makes it safer than L-tryptophan which was synthesized by bacteria. 5-HTP has been prescribed for insomnia for years and it is also used to boost weight loss. It is still available as an over-the-counter supplement and, in small trials, minimal appetite reduction and weight loss (averaging 4.9kg (11lb) in 12 weeks) occurred with daily doses of 600–900mg but it should be used with caution. Impurities called 'Peak X' were found in 5-HTP in 1998 which was also found in one case of EMS in 1991. Because 5-HTP is essentially a natural anti-depressant it should not be taken with anti-depressants, weight-control drugs, or substances known to cause liver damage. People with liver disease may not be able to regulate 5-HTP adequately and some reports link 5-HTP to a scleroderma (auto-immune disease) -like condition. Side effects are nausea, headache, sleepiness, muscle pain and anxiety.

PPA/EPHIDRINE(MaHuang/ephedra/phenylpropanolamine/pseudoephedrine/phenylpropanolamine/herbal fen-phen) The ephedra alkaloids include ephedrine, pseudoephedrine and phenylpropanolamine (PPA), all of which possess

I went to a private slimming clinic to get diet pills. I only took a few but they made me feel quite dizzy, and I found I couldn't concentrate at work. My boyfriend noticed a change in me and we kept arguing. When he found the pills he went mad and threw them away. Probably a good thing really.
Sally, 50, UK

I have been taking creatine to build up muscle mass for a couple of months now. I think it is working and I certainly feel that I have more stamina at the gym. Obviously I am a bit worried about long-term health effects but I am 25 and I need to get myself into peak physical shape before I am 30.
Nicki, 25, US

I have used both laxatives and diuretics to lose weight. At one point I was doing about 25 senna tablets a day because you lose sensitivity to them so you have to keep increasing the quantities. I was in almost constant pain with cramping and I began to bleed. At the chemist they realized that I was buying too many and they stopped selling them to me but I just went to other shops.
Olivia, 35, UK

stimulant properties similar to those of addictive amphetamines. PPA used to be found in a number of over-the-counter nasal decongestants and was the active ingredient in Dexatrim and Acutrim slimming pills. However in November 2000 the FDA announced a ban on the use of PPA in products sold without a doctor's prescription after the chemical was found to be linked to an increased risk of haemorrhagic stroke. Given that the FDA's Office of Over the Counter Drug Evaluation found only about a half pound greater weight loss per week using PPA than placebo the product is no great loss to dieters.

Though PPA has been withdrawn, the herbal equivalents are not regulated and remain available. Ephedra, also known as MaHuang, is a strong stimulant found in popular herbal phen-fen weight loss supplements. Many states in the US have banned MaHuang, though you can still buy it in the UK and the US. MaHuang can suppress appetite, but there is no substantial clinical evidence that it is either safe or effective for weight loss.

Ephedra compounds have been associated with many dangerous side effects including high blood pressure, increased heart rate, heart palpitations, seizure, stroke and even death. They pose a particular hazard for people with conditions such as glaucoma, heart disease or high blood pressure or those taking antidepressants. Because many of the complications occur when the dose exceeds 24mg per day, labelling now instructs consumers not to take ephedra products for more than seven consecutive days to discourage long-term use for weight loss. According to the FDA, dietary supplements containing ephedra have been linked to 117 deaths in the US and there are a further 18,000 reports of other medical problems so they advise against using any of them at any time. Synthetic ephedrine (ephedrine hydrochloride) is also banned from dietary supplements because it is registered as a drug.

PYRUVATE Several small US studies have shown that pyruvate supplements can help to increase weight loss, but the studies were carried out in very exclusive circumstances and the doses used were extremely high – 22–28g (1oz) several times a day compared to a recommended dose of 500mg–1g three times a day. No studies have been carried out on its safety for long-term use and any commercial product is likely to contain minuscule amounts of the ingredient.

STARCH BLOCKERS These promise to impede starch digestion and were popular in the late '80s and early '90s. British research shows they don't work and can cause side effects such as nausea, vomiting, diarrhoea and stomach pains.

The future of anti-obesity medications

While governments scratch their heads and wonder how to tackle the problem of obesity, scientists and the pharmaceutical industry are scrambling to find a cure. The huge market potential for a drug that helps people lose weight has made the development of new anti-obesity products a major priority and positive results in pre-clinical research have seen the number of drugs in development rise three-fold over the last seven years.

Early research into anti-obesity drugs centred on leptin, a hormone produced by fat cells in the body. If fat mass increases, the body produces more leptin (p.11), so scientists thought that it was a messenger that told the brain to stop eating. It was originally thought that giving leptin to the obese would help them to stop eating, but it turned out that obese people already have high leptin levels and it didn't stop them eating because they have developed leptin resistance. Leptin is, in fact, the evolutionary control that allowed us to get fat in the summer so that we wouldn't starve in the winter when food was more scarce (p.66). It reassures the brain there is enough fat to get pregnant, etc., but it doesn't control weight.

Further research centred on ghrelin, a hormone from the stomach that signals when the stomach is empty, increases food intake and body weight in rats, and increases appetite in humans. Scientists believe that if they can make a drug that blocks the action of ghrelin in the brain, it may reduce appetite and body weight. Ghrelin was identified in 1999, and since then, over 400 papers have been published on it. As a number of patents have already been filed, a drug may soon emerge as a pharmacological option in the treatment of obesity.

In the UK, research by Professor Steve Bloom's Endocrine Research Unit at the Hammersmith Hospital has demonstrated the impact of the hormone PYY3-36, which is released after eating and tells the brain that the stomach is full. Giving PYY3-36 as an injection effectively 'turns off' hunger and reduces the amount of food subjects eat. At present, only short-term effects have been proven and other scientists have struggled to replicate the initial findings but his research continues.

Most recently French scientists have been working on a pill called Rimonabant, that helps people quit smoking and slim down at the same time by blocking the circuits in the brain that control the urge to eat and smoke. The drug works by shutting down the endocannabinoid system in the brain which regulates hunger and other cravings in the brain (The drug marijuana makes people ravenous by stimulating this same circuitry). As with the PYY3-36 hormone, it is thought that eating too much and smoking over stimulate this system and as gradual tolerance builds up people eat and smoke more, and more.

Many people can't manage slimming and hate jogging. For them we need some easy way forward. To fool the brain that you have just eaten a meal is one safe way. An injection of the hormones that tell the brain that your belly is full stops hunger most effectively. What we now have to do is to make it into a convenient, everyday medicine.
Prof. Steve Bloom

My weight has ballooned since I quit smoking but I cannot seem to shift a pound, even when I eat hardly anything. I have monitored my food intake and I guess I am using coffees, sodas, hard candy and gum as a way of getting over smoking, so, even though I don't feel I am eating that much more, every coke and every sweet is adding to my weight. I realize that I need sugar as much as I needed cigarettes. I have swapped to black coffee, diet soda and sugar-free gum. I have even found sugar-free lollies. Not very healthy I know, but I have to have something in my mouth. I wish there was a way of switching everything off. I cannot cope with my cravings.
Monica, 35, US

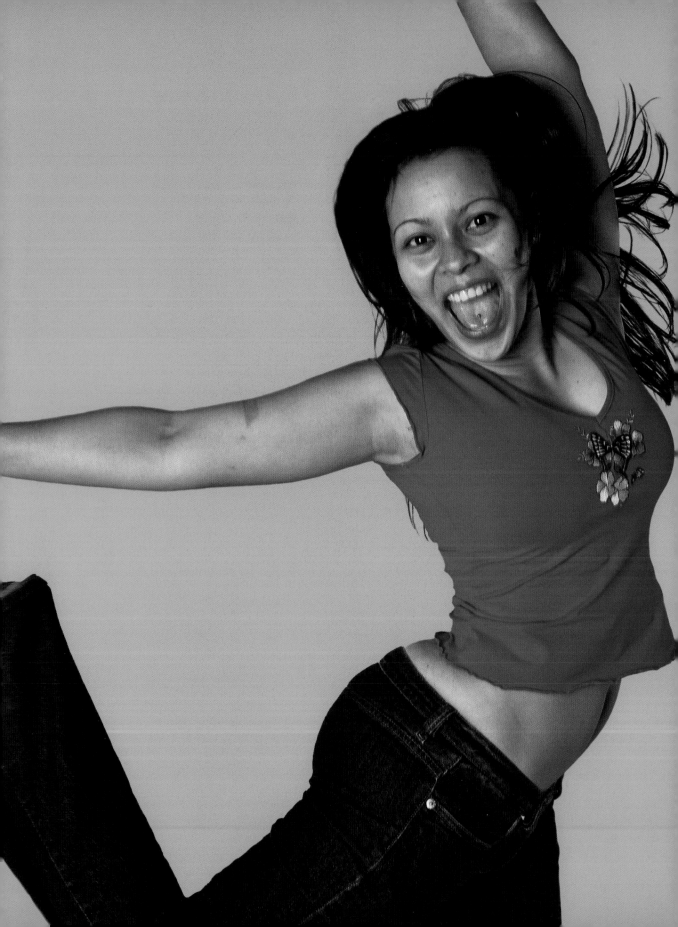

THE
Fitness
CHAPTER

From smelling salts to jogger's nipple

Everyone knows that exercise is the key to health, happiness and longevity. Medical research, government health advice and, of course, the sports industry, have been drumming the message into us for years. But statistics suggest that either something is wrong with the message, or something is wrong with us, because despite the media hype and the unavoidable guilt-inducing medical evidence, only 25% of women do enough exercise. The rest of us don't exert ourselves enough to see any positive health benefits and 26% of women do absolutely nothing at all.

There are a number of reasons for female inactivity. Sloth *is* one of them, no doubt, but the issue is more complex than laziness. Mixed media messages urging physical activity clash with a gender history which, until relatively recently, demanded precisely the opposite. Historically, female physical fitness was considered to be of very little importance. In fact, sport was actually thought to be detrimental to female health and fertility. Modesty took precedence over mobility and female sporting ability just wasn't taken seriously.

In fact, athleticism in women was viewed with some suspicion. Professional sports women were seen as masculine, lesbian even, and this didn't broaden their appeal to either sex. Male standards of strength, speed and competitiveness set the measure of athletic success and female achievements were continually undermined in comparison. Women struggled for equity, sponsorship and recognition in an arena almost entirely dominated by male athletes, managers and promoters. So it was hardly surprising that women, of the common or garden variety, saw sports as a vocation for a select few, and a fairly masochistic select few at that.

However, despite the fact that female physical fitness was marginalized, the average woman in the 1920s, for example, was much fitter than her contemporary counterpart today. Soaking, scrubbing, wringing, lifting, hanging and walking did wonders for upper body strength, flexibility, stamina, muscularity and cardio-vascular fitness. But by the 1950s the arrival of affordable 'energy efficient' hoovers, washing machines, tumble dryers and mixing machines had gradually begun to eliminate opportunities for domestic physical exertion. And within 20 years, 'ease' had begun its uneasy relationship with inactivity, obesity and ill health.

The 1960s did little to promote female physical activity, but the era did a lot to cultivate negative female body image. Sixties models were pubescent waifs with Bambi eyes, stick legs, flat chests and mini skirts – a shape our mothers, real women, would never come close to - and a proliferation of new media broadcast this new boy shaped ideal at every opportunity. The birth of feminism in the 70s managed to disguise some of the disquiet that had begun to unsettle the female psyche. But it wasn't enough. Women were desperate to think more of themselves. But when they took off their kaftans they were desperate to see less of themselves. When aerobics queen Jane Fonda and hip and thigh eliminator Rosemary Conley sold working out as weight loss, and discipline as empowerment, they put their finger on the pulse of female paranoia and created a lucrative straitjacket for a gender still struggling to get to grips with relatively new-found freedoms. 'Feel the burn', 'No pain, no gain', 'Work it baby' – the masochistic slogans of punishing aerobic regimes, preached a doctrine that women intuitively understood. Working out was just another, more exhausting, form of dieting. And inevitably, viewed as an optional punishment on top of low calorie, low fat and low self-esteem, many women have, quite understandably, declined the invitation to 'just do it'.

For a huge number of women exercise is still a reactionary response to concerns about weight. And, as such, the motivation to get fit only lasts as long as the willpower to diet. Negative associations – feeling guilty about being lazy and unfit or feeling 'less than' for carrying extra weight – are a disincentive, and going to the gym simply highlights physical shortcomings that can otherwise be disguised by wearing black and avoiding horizontal stripes. More importantly, excercise doesn't deliver what women really want from it. Weight loss. Though it does help people to get slimmer, results take time and given the choice between pounding a treadmill five hours a week, 52 weeks a year, or one 24-hour stint in a liposuction clinic, a generation of women reared on 'fast' have become increasingly inclined to choose the latter.

When it comes to exercise, the enduring link between fitness, fatness and self-flagel-lation has distorted female perspective. But the real fitness message is actually very simple. Regular exercise = strength, stamina, health, longevity and a better quality of life. Women who exercise through and into later life remain more mentally and physically alert. They maintain their physical independence and enjoy a greatly extended and healthier old age. Unfortunately, up to 75% of women have, as yet, failed to take this in. General levels of female exertion are at an all-time low and unless women, all women, start to take personal responsibility for their health, the 'have it all' generation face a retirement plagued by immobility and obesity. Anyone who is over 50, inexperienced, injured or unhealthy should consult their GP before begining a fitness programme, but ill health shouldn't be used as a way of avoiding exercise. This chapter steers clear of anything complicated which would be better and more safely taught by an instructor and instead, concentrates on low tech, low cost, flexible exercise options. Ultimately, the most important consideration with any fitness regime is not whether you can do it, but whether you can sustain the programme long term.

When I was in my 20s and 30s I went to the gym quite regularly. I was only really concerned about weight and I had absolutely no interest in the health benefits. But I think that the exercise I did then has stood me in good stead because I still don't go to the gym very often but I seem to be able to maintain a reasonable level of basic fitness. Even though I am nearly 40 I know that I could get fit in about six weeks if I went to the gym three times a week.
Cammila, 39, UK

I LOVE the rush of endorphins when you have a really tough workout. I really sleep better and have more energy when I exercise regularly.
Rachael, 26, Aus

I think I am doing pretty well for someone who used to avoid physical exercise like the plague. As I've gotten older I have realized that if I want to maintain my busy lifestyle I have to do something to keep my energy up and keep myself in shape. So I go to a women's gym somewhere between three and five days a week and I do a lot of heavy lifting and construction type work at the theatre where I am company manager.
Jen, 27, US

Why exercise?

IT STRENGTHENS YOUR HEART Regular physical exercise raises your heart rate and reduces stiffening of the arteries, a major cause of high blood pressure, which can lead to heart disease and stroke. It lowers your resting heart rate by allowing your heart to pump more blood per beat, which means your heart is not working as hard when you are at rest. It also lowers or helps control your blood pressure. Results from the largest study to ever examine the association between physical activity and stroke in women found that by adding 30 minutes of moderate to vigorous exercise to a woman's daily routine, her risk of stroke would be decreased by 20%. The same amount of exercise would decrease a woman's risk of ischaemic stroke, the most common type of stroke by 30%.

IT BOOSTS YOUR IMMUNE SYSTEM Excercise increases levels of HDL, good cholesterol and reduces circulating levels of triglycerides, the amount of free fatty acid found in the blood. It increases insulin sensitivity to protect against type-2 diabetes (adult onset diabetes) and reduces your risk of developing colon cancer and breast cancer. It can lower the risk of severe intestinal bleeding in later life by almost half. It helps to relieve and prevent migraine headache attacks, symptoms of PMS and reduces the likelihood of a difficult menopause.

IT MAKES YOUR LUNGS MORE EFFICIENT Exercise improves your body's ability to take in oxygen and deliver it to your working muscles (defined as your VO2 max). This measure is generally regarded as the best measure of your physical fitness level. Aerobic exercise improves blood flow and oxygenates the skin so that it maintains a healthy glow, stays firmer and doesn't age as fast. And the better you look the better you feel. As you get fitter, people will compliment you on your toned physique and rosy complexion and this will motivate you and give you increased confidence.

STRONGER MUSCLES AND BONES Exercise can help increase muscular strength and endurance. It improves stamina and your ability to do continuous work. It increases or maintains your bone mineral density to prevent osteoporosis and ease or eliminate the pain of arthritis. It provides protection against injury and maintains or improves joint integrity. It improves your balance and coordination, which means you are less likely to have an accident and injure yourself. And if you have an accident, a fitter body has a better capacity for healing.

IT IMPROVES YOUR MENTAL HEALTH More than 150 US studies show that regular exercise combats stress and anxiety. It decreases the likelihood that you will suffer from depression or insomnia and improves your overall quality of life. Feeling fitter boosts your self-esteem and confidence. It teaches you about motivation, setting goals and commitment and it can help your efforts to stop smoking, too. In a six-month study of previously sedentary men and women over 60, those who walked three times a week scored 25% better on memory and judgement tasks and there is some evidence that it may protect against Alzheimer's. Exercise gives you time to think and come up with new ideas. In studies, people who did aerobic exercise scored much higher on creative tests than people who watched a video. And exercise is a good outlet for anger, so you are likely to be calmer in your day to day life.

IT IMPROVES YOUR PHYSIQUE Increased body mass index (BMI) is associated with an increase in morbidity and mortality. Exercise helps you develop more muscles and lowers your BMI (p.16). This increases the speed of your metabolism and helps to prevent weight gain. For every 900g (2lb) of muscle you carry, you burn an extra 20 or 30 calories per day. Being physically fit puts you in tune with your body and your physical capabilities. It helps you to transform your body shape by firming up your butt, your stomach, your thighs, your upper arms and your jawline. Fit people have better posture, which means they stand taller, and look thinner.

AND IT HAS SOCIAL BENEFITS TOO The fitter you are, the broader your sporting options will be. You can take up a range of challenging activities from hill walking to parachuting and conquering new challenges will give you an enormous sense of achievement. Taking up new activities will inevitably bring you into contact with new people and working out or playing sports with friends transforms the experience into a social event. Your interest in exercise will be a good influence on your family, too. You will be able to keep fit with your partner and encourage your family to cycle or play sport instead of lounging in front of the TV. And recent research indicates that an interest in sports and exercise has been linked to lower pregnancy rate in teens.

Older women who are physically fit enjoy life more. They have a better social life because they are more mobile and active and they can be more involved grandparents if they choose to be. But they may be too busy working. Experience combined with good health makes older women model employees. They are less likely to get ill, they have more energy at work and they are less likely to suffer from back strain or carpal tunnel syndrome.

REMEMBER Experts believe that a good 70% of what we think of as normal ageing is really a result of inactivity – laziness – and poor lifestyle choices such as exposure to the sun or poor diet.

I am of average fitness but I have only been regularly going to the gym for about a year now. Exercise has a very positive effect on my energy levels but it has also boosted my self-esteem.
Michaela, 31, NZ

I always have to motivate myself to start but I always feel great afterwards – not just from the endorphins but it gives me a real smug 'I did it' feeling when I've managed to get off my backside and actually do something!
Tammy, 25, UK

I suffer from severe depression and exercise is the only way I can alleviate it without taking pills. When I feel low and dead it is a real struggle to make myself go to the gym but once I am there I go into a sort of trance on the treadmill and it is as if I start to feel my body and my nerve endings again. It doesn't take much. If I sweat for half an hour, it is better than ten doses of Prozac.
Sarah, 38, US

I worry a lot about my health and get paranoid that I have cancer or something, but when I work out I feel absolutely sure that I am completely healthy.
Rose, 48, UK

Fitting in fitness

Change your life

Make exercise a mental and physical priority.

Wake up half an hour earlier in the morning to exercise. If you can't do that try to block out the same time period every day for exercise and don't let anyone or anything intrude on it.

The average adult spends 16 hours a week watching TV. Cut your viewing by 30 minutes a day and work out instead.

A power walk (15 minutes there – 15 minutes back) to buy your lunch covers your daily exercise quota.

Instead of chatting with friends while snacking at the kitchen table, get out and have a chat while you walk around the park.

If you are going out to dinner, walk to the restaurant or walk home afterwards.

Walk, run, cycle, skate, or use a microscooter to get to and from work.

If you really can't get out of the house to workout, invest in some equipment for your home. Set it up in front of a TV, play music or read to help you pass the time.

Lack of time is the number one reason most women give when asked why they don't exercise. And a very valid reason it is too. Keeping fit quickly crawls down the list of priorities for anyone with a full-time job. And because most women are also responsible for the unwritten, unrecognized roles of primary care giver, domestic organizer, chauffeur, cleaner, chief cook and bottle washer, their 'free time' is generally spent looking after everyone else rather than looking after themselves. With precious little 'me time' available, when women do unwind they would generally prefer to relax rather than run up a couple of hills. The boom in pampering, the profligation of spas and salons, even the increase in female alcohol consumption, are evidence of a gender that is suffering the corrosive effects of 'making, doing and giving' 24/7. However, aromatherapy and alcohol provide a very temporary balm. To strengthen their core, their hearts, lungs, bones and brains, women need to swap essential oils for exercise. When it comes to fitness, most women are not trying to win the marathon, they are aiming to cover the minimum quota required to maintain a decent level of fitness, keep their inner fat person at bay and alleviate daily stress. Government guidelines on how much is enough seem to change on an annual basis but any woman who has time to watch 'Friends' has time to either do two 15-minute exercise sessions or one half-hour exercise session every day.

Fitting a tamper-proof routine into your weekly schedule that won't be messed about by work, kids or social commitments is hard. Eventually, many women find that the only way to ensure they actually stick to some sort of programme is to set their alarm half an hour earlier and get out of the house before anyone notices they are gone. This is a discipline made more difficult by insomnia, hangovers, kids that don't sleep, jet lag or relatives sleeping over, but in general, there are fewer intrusions on your time in the early morning. In terms of safety, in the summer when it gets light earlier you can probably plan to be out for a walk or a run by 6.00am. As the winter approaches and mornings are darker you should schedule your half hour slot for later in the morning when it is lighter or fit it in at lunchtime.

If you're not good at getting up in the morning, walking to and from your office at a brisk pace five mornings a week will cover your fitness quota without taking much time out of the working day. If you can't manage the whole journey, take the bus half way and walk the rest. Women who don't work but have kids at school should realistically be able to find half an hour each day to exercise. Home-based programmes during nap time are a good option for women with small babies, as is a brisk 30-minute walk while pushing a buggy. Whatever exercise option you choose, remember that over time, you don't need to work out for longer, you just need to work harder during your routine. Time yourself, measure your distances, do more reps per minute and gradually up your pace and push yourself harder.

Do you even remember the way to the gym?

How many women have nursed a New Year's day hangover by polishing their shiny new pledge to fitness. Resolute and unstoppable, they sign up to a gym, work out religiously three times a week and then crash and burn after two months when they realize that they hate exercise, they still weigh as much and they are paying for a membership that they haven't used for weeks.

For many women, joining a gym can actually have a negative impact on general fitness because, psychologically, exercise is then isolated to one specific location. The 'I didn't make it to the gym so I couldn't work out' mentality does nothing to encourage women to address their general levels of inactivity. And guilt about not using an expensive membership eventually leads to more than a quarter of all gym members giving up. Gym goers are generally under 45, single, ABC1s, currently working, with a household income of £30,000+. That profile describes a relatively small group of women and a survey by MORI in the UK shows that 'lapsed gym-goers are more likely to be parents with children currently living at home'. Widening facilities at clubs to include crèches and other family facilities/activities would undoubtedly make it easier for women to get to the gym, but if this ever happens, it will cost money and many gyms are already prohibitively expensive.

Public leisure centres are obviously a cheaper options but few women enjoy wrestling for a turn on oversubscribed equipment, so most join commercial gyms – which charge higher premiums for use during peak (convenient) times. The upshot of this is that a huge number of women sign up to clubs as off-peak members and then never use them because the hours just don't fit in with their commitments at work and at home. Before you part with registration fees, weigh up whether your schedule will allow you to really get your money's worth. If you can afford the fees and find the time, a good gym provides state-of- the-art equipment and a level of support that you won't get elsewhere. Most gyms offer fitness assessments, which will help you establish how hard you can work without hurting yourself, and will design personal fitness programme for you. Women who are overweight, over the hill, unwell or unfit can find the prospect of huffing and puffing on a treadmill next to work-out-Barbie quite intimidating, but those who lack confidence or self-discipline can find that booking a few sessions with a personal trainer is a great incentive. Personal trainers will monitor progress, push you harder than you might push yourself and devise an individual trsining programme for you to follow when your course is finished. The real merit of gyms, though, is the fact that most of them provide a wide range of classes from kick boxing to yoga to spinning. Women who connect into group activities find that a good teacher, friendly competition, companionship and mutual encouragement are a much greater incentive than scary medical statistics.

When I exercise I feel absolutely knackered coz I'm a daft bugger that is convinced there is a supermodel's body inside of me and I always overdo it.
Caroline, 40, Aus

When I first started I never wanted to go but if I'd promised to meet my friend there, I would go even if I didn't want to because I knew she would be waiting. It's that first bit of motivation that you need. Once you are there you can have a chat and a laugh and then you will feel so much better for having made the effort.
Tammy, 25, UK

When I was single, I exercised almost daily at home: doing sit-ups or yoga. Much as I hate to admit it, I feel less inclined to do so with my partner present.
Frances, 30, UK

I joined an expensive local gym and went to it only four times in the whole year. I worked it out. It cost me £150 per swim. I could have gone to the south of France.
Petra, 28, UK

If gyms were more child friendly it might be easier for women to use them.
Alex, 32, US

The heart of the matter

I am anti-fitness. I hate going to the gym and I very rarely exercise. When I am sad, my boyfriend tells me that if I go to the gym or go for a swim, it will cheer me up. I know it is probably true and when I do get around to doing anything I do actually feel better, but I find it annoying that there always needs to be a physical reason for the way I feel. I think attitudes to fitness and wellbeing are not so much social as cultural. American or Australian girls seem to be more sporty and balanced than European girls. Maybe Europe is just too wrapped up in psychology. Women have a tendency to be more thoughtful than men and, historically, they have been more 'indoors' than men, who are 'outdoors'. Because they spend more time at home they have more time to think about things but I don't necessarily think that it is good for us. As a gender, women don't take the same physical risks as men because traditionally they have been homemakers and have had to take care of kids. Men take more risks, drive faster, play dangerous sport. Men die younger. Women with children can't afford to.
Cateriona, 29, Italy
(Pictured right)

HOW FIT ARE YOU? Before you embark on a fitness programme you should establish your basic level of fitness and work out your resting heart rate. Your resting heart rate or pulse is the number of times your heart beats per minute. The fitter you are, the lower your heart rate will be – apparently Bjorn Borg had a resting heart rate of 30 beats per minute! Your resting heart rate will be faster if you are nervous or if you have drunk a lot of coffee or smoked. Certain medications such as asthma inhalers or cough medicines can speed up your heart rate too.

SAFETY Knowing how to measure your heart rate allows you to establish whether you are working too hard or not working hard enough when you exercise. The 'no pain, no gain' approach can be very damaging, particularly for women who do nothing for ages and then put a huge amount of pressure on themselves in a short space of time. Everyone has off days and trying to force yourself through a routine when you don't feel great is not a good idea. Measuring your pulse lets you know if you are pushing your heart rate too high and need to slow down a bit or not working hard enough and need to speed up.

TO FIND YOUR RESTING HEART RATE The best time to get a true measurement for your resting heart rate is before you get out of bed in the morning. Look at your hand with your palm facing up and find your radial artery, a faint blue vein that you should be able to see through your skin on the thumb side of your wrist. Using your middle and index fingers (not your thumb as it can have its own pulse) place your fingertips over the vein and see if you can feel a light palpitation. Don't press too hard or you could block the artery and you won't feel anything at all. After finding your pulse, look at the second hand on your watch and count the number of beats in one minute. (Those with a low attention span can count the number of beats in 6 seconds and add a zero.) This number of beats per minute is your resting heart rate.

AVERAGE HEART RATES An average resting heart rate score of 60 is excellent and means you are very fit, 60–69 is considered good, 70–79 is average, 80–89 is fair, 89+ is poor and means you are very unfit. But don't panic. As soon as you start exercising your resting heart rate will gradually drop, which is a good thing. If your resting heart rate drops from 90 beats a minute to 80 beats a minute, it means your heart only needs to beat 80 times to push the same amount of blood around your body and in the long run this saves your heart from wear and tear.

TARGET HEART RATES Once you know your resting heart rate you can work out your target heart rates. This helps you to monitor how hard you are working while you exercise. To work out effectively, you need to elevate your heart

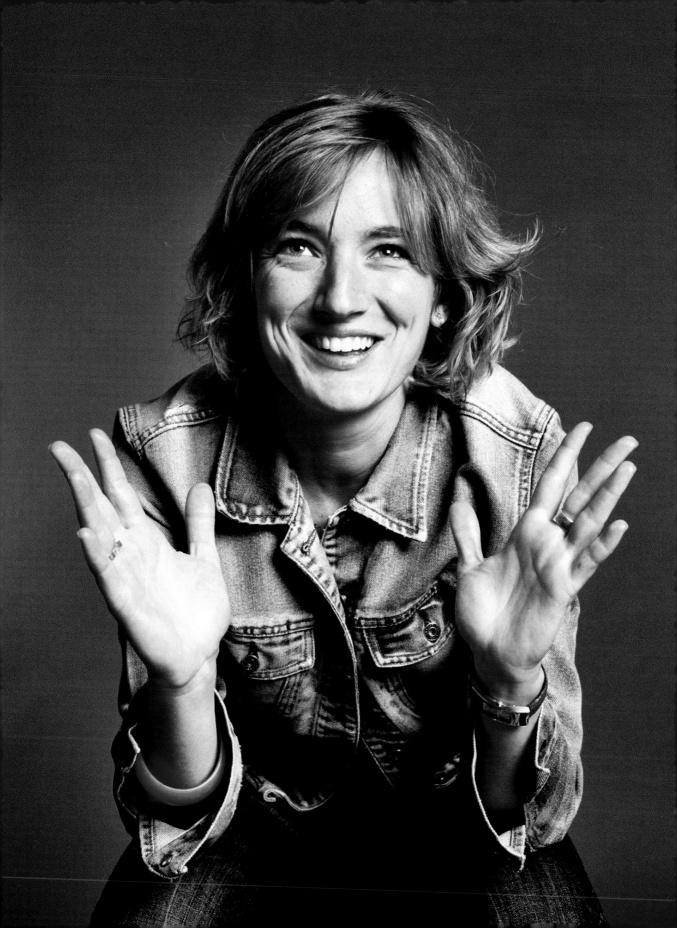

Aerobics: 342 calories

Boxing: 225 calories

Cross country skiing: 200 calories

Cycling at 12mph on the flat: 283 calories

Football: 180 calories

Golf: 150 calories

Horse-riding: 142 calories

Ice skating: 120 calories

Rowing machine: 208 calories

Rugby: 190 calories

Running: 10-minute mile: 365 calories 8-minute mile: 446 calories

Skipping 60–80 skips per minute: 286 calories

Snowboarding: 120 calories

Squash: 280 calories

Swimming: 248 calories

Tennis Singles: 232 calories Doubles: 125 calories

Versa climber: 375 calories

Water aerobics: 140 calories

Walking 20-minute mile on flat terrain: 120 calories 20-minute mile on hilly terrain: 162 calories.

Weight training: 378 calories

rate, but there is a minimum and a maximum range within which you should be working to improve your current levels of fitness. If you are a beginner and starting out on a fitness programme, you should be aiming to work at the lower end of your target fitness zone. As you get fitter, you push yourself harder and eventually you should be working at your maximum target zone. Ultimately, it's not how fast you can do something but how long you can do it for that counts. As long as you keep your heart rate up it doesn't matter whether you jog a lap of the running track, then walk for a few minutes, then jog again. Keeping your heart rate up for 30 minutes, even if you are walking for 15 of them, is much better for you than burning around for two laps and then collapsing in a sweaty heap.

TO FIND YOUR MINIMUM TARGET HEART RATE

Subtract your age from 220 e.g. 220 − 35 = 185. Then subtract your resting heart rate from your result, e.g.185 − 70 = 115. Multiply your second result by 0.5, i.e. 115 × 0.50 = 57.5. Then add your resting heart rate to that figure, i.e. 57.5 + 70 = 127.5. This figure is the low end of your target heart zone and the figure you should be working above if you are embarking on a new fitness programme.

TO FIND YOUR MAXIMUM TARGET HEART RATE

Subtract your age from 220, e.g. 220 − 35 = 185. Then subtract your resting heart rate from your result, e.g. 185 − 70 = 115. Multiply your second result by 0.85 i.e. 111 × 0.85 = 97.75. Then add your resting heart rate to that figure, i.e. 97.75 + 70 = 167.75. This figure is the high end of your target heart zone. If you are working at this level you are pushing yourself as hard as is healthy. What you will find is that over time, as you get fitter, your resting heart rate will drop and you will need to revise these figures.

CARDIAC HEART MONITORS Measuring your pulse is a bit of a pain, not particularly accurate and virtually impossible to do while you are exercising, so although you don't necessarily need gadgets like heart monitors, they can be a great incentive to exercise because they help you to track physical improvement. The basic models are all a beginner will need and they are not particularly expensive. The most accurate versions have a strap that fastens around your chest and places an electrode over your heart. The strap feeds information to a digital read out, usually a watch, which you wear around your wrist while you are working out. Some companies make special sports bras with loops to hold the chest strap in place, though once you start sweating the electrode sticks to your skin anyway. If you are considering buying a heart monitor, you need to think about where you will be using it as electromagnetic interference in gyms can reduce accuracy. Newer models have in-built devices to counter this.

How much is enough?

START SLOWLY If you have not exercised for some time, it is very important that you build up over a period of weeks. This might, for example, mean starting out with five minutes at first and pushing it to ten when you feel ready. Eventually you are aiming for a target of 30 minutes to one hour of exercise per day. Though the 30 minutes can be broken up into three ten-minute blocks, it is probably best to just get it over with in one session if you can. If you want to manage or lose weight you should increase that time to one hour a day, five days a week. However, unless it is part of a calorie-controlled diet, exercise alone will not be enough. Remember, what constitutes a strenuous, moderate or mild exercise work load for you will depend on your current state of health and fitness. If you are an Olympic 10,000m sprinter, jogging one mile in five minutes would count as mild activity. However, for most of us this would be either very strenuous or not possible. If you overdo it at the beginning, you risk hurting yourself.

TRAINING ZONES Once you know your resting heart rate and your maximum heart rate, you can work out your percentage heart rate and plan your training around how hard and how long your heart should be working.

HEALTHY HEART ZONE/WARM UP 30 minutes exercise at 55% of maximum heart rate is probably the best zone for older women or those who are just starting a fitness program. To find your healthy heart percentage heart rate divide your maximum heart rate by 100 and then multiply that figure by 55 (e.g. pulse/heart monitor display of 92 bpm for a 35-year-old with a resting heart rate of 70). It can also be used as a warm-up zone once you get fitter. It is essential to warm up and cool down before and after you exercise. Starting or stopping abruptly when exercising increases the probability of muscle soreness, cramps and injury. Begin all exercise sessions with stretching and gradually reduce the intensity at which you are working by about half for five to ten minutes at the end.

TO IMPROVE HEALTH AND FITNESS 30 minutes exercise at 60–70% of your maximum heart rate provides the same benefits as the healthy heart zone, but is a little more strenuous, so it burns more calories. To find your training percentage heart rate divide your maximum heart rate by 100 and then multiply that figure by 65 (e.g. pulse/heart monitor display of 109 bpm for a 35-year-old with a resting heart rate of 80). This zone is good for burning stored fat because it is not intense enough to draw on your muscles, glycogen reserves. It improves your general levels of fitness, increases your aerobic capacity, helps decrease blood pressure, cholesterol levels and risk of degenerative diseases such as osteoporosis and cancer. As this level is not too strenuous it has a low risk of injury and is easier to sustain over a long period of time.

Your body is where you live. You need to look after it in the same way you look after your house, your car or the clothes you wear.
Anne, 58, UK

I find the gym so boring. The repetitive nature of using machines to exercise makes me feel like a robot. I wish we all played games in the community like rounders or tennis like they used to in the old days.
Natasha, 28, Pakistan

I think boys tend to have a more pragmatic approach to life. They separate the body from the soul, whereas women don't see an immediate cause and effect between how they feel physically and how they feel emotionally. Men are more primal, they eat, they sleep they have sex. If a man feels down, he will do some sport or go out with his mates. Women tend to be more analytical about things. When a woman feels down, she will sit at home and worry about the issue instead of finding immediate ways to make herself feel better. We over complicate things I suppose.
Beverly, 25, UK

If you are so out of breath that you can't speak, you are working too hard. If you can hold a conversation but feel like you are working out, then you are probably going at the right pace. If you can sing along to your Walkman, then you need to step on it.

Rate of Perceived Exertion (RPE)

This system is based on your own personal rating of how hard you feel you are exercising. Doctors often use it to get small children to describe the intensity of pain as in, 0 = no pain, 10 = really bad pain.

In terms of exercise you assign a number from 0 to 10 to rate your exercise intensity as in, 0 = feet up, 10= close to death.

A major benefit of this system is that it gets you in touch with how you feel while you're exercising and you don't need any special equipment.

If you have a heart rate monitor or enjoy counting your beats, you can use RPE along with your heart rate. Try comparing your perception of exercise intensity to your cardiac reading.

TO MANAGE YOUR WEIGHT 60 minutes exercise at 70–80% of your maximum heart rate means you are working in your aerobic zone. This zone will help improve your cardio-respiratory system and help you burn more calories while you work out. To find your aerobic percentage heart rate divide your maximum heart rate by 100 then multiply that figure by 75 (e.g. pulse/heart monitor display of 125 bpm for a 35-year-old with a resting heart rate of 80). Cycling or jogging should be at a pace you find 'somewhat hard'. The fitter you get, the faster your metabolism will be, and you will continue to burn calories after exercising.

TO LOSE WEIGHT 60 minutes exercise at 80–90% of your maximum heart rate will improve your oxygen uptake and give you an improved VO2 max (the highest amount of oxygen one can consume during exercise), and boost your cardio-respiratory system. It will help you to fight fatigue, improve your endurance and build muscle, making you look more toned. To find your cardio-respiratory percentage heart rate divide your maximum heart rate by 100 and then multiply that figure by 85 (e.g. pulse/heart monitor display of 142 bpm for a 35-year-old with a resting heart rate of 80). This zone burns less stored fat and uses more carbohydrate and glycogen, but after you finish your workout your fat reserves are burned to replace the glycogen you have used. Intersperse fast pace walking or jogging with higher intensity running, cycling, step or aerobics to build muscle. The more muscle you have, the higher your metabolic rate, so you are less likely to plateau when dieting.

RED LINE (MAXIMUM EFFORT) Working at 90–100% of your capacity is the hardest you should work. To find your red line percentage heart rate divide your maximum heart rate by 100 and then multiply that figure by 95 (e.g. pulse/heart monitor display of up to 159 bpm for a 35-year-old with a resting heart rate of 80). This zone burns the highest number of calories, but it is very intense and most people can only stay in this zone for short periods. Only train in this zone if you are in very good shape and have been cleared by a physician to do so.

SEEING IMPROVEMENT When you start exercising, your body has to work hard to keep up with the demand for blood and oxygen during exercise. Over time your aerobic system becomes more efficient and the same level of exercise won't push your heart rate up as much so you can increase the intensity of your work outs. You can also monitor improvement by checking how long it takes for your heart rate to drop back to normal after you stop exercising. The fitter you are, the faster the fall. Measure your heart rate immediately after you stop exercising (e.g. 90 beats per minute) and then 60 seconds later (e.g. 70 beats per minute). Your heart rate should drop 20 beats in the first minute but people who are very fit can drop their heart rate by 40 beats in 60 seconds.

Fitness in 15-minutes

Doing the following routine as soon as you wake up every morning will improve every aspect of your physical fitness. You don't need any equipment and you can do all the exercises while you are still in your pyjamas. The exercises are simple but as a combination they work on strength, speed, co-ordination, stamina and flexibility. Start slowly, concentrate on form and breathe deeply. It is better to do two repetitions correctly than ten incorrectly. As with any of the exercises described in this book, if you have any serious health problems, back problems or heart problems, check with your doctor before you attempt anything strenuous.

SIXTY SECONDS OF PRESS-UPS In women, muscle mass declines as we age, particularly in the upper body which tends to be ignored during exercise. Doing the following exercise for one minute every morning will help maintain strength in your arms and shoulders. As you get better at them, try doing more in 60 seconds rather than extending the time, but don't compromise your form. Lie on your front. Place both hands flat on the floor with your thumbs directly under your shoulders and your elbows bent. Keep your toes flexed on the floor and push through your palms to raise your upper body. Your back should be flat so keep your stomach and back muscles taut and in line with each other. Your bum should not be sticking up in the air. When your arms are fully extended don't lock your elbows. Now lower your body slowly back down to shoulder level and repeat as many times as you can. Work slowly, a maximum of one press-up in three seconds.

SIXTY SECONDS OF SQUATS These measure lower body strength but women's thighs and calves are generally stronger than their upper bodies so you should be able to do quite a few. Doing 40–60 squats for one minute every morning will keep your thighs and buttocks toned. Stand with your feet hip width apart. Now bend your knees (which are facing forwards) and lower your bottom as if you are going to sit on a chair. Your knees should not go forward further than your toes and your thigh should be parallel with the floor. Now raise back up and repeat.

FIVE MINUTES OF STEP-UPS This improves cardio fitness, muscle strength, speed and co-ordination. Five minutes step work will get your heart pumping and improve overall fitness. Find a step about 12–20cm (6-8in) in height, or use the first step of the stairs. Step up with your left foot, then raise your right foot to join it. Take your left foot down and then the right. Repeat for five minutes.

SIXTY SECONDS OF TOE TOUCHING This exercise stretches the muscles at the back of the legs and lower back. Sit on the floor with your legs outstretched in front of you and your feet flexed towards the sky. Bending slowly forwards from your hips reach towards your toes and see which part of your leg

I just find it so hard to get a routine for fitness. I do enjoy going to yoga at the gym but something always gets in the way and to be honest I feel guilty if I take time out for myself so I let everything else take priority. It didn't really matter when I was younger but I feel that the rubbery tyre around my middle is here to stay now and that frightens me. If I don't do something and fast it will be all downhill from here.
Erica, 43, UK

Since my husband retired we have started walking in earnest. We wake up every morning at 7.30 and hike for an hour to a little cafe, where we have breakfast and read the papers. Both of us are fitter now than we were ten years ago and our early morning walk just sets us up for the day.
Vera, 64, NZ

I do a home exercise programme every morning for 20 minutes because it is the only way I can ensure that I actually get it out of the way. If I can manage to do a walk later in the day then that's great, but at least I know I am doing my little bit to protect myself against decrepitude.
Helga, 61, Holland

or foot you can actually grasp – not touch. Grip and hold for ten seconds. Breathe out as you stretch forwards and gradually try to improve your stretch. You should eventually be able to wrap your hands around the soles of your feet. Repeat three times on each side.

TWO MINUTES SIT-UPS Sit-ups improve abdominal muscle tone, a must for all women. Incorporating 40–60 sit-ups into your morning routine will make a huge difference to your shape. Lie flat on the floor on your back with your knees bent and your feet flat on the floor. Place your palms on your hips and run them slowly up to your knees, pulling yourself up with your stomach muscles.

SIXTY-SECOND BACK SCRATCHER Maintaining movement in the upper body and shoulders is particularly important for women who spend a lot of time working on computers. You should try to do this exercise a couple of times on each side every morning though you may find one side is easier than the other. Sit with your back straight and your legs stretched out in front of you. Stretch up with the right arm and bend it behind your head as if you are trying to scratch your back, in-between your shoulder blades. Then reach your left arm behind your back to touch or hold the right hand's fingers. Do this on both sides, holding for 30 seconds, breathing deeply.

SIXTY-SECOND BACK STRETCH Back stretching gives a gentle stretch to the muscles of the back and neck, releases toxins and relieves stiffness in the spine. Sit with your back straight and your legs straight out in front of you. Place your right hand palm flat on the floor behind you by your spine and then twist your head and shoulders so that you are looking over your right shoulder, keeping both buttocks on the floor. Hold the pose for 15 seconds each time and do two twists on each side.

TWO-MINUTE BALANCE After the age of 40 balance begins to decline. If you don't incorporate balancing exercises into your workout programme, the deterioration occurs even earlier. To improve balance, stand up straight, arms down by your sides. Now move your weight onto your right leg and bring your left knee up to hip height and hold, for one minute, keeping your arms by your side. Repeat on the other side.

ONE MINUTE SITTING CROSS-LEGGED This position helps to maintain hip flexibility and gives a gentle stretch to the muscles of the lower back, upper thighs and buttocks. Try to sit cross-legged when you are watching TV or whenever the opportunity arises.

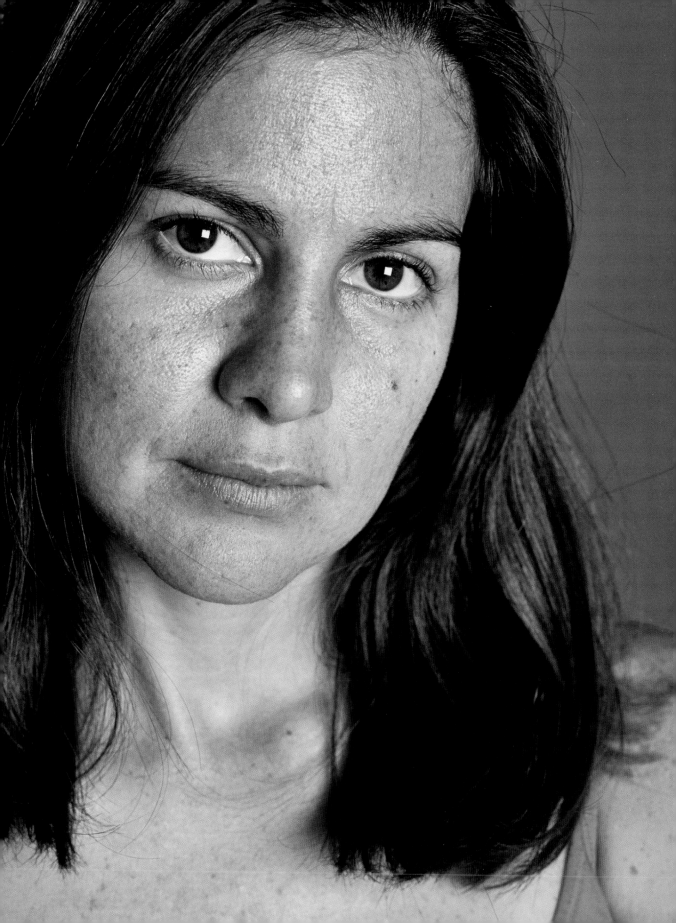

Test your fitness age

THE TEST To do the tests you will need a friend, a watch with a second hand or a stopwatch, a ruler, a pen and some paper. To work out your score, write down your real age, then do the first test and add or subtract your score from your real age. Do the second test and add or subtract your score from your first result. Carry on adding or subtracting from the previous result and you will be left with your fitness age. If you find any of the exercises too strenuous, stop. It probably just means that you are desperately unfit but you ought to see a doctor to establish that there is nothing physically wrong and get some advice on the kind of routine that would be suitable for you. Refer to the page numbers in brackets to find the BMI chart, how to measure your heart rate and how to do the exercises correctly.

1. FIND YOUR RESTING HEART RATE (P.110) • *Under 65: subtract five years from your real age* • *66–89: do nothing* • *80–90: add two years to your real age*

2. BODY MASS INDEX (P.17) • *Under 18.5: add two years to the result you got in question 1* • *18.5–24: do nothing* • *25–30: add two years to the result you got in question 1* • *Over 30: add four years to result 1.*

3. HOW MUCH DO YOU SMOKE EACH DAY? • *20 or more: add five years to result 2* • *less than 5: add two years to result 2* • *Non-smoker: do nothing.*

4. HOW MUCH DO YOU DRINK EACH DAY? (P.63) • *Nothing all week, then 20 units at the weekend: add five years to result 3* • *Approximately 4 units: add two years to result 3* • *Under 2 units: do nothing*

5. PRESS-UPS (P.115) How many press-ups can you do in 60 seconds? Get your partner to time you. • *0–2: add two years to result 4* • *2–5: do nothing* • *6+: subtract two years from result 4.*

6. SQUATS (P.115) Women generally have stronger lower body strength so a poor squat score implies lower levels of all-round fitness than a poor score at press-ups. How many can you do in 60 seconds? • *0–20: add five years to result 5* • *20–40: do nothing* • *40–60: subtract two years from result 5.*

7. STEP-UPS (P.115) This tests your stamina and speed. How many can you do in 60 seconds? Get your partner to time you. • *0–20: add five years to result 6* • *20–30: add two years to result 6* • *30–40: do nothing* • *40–60: subtract two years from result 6* • *60+: subtract five years from result 6.*

8. TOE TOUCHING (P.115) This tests your flexibility and muscular stiffness. How far can you reach when you try and touch your toes? • *Between knees and calves: add five years to result 7* • *Between calves and ankles: do nothing* • *Toes: subtract two years from result 7.*

9. SIT-UPS (P.116) To test your abdominal strength. How many can you do in 60 seconds? Get your partner to time you. • *0–10: add five years to result 8* • *20–30: do nothing* • *31–50: subtract two years from result 8•*

10. BACK SCRATCHER (P.116) To test shoulder flexibility. Hold the pose for 20 seconds. • *Hands more than 5cm (2in) apart: add two years to result 9•* *Can just about touch the bottom of your fingers: do nothing* • *Can hold your hands on both sides: subtract two years from result 9.*

11. BACK STRETCH (P.116) This tests your spinal flexibility. You need to hold the pose for 20 seconds. • *Couldn't twist your shoulders at all: add five years to result 10•* *Can twist but not hold the look over your shoulder for the whole time: do nothing• Can do the pose easily: subtract two years from result 10.*

12. BALANCE (P.116) How long can you stand on one leg? Hold the pose for 60 seconds. Time your partner with a stopwatch and get them to time you. • *Wobbled before 30 seconds: add two years to result 11• Can hold for 30 seconds to a minute: do nothing* • *Can hold for more than a minute: subtract two years from result 11.*

13. REFLEXES Our brain cells deteriorate as we age and this means our reflexes decline too. However, this occurs less in people who are physically fit. To test your reflexes, stand facing your partner, hands extended 15cm (6in) apart. Get your partner to drop a ruler vertically between your hands five times making sure they start from the same height every time. How many times did you catch the ruler? • *Nil: add five years to result 12* • *1 or 2 times: add one year to result 12* • *3 times: do nothing* • *4-5 times: subtract two years from result 12.*

14. CROSS-LEGGED (P.116): To test your hip flexibility sit cross-legged for sixty seconds. • *Knees more than 12.5cm (5in) off the floor: add five years to result 13* • *Knees 6 cm (2½in) from floor: do nothing* • *Knees touching floor: subtract two years from result 13.*

Being unfit and over weight is a psychological by product of not liking yourself. You can't like yourself much if you are not prepared to take care of your body. If you are very out of shape, starting can be intimidating. It is like standing at the bottom of a mountain looking up. But as soon as you get into training it gets easier. Before you know it, you are half way up the mountain looking down. You become a lot more conscious of your whole body and you spend more time grooming and feeling positive about yourself. Women who feel that getting fit or losing weight is an impossible task put themselves at the bottom of the pile of their 'to do' list. And then they never do anything about it. I started to get fit because I felt I was not making myself a priority. I knew I was still young and I wanted to take more care of myself. I was spending too much time working and neglecting my fitness levels. Luckily I am single so I didn't have to ask anyone's permission to take time out for myself. And once I made time for it I found that I was able to work better and I had loads more energy.
Antonia, 32, UK

Results

Everything about me feels better when I exercise; my body, my mind, my skin, my libido and I also sleep a lot better. My main way of keeping fit is walking. I try to walk everywhere. I think I was addicted to exercise in the past, but I am not any more. I just couldn't keep up with it any more. It was taking over everything, mentally, physically, socially.
Sari, 24, UK

I think I am moderately fit (but only just): I walk to work every day (for 40 minutes) and often home again in the evening. I think I could do more exercise, but find that doing this amount (which is probably a minimum) at least keeps me feeling slightly active. I feel much better if I do a degree of exercise – partly because it gets me out of the class-room where most of my day is spent teaching, writing or working at a computer. I also find I sleep better if I am physically, as well as mentally, tired.
Frances, 30, US

I had a fitness test at my gym and I scored well except in lung capacity. I am now working on specifically aerobic tasks.
Susie, 28, UK

MORE THAN 10 YEARS OLDER THAN REAL AGE The bad news is that you are likely to suffer from age-related problems such as weight gain, backache and breathlessness sooner than you should. The good news is that it is never too late to start exercising and if you begin a regular exercise programme today and do this test again in 12 weeks you should see a marked improvement.

LESS THAN 10 YEARS' DIFFERENCE If you don't do any exercise and you manage to come in with less than 10 years' difference, count yourself lucky. You obviously have a natural level of fitness that would be easy to boost with a little more input. If you do exercise and this was your result, chances are one element of your fitness is letting you down. You may be strong on stamina if you run, but poor on flexibility and balance. You need to vary your exercise programme and combine yoga or strength training with your aerobic work.

ROUGHLY THE SAME AS REAL AGE This means you are performing as expected for your age but don't get complacent. If you don't start to build stronger muscles and boost your cardiovascular system now your fitness levels can easily slide. Try and up your general activity levels by taking the stairs or playing football with the kids.

YOUNGER THAN REAL AGE Way to go girl. You are obviously an active and energetic person who is keeping in shape. Keep it up and remember to increase your pace and push yourself a little harder as soon as your exercise routine starts to become repetitive or less challenging.

IMPROVING YOUR SCORE You don't need to do a huge amount to keep your heart, lungs, muscles and bones in good condition. Follow the 15-minute fitness programme (p. 115) every day, add a brisk walk, a three mile run or a cycle daily for 12 weeks, and you will see a big improvement in your general fitness level. The short-term benefits of increased fitness are better muscle tone, a lower resting heart rate and faster metabolism. In the long term you will cut your risk of stroke, type-2 diabetes, coronary heart disease, osteoporosis and some cancers and keep your weight in check.

If you haven't exercised for a while, if you haven't been well, or you are over 60 years of age, it is best to start out with low-impact exercises such as walking or swimming. However, if you did well in the fitness test and think nothing of zooming up and down flights of stairs, digging out the flowerbeds, walking the dog, scrubbing the floor and carrying a small child around, then chances are, you are a lot fitter than you give yourself credit for.

Fat burning

JUST DO IT To lose body fat you must burn up more calories than you eat. Exercise creates an energy deficit which prompts your body to take fat out of storage and convert it back into energy, meaning you lose weight. How you choose to increase your energy expenditure doesn't matter. Basically all exercise burns calories, and all exercise will contribute to fat loss as long as you don't increase your calorie consumption too.

FAT V. GLUCOSE Physical activity uses both carbohydrate and stored fat as an energy source (p.36). Fat is a good source of fuel during low-intensity exercises when your breathing rate and oxygen use can keep up with the demands of the exercise. This type of exercise is often referred to as 'aerobic' meaning 'with oxygen'. During light or low effort exercise such as walking, fat is the primary fuel source, supplying about 60 to 70% of the calories burned (glucose stores provide the difference). But as you increase your exercise intensity, e.g. increase pace from a walk to a run, you burn proportionally more glucose and less fat. At very high intensity, i.e. sprinting, when breathing rate or oxygen needs fall short of the energy demands of the exercise, carbohydrate is the only fuel source. This type of high-intensity exercise is called 'anaerobic', or without oxygen.

FUEL EFFICIENCY Low-intensity exercises like walking are easier to do, especially as you start a fitness program, and you'd be forgiven for concluding that they are a better way of burning fat and losing weight. But how many total calories you burn during an exercise activity also depends on your fitness level. As you get fitter, your muscles become better fat burners so that at a given running pace, you burn more fat and less glucose than when you were less fit and running at the same pace. When you raise your fat-burning ability, you increase your ability to exercise for a longer period. Your muscles and liver store enough glucose and glycogen to fuel between 90 minutes and two hours continuous exercise. If you can burn fat while you run, you reserve your glycogen stores, allowing you to run for longer.

REV UP YOUR METABOLISM What your body burns as fuel after you work out also contributes to fat burning. Following a high-intensity exercise programme your body continues to burn fat to compensate for the glycogen that has been used up. This revved-up fat burning can continue for more than 24 hours, depending upon your levels of exertion. Also, high-intensity exercise burns more calories per minute than 'slow' activities so you use more calories in a shorter space of time. And the more muscle you have, the higher your metabolic rate or speed at which you burn up calories. For every 990g (2lb) of muscle you carry, you can burn up an extra 20–30 calories per day. It's not a huge amount but over a year it adds up to 9125 calories – enough to help you lose 1.3kg (3lb).

In my 20s I liked my body a lot as I was very fit. But I developed a back problem in my late 20s – due to an unscrupulous employer – which I still have to this day. Obviously, it doesn't improve with age and it can be quite debilitating at times. I am a dress size larger than I was ten years ago, although much of this has to do with the fact that I don't take nearly the amount of exercise that I used to. I have to admit that mainly this is down to my own lack of planning; but sometimes it is due to back pain. I wouldn't say that personal appearance becomes less relevant as one gets older, but one concerns oneself more with health and how one is feeling, rather than how one is looking. I wouldn't say I'm sloppy about my appearance. I do make an effort for work and when I am going out somewhere but I have never been the kind of person that feels she has to be made up to the nines every day. Caroline, 40, UK

Swimming at high school changed my life. I finally found something I was good at. I could escape from my deadbeat family and train in the pool all day. Shanaz, 34, US

CYCLING Most adults give up cycling as soon as they get their first wage packet. Associated with students, couriers and the occasional elderly gent, cycling isn't viewed as an appropriate mode of transport for women wearing make-up. But why not? It is faster than public transport, it is environmentally friendly. And it is precisely the sort of daily activity that would boost our baseline fitness levels if we bothered to incorporate it into our daily lives.

Cycling is not a load bearing exercise so it needs to be combined with resistance training, walking or running. However, it is great for boosting cardiovascular fitness and is easier on the joints so it is good for older, less mobile people. Two 15-minute cycling trips a day will cover your basic exercise quota and get you to work on time too. Traffic can be a problem but the more that people cycle, the more pressure there is on local councils to expand safer cycle lane programmes. If you are going to ride outside you will obviously need a helmet, lights and a reflective jacket. Make sure your saddle is in good repair and the right height – your leg should extend fully at the base of a revolution. Never cycle under the influence of alcohol and follow the rules of the road. Thirty minutes of cycling at 12mph burns 283 calories and on a hill you burn an extra 22 calories per mile.

SWIMMING Swimming is the ideal activity for people who can't bear the joint stress of jogging. And for the very overweight, it is probably the best way to get back into exercise because body weight is suspended. It provides a total body cardiovascular workout, however the down side of swimming is that bone density is directly related to load bearing exercises so it needs to be combined with weight training, running or walking. Unfortunately, swimming may not be suitable for asthmatics or those with respiratory problems as recent research has found a direct correlation between the huge rise in childhood asthma and the chlorine in swimming pools.

Water is 1000 times denser than air and provides up to 12 times the resistance that you would get from working out on land. Swimming works out all the muscles in your body and the faster you go, the harder your heart works.

If you are a beginner, don't rush things. Start with a 30-minute session three times a week and concentrate on increasing the number of laps you do rather than extending the time period. During the first week try swimming for one length and resting for 30 seconds. Repeat this up to ten times. Vary your strokes because each stroke works different muscle groups. Stick to this easy routine for a few weeks or until it becomes too easy, then gradually increase the lengths and decrease your rest times. Never increase the number of lengths by more than 10% at a time; i.e. go from 10 to 11, not 10 to 15. This will stop you overtraining and injuring yourself.

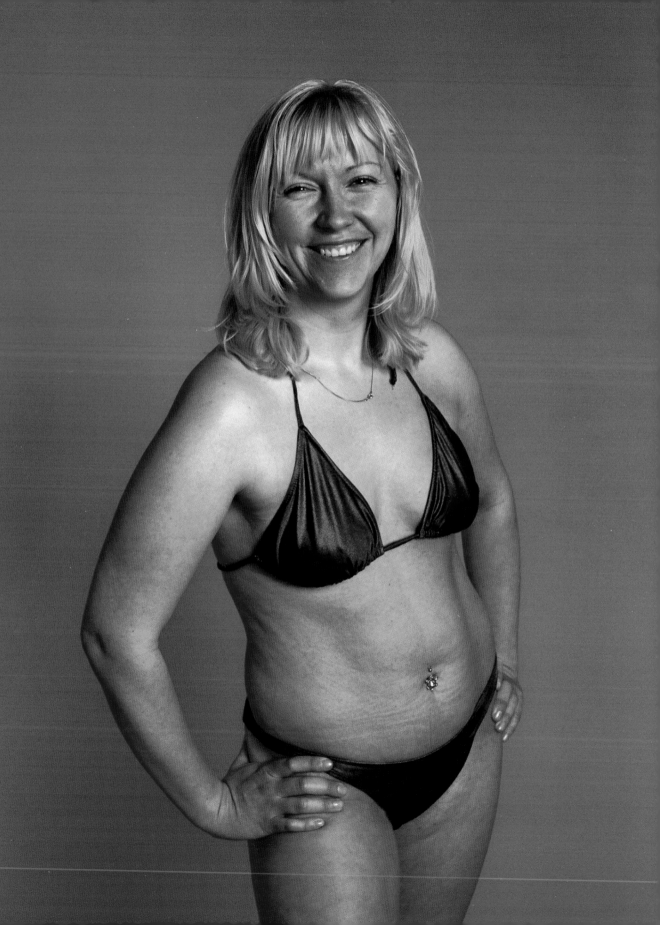

Initially it is best to feel that you are more than capable of the level you are at. Swimming is far more technical than other activities but most pools run classes for beginners, intermediate and advanced swimmers. Using floats and flippers can increase the intensity of the exercise and many gyms run water aerobics classes, which combine resistance work with lengths. Most pools hold sponsored swims, which can give you a reason to train and if you haven't done your swimming badges you could even sign up to get through the tests, learn how to lifesave or become an instructor. Swimming for 30 minutes at a reasonable speed burns 248 calories whereas 30 minutes of water aerobics only burns 140 calories.

TRAMPOLINING   Trampolining is a low-impact aerobic exercise that exercises virtually every major muscle in the body. It improves co-ordination, stamina, muscle development, and aids the cardiovascular system and burns the same amount of calories as running. It is extremely low impact to the knees and spine and should be combined with resistance training to form a complete workout. You can intersperse jumping with running on the spot and hold light weights in your hands to work your upper body too. You can set a mini-trampoline up anywhere, even in front of the TV. Try and do three ten-minute sessions or one 30-minute session every day. Trampolining for 30 minutes burns up to 400 calories.

WALKING   Brisk walking is one of the easiest ways to integrate exercise into your daily routine and it is also one of the few exercises that kids can do with you from an early age. Some years ago, a US study found that 80% of people who are successful in maintaining long-term fitness and weight loss use walking as their main form of exercise. And a study of men and women in their 70s found that following a walking programme reversed more than 20 years of declining lung capacity, while another found that elderly people who walk several times a week decrease their risk of hip fractures, arthritis and osteoporosis by up to 50 per cent. Other walking related research shows that mortality is halved in retired men who walk more than two miles every day and people who walk regularly show decreased aerobic deterioration and reduce their chances of developing Alzheimer's disease. So, walk to work, walk around the park, get a dog, join a rambling association, sign up for a sponsored walk or book a walking holiday in the Himalayas. And get moving.

Women who wear high heels a lot during the day should make sure to stretch their calf muscles before walking to avoid damaging their Achilles tendon. Stand facing a wall with your hands flat against it, arms straight, one leg bent and the other leg stretched about three feet behind it with both heels flat on the floor. Press against the wall until you can feel the stretch in the back of your leg from the tendon to the back of the knee. Then do the other leg.

Many people walk incorrectly and this can lead to back problems, so stand straight, don't bend forward, relax your shoulders, widen your chest and pull in your stomach. Keep your head and chin up and keep your hands relaxed. As you walk, swing your bent arms backwards. On the downswing your hand should brush against your hip. Keep your hips loose and push off from your toes and the ball of your foot and land heel first. If you want to exercise your upper body too, try holding light hand weights while you are walking.

Start with ten-minute walking sessions at a brisk pace. Do this every day for two weeks, then increase your walk by a further five minutes per day, but don't drop the pace. When your time increases to 20 minutes a day and you are going at the correct pace, you should be covering a mile of ground (measure your route by driving around it).

The brilliant thing about walking is that you don't really need any equipment and you can do it anywhere. A good pair of comfortable walking shoes will last years but a pair of trainers is fine for anyone walking on the flat. If you plan to hike on more rugged terrain, you will need to buy a walking shoe with treaded soles and heel and ankle supports.

You might want to invest in a pedometer, a small clip-on device that tracks the distance you travel by sensing your body motion and counting your footsteps. The count can be converted into distance if you know the length of your usual stride, though more sophisticated pedometers will do this for you. You can wear a pedometer all day, every day and record your total steps or you can just use it to gauge steps on a walking workout. The display should be easy to read without removing the unit from your waistband and it should be protected so that bumps don't re-set the count. The simplest, and cheapest, pedometers only count and display steps and/or distance but this is generally all that you need.

The recommended number of steps per day is 6000 for health or 10,000 for weight loss. If you walk 6000 steps in an average day, try and up this figure by 500 steps daily for a week. The following week add a further 500 steps daily and keep going until you are averaging 10,000 steps per day (three hours trudging round a shopping centre = 3000 steps). For weight loss, an uninterrupted walk each day of 4000–6000 steps is recommended, but you can increase your daily steps by walking as often as possible throughout the day. You might want to invest in a pedometer to check your distance and speed – you should be travelling at 3–4 miles per hour. Walking a 20-minute mile on flat terrain burns 120 calories, on hilly terrain a 20-minute mile burns 162 calories.

How much do people walk in a day?

A study by the Department of Physical Activity and Sports Studies at University College, Worcester, measured the number of steps taken by a group of volunteers. The greatest number of steps recorded in one day was 31,000 by a chef. The least recorded was 300 by a student. The average number of steps for those with sedentary jobs was 3000–4500 but people with a sedentary job who took a regular walk averaged 7000 steps a day. People without cars walked on average between 6000–7000 steps per day.

A failed tip ... Bought my mum, a self-confessed cakeaholic, a book on rambling and cafés, hoping she would take up walking if there was a cream cake incentive at the end. It failed. She just drove straight to the café every time!
Caroline, 40, Aus

When I crashed my car I didn't buy a new one and now I find that I am walking a lot more and my fitness has really increased.
Phoebe, 39, UK

Heart pumping

All exercise is beneficial, but to improve the strength and capacity of your heart (and lungs) you need to step up the pace. Running, swimming, cycling, step and walking at faster speeds will give your heart a harder work out. But skipping, hula hooping and rowing are good alternatives too.

HULA HOOPING Hula hoops were first produced in the US in 1958 by Wham-O Manufacturing and within a year more than 100 million were sold worldwide. These days it is a very underrated fitness activity, but it is absolutely great for the waist and hips, which are notoriously difficult to work out. It's also brilliant for your rhythm, timing and balance too. Though it takes a while to learn how to do it, anyone who practises enough will eventually get the hang of it. Large children's hoops are the cheapest option for beginners, though adults generally find it easier to control sports hoops, which are bigger and slightly heavier.

Hula hooping is deceptively exhausting. It doesn't feel that strenuous at first but keep the hoop going for more than five minutes and you will feel the burn in your heart, your lungs and your waist. Gradually build up your time to a maximum of ten minutes. Before you start a hula hooping programme, measure your waistline. Do ten minutes twice a day for eight weeks and measure your waist again. Hula hooping for ten minutes burns 70 calories.

JOGGING Though walking is an effective way of keeping fit and burning fat, the faster you go and the harder you work, the more you elevate your heart rate and boost your aerobic capacity. Jogging is an anywhere, anytime, fitness programme. All you need is a jogging bra and a pair of lightweight, flexible, cushioned, running shoes. Good sports stores will video your running style in order to recommend the most appropriate shoe. To run correctly you need to keep your head up, your shoulders relaxed, and your abs pulled in. Don't arch your back and keep your arms close to your body, swinging back and forth as you run. Push off from the balls of your feet and land heel first, then roll through to your toes and push off again.

Running is an excellent cardiovascular exercise and because it is high impact and load bearing it is one of the best activities for strengthening bones and avoiding arthritis, rheumatism or osteoporosis. However, this is also one of its downsides. Because it can be quite hard on the joints, some people experience joint pain, ankle, knee or lower back pain. (If running hurts or you feel it puts too much pressure on you, you are better off sticking to power walking or cycling.) Joining a running club or signing up to do a 5k run can be a great training incentive and it's a good way of meeting people too. Start your running programme with alternated running and walking and don't push yourself too hard initially. In your first week or two, intersperse five minutes of running with two minutes of walking for up to 15 or 20 minutes. As you gradually increase your running time, you can decrease your walking time. Eventually you should be able to run continuously for 20 minutes or more. Increase your speed gradually but don't increase your mileage by more than half a mile in one jump or you risk injury.

Recently an eminent plastic surgeon suggested that running is a primary cause of skin ageing and wrinkles because the facial skin is pulled away from the muscles supporting it with the impact of each step. However, many other experts disagree with this theory and it will not be relevant to women who run moderate amounts. Running three times a week is plenty and you should alternate it with strength training to give your whole body a workout. Thirty minutes running doing ten-minute miles burns 365 calories. Thirty minutes running eight-minute miles burns 446 calories. Thirty minutes' tennis burns 232 calories.

ROWING Rowing is the most complete exercise form in terms of muscles, heart and lungs so if you do plan to invest in a large piece of exercise equipment for your home, a rowing machine is probably your best buy. It works out all the major muscle groups, doesn't jar the joints and provides a great cardiovascular workout too. The downside is that the machines take up quite a bit of space. They are about 1.8m (6ft) long and can weigh anything from 13.5–54kg (30–120lb). Most are stored standing up, but if your machine is heavy you are probably better off finding a permanent home for it and leaving it set up, preferably in front of a TV. Do two 15-minute rowing sessions a day five times a week and aim to increase your speed gradually. Thirty minutes on a rowing machine burns 208 calories.

SKIPPING A simple skipping rope is a low cost, flexible way of improving aerobic endurance, boosting cardio-respiratory fitness and improving flexibility and co-ordination. It is absolutely exhausting so you will probably only be able to do several short bursts at first. Begin by trying to skip for three consecutive minutes with a one-minute rest period. Repeat this sequence four times, twice a day, for the first couple of weeks, or until it becomes easy. Gradually increase the length of time you skip in increments of 10% and cut the rest time by 50 per cent. Two 15-minute sessions may be easier than one 30-minute session. Combine skipping with swimming, hula hooping, running and weight training for a full body work out. Skipping is a high impact exercise so practise on a cushioned surface such as grass, carpet or a yoga mat to avoid joint injury. Twenty skips five times a day subjects your spine and hips to 100 high-impact jolts, which will keep your bones strong. Skipping at 60–80 skips per minute for 30 minutes burns 286 calories.

I am very strong, physically. This is due to both my build and the fact that as a child I did lots of ballet, climbing, etc. and through to my early thirties I had a very good exercise regime. However, it has all rather gone to pot over the last five years, so I'm not as fit as I should be. I still feel great if I exercise REGULARLY, but not if I do it in bouts. I have a back problem and find that a continuous problem. A swimming and yoga exercise plan increases my suppleness and decreases the pain. But unfortunately, I know that I don't take nearly enough exercise on a regular basis to keep it at bay.
Fay, 55, UK

I have very limited use of my legs as a result of a car accident when I was in my mid-30s. I can walk a little but I need assistance and I can't exercise. When I see able-bodied women who are overweight and unfit I want to shake them because if I could walk, let alone run I would do so all the time. They have the full use of all their limbs yet they do nothing with them. I suppose it is an age-old story but it is not until something is taken away that you really appreciate it. Mobility is irreplaceable.
Fran, 63, UK

Bone building

By around the age of 35 female bone density begins to decrease by about 0.5–1% each year. And this figure doubles in the first five years after the menopause. Women are three times more likely than men to be affected by osteoporosis, osteoarthritis and rheumatoid arthritis and the pain of these debilitating conditions makes exercise a very low priority. However, studies consistently prove that exercise, particularly load bearing and resistance activities, are hugely beneficial in both the prevention and alleviation of joint and muscle pain. Inactivity might seem like short-term pain avoidance, but in the long term it does more damage because it weakens the muscles, stiffens the joints and reduces mobility and energy levels. People who don't exercise also lose 30–40% of their strength by the age of 65. By the age of 74 years more than two-thirds of women can't lift an object heavier than 4.5kg (10lb). The gradual slide begins in your early 20s as muscle mass to fat ratio declines. But you *can* halt the process. By lifting weights you can double or triple your strength within 12 weeks. And if you get into a regular exercise routine, you can decrease bone loss by about 50 per cent.

WHAT SHOULD I DO? You really need to do a mixture of aerobic endurance, stretching and strengthening exercises. Aerobic endurance improves cardiovascular fitness and helps you to control your weight (extra weight puts additional pressure on many joints). Stretching and strengthening exercises help maintain normal joint movement, relieve stiffness and increase the flexibility of muscles, tendons and joint capsules. Though swimming and cycling are generally easier for people with mobility problems because their body weight is supported, bones only respond by building themselves up when they have to support your weight, so 'load bearing' exercises such as walking or running are more effective. This really is rocket science. The relationship between bone density and pressure was discovered when the first astronauts in space were found to have experienced significantly decreased bone density having spent so long in zero gravity without any weight on their bones. Now astronauts who go into space have to spend several hours a day exercising.

RESISTANCE TRAINING Resistance training helps reduce body fat and increase the amount of lean muscle you carry. If you attend a gym, an instructor will take you through free weights and show you how to train, but women who can't, or won't, make it to the gym can develop their strength by doing resistance training and stretching (p.130) at home. The idea is to develop strength and resistance in your own muscles by doing repeat exercises (reps). More frequent repetitions with lighter weights is better for your body than fewer reps with heavier weights. In a controlled study in the US, a 12-week weights programme more than doubled the muscle strength of some women aged 64 years and over.

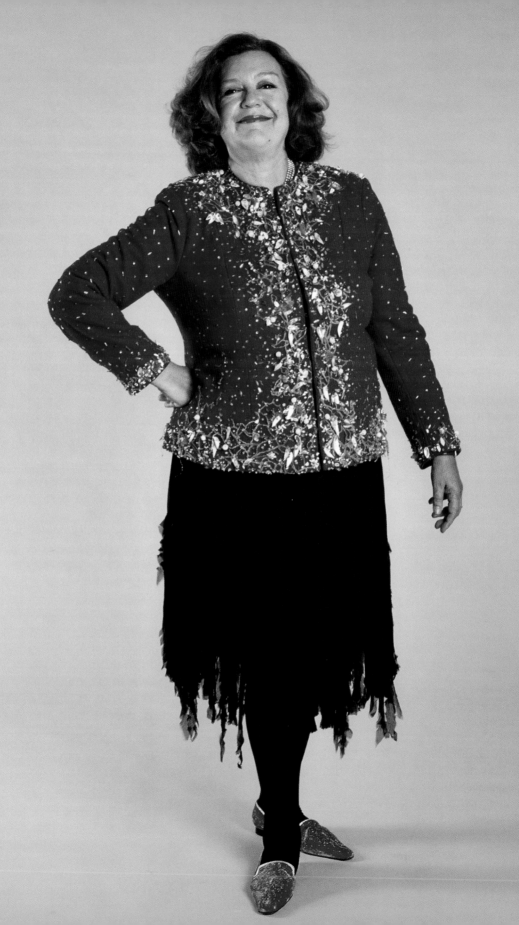

Muscle strengthening

SQUATS (P. 1 1 5) Hold the pose for 30 seconds building to 60 seconds as you get better. Do 25–50 reps night and morning to tone bum and upper thighs.

CALF AND SPINE STRETCH Use a yoga mat or a bath towel to sit on. Sit with your legs straight out in front of you. Loop a wide belt around the ball of one foot and straighten your leg. Stretch your body forwards, down towards your knee, pulling tighter on the belt and using your foot as resistance. Hold the pose for 30–60 seconds and repeat on other leg. Do 25 reps on each leg.

TORSO TIGHTENER Stand against a wall, back flat, arms straight up above your head holding each end of a taut tea towel. Pull on the ends of the towel as you bend your upper body slowly to one side. Hold the pose at about 45 degrees for 5–15 seconds. Do 25 reps each side.

LEG AND SPINE STRETCH While standing, rest your heel on a table at hip height. Straighten your leg. Bend forwards, with your face close to your knee and hands close to your ankle. Hold for 30-60 seconds. Do 10 reps on each leg.

UPPER ARM LIFT If you don't have dumbbells, tins of food or small jars of sugar or dried beans make excellent hand weights. Hold them in your hands, palms facing your hips with your arms by your side. Now slowly raise your straight arms to shoulder height and bring them back down again. Do 25 reps with both arms at the same time. Hold the cans in your hands, with your hands facing forwards and your arms by your side. Bend your elbows and bring your weights up towards your shoulders until your lower arms are parallel with the floor, no higher. Keep your elbows close to your sides. Do 25 reps with both arms at the same time.

LEG WEIGHTS Use an old pair of nylon tights as ankle weights. Cut off the legs and fill each with 900g (2lb) of rice, lentils, dried beans or sand. Tie each end, leaving material over to tie around your ankles. Wear them while doing your chores.

BABY SPLITS Lie on your back, making sure your lower back is flat on the ground. Bend one knee and keep the other leg straight. Lift the bent leg as high as you can off the ground and hold it there for 60 seconds, making sure the other leg stays flat on the ground. Repeat using the other leg. Do 25 reps on each leg.

INNER THIGH STRETCH Lie on your back with your knees bent. Pull your feet in until they touch your buttocks. Turn your ankles so that the soles of your feet are touching each other and let your knees fall out to the sides. Keep the base of your spine flat to the floor. Hold for 60 seconds.

SPINAL TWIST Lie flat on your back with your arms out at shoulder level. Bend your knees and, keeping them together, lower both your legs to the floor on the right side keeping both shoulders on the floor. Turn your head and look to the left. Hold the pose for 60 seconds. Then repeat in reverse. Do two reps.

TENSION CONTRAST Lie on your right side with arms out above your head. Tense your entire body so it is stiff as a board. Relax completely, letting your body fall either forwards or backwards as it loses balance. Repeat on the other side.

Stress busting

In a six-year study of medical expenditure on more than 46,000 workers, depression and unmanaged stress emerged as the most costly risk factors. Regular physical activity has been shown to help counter the damaging effects of stress and increased anxiety levels but many people find it difficult to fit exercise in during the day. This workout is designed to be carried out at your office desk and takes less than a coffee break to accomplish. Doing it regularly can help relieve tension, stiffness and RSI.

NECK STRETCH Roll the head slowly in a semi-circle around the bottom of the clock and then back again. Then roll the head in a semi-circle around the top half of the clock. Do not make a full circle by tipping the head back. Close your eyes and feel the stretch. Repeat ten times for each half of the clock.

SHOULDER LIFT Hunch the shoulders as high as possible (contract) and then let them drop (relax). Inhale on the lift; exhale on the drop. Do seven reps.

LOWER BACK STRETCH Stretch your lower back by gently bending forwards and pressing your chest into or close to your thighs.

TRUNK STRETCH AND DROP Stand on tip toe and reach as high as possible; stretch every muscle, then collapse forward letting your knees flex and trunk, head and arms dangle freely to the floor. Inhale on the stretch and exhale on the collapse. Repeat two or three times.

TRUNK SWINGS Remain in the 'drop' position and with a minimum of muscular effort, set the trunk swinging side to side by shifting the weight from one foot to the other. Keep the entire body (especially the neck) limp. Repeat three times.

LEG STRETCH In your chair, extend your legs in front of you, lean over on your chair and reach your arms towards your feet. You can increase the effectiveness of this stretch by flexing your feet and lifting your toes up in the air.

HAND AND FOREARM Contract your right hand, making a fist; hold for three counts; relax on six to ten counts. Repeat, then do left fist, then both.

BICEPS AND TRICEPS Hold your arms out to the sides at shoulder level parallel with the floor. With your fists facing towards the ceiling, bend your elbows and contract your biceps; hold, relax and do five reps. Repeat, but this time with your fists pointing down towards the floor, bend your elbows and contract your triceps at the back of your arm; hold, relax, and repeat five times.

THIGHS AND BUTTOCKS While sitting, squeeze your buttocks together and push your heels into the floor; hold for three counts; relax for six to ten counts.

CALVES Pull instep and toes towards your shins; hold for three counts, relax and repeat.

GRIP STRENGTHENER Make your own stress ball. Squeeze a ball, or a tightly rolled up pair of socks in each hand. Do 25 reps on each hand.

I am interested in the totality of wellbeing. Being well in oneself doesn't just mean physical health, it means emotional wellbeing too. It is ironic that there is so much focus on physical health and wellbeing but only within the context of our unnatural, unrelaxed and stressed lives. Good health and happiness is a natural function. It's a balance, not something we should have to strive for. If we were not working so hard and just being as we should be, we wouldn't have to work at keeping fit. The pressure to succeed starts as soon as we are born now. As children we have to learn to read and write even though we are not ready to do anything other than play with our toys.
Phoebe, 47, UK

Stress has been a major part of my life for the last ten years. I used to run on adrenaline. I was unhappily married so I worked too hard to get away from him, from home. I tried to do yoga and Pilates as a way of unwinding but what I really needed was a divorce. I finally did it two years ago. Since then my mind and body have altered beyond recognition.
Esther, 34, UK

Mind expanding

The link between mind and body was accepted in ancient India, the birthplace of yoga, thousands of years ago. It has taken a while for Western fitness experts to embrace the idea. But now the concept of holistic health and fitness is rapidly gaining in popularity. Yoga and Pilates appeal to women because they are not competitive or aggressive and the challenges and pleasures they present are derived from skill and self-possession. Because classes involve relaxation and meditation, they have a nurturing aspect that appeals to women and as such, they appear to be viewed more as a way of life than an exercise programme. However, the sudden growth in popularity has meant that demand has outstripped the supply of good teachers. Yoga's governing body, the British Wheel of Yoga (BWY) admits that only half the estimated 10,000 people now teaching yoga are properly qualified. There are a plethora of yoga training schools where anyone can pick up a certificate to teach within a month, but the BWY says tutors should study for four years before they are fully qualified. Many instructors are simply good students who fall into teaching when they stand in for an absent teacher, but being good at yoga doesn't necessarily make someone a good teacher. A good yoga teacher helps to put you into the right poses and doesn't spend the class showing off how easy it is for them. There are many forms of yoga Some are more dynamic, others are more meditative. Choose the class that suits your needs and fitness levels.

ANANDA Great for beginners. Requires less strength and flexibility.
ANUSARA A relatively new form of yoga, quite hippy dippy and spiritual.
ASTANGA Sometimes called power yoga, this is the most physically demanding in terms of strength, flexibility and stamina. Not for beginners but an incredible workout that leaves you feeling totally relaxed.
BIKRAM Here, 26 poses are performed in a room heated to 100 degrees. Hot and hard as hell and quite likely to make you feel sick until you get used to it. Not an option for anyone with high blood pressure or breathing difficulties.
INTEGRAL Lots of chanting and meditation with easier postures.
IYENGAR Iyengar yoga teachers have to do a specific qualification so they tend to be quite good. Uses blocks and belts with heavy focus on body alignment.
KRIPALU A more meditative style of yoga that emphasizes alignment, co-ordination and breath. Students learn the postures and progress to sustaining them.
KUNDALINI One the first Western yoga styles. It's designed to increase energy levels and most of the poses are based on flexibility.
PILATES Designed by Joseph Pilates, a former gymnast to help injured dancers. It develops strength, flexibility and muscular endurance, co-ordination and good posture and is very safe. Gyms offer Pilates classes on floor mats but some run classes on special Pilates machines. Like yoga, it is a perfect workout for women because it concentrates the mind and is continually challenging.

Exercise addiction

Though there are certainly worse things you could be addicted to, when exercise becomes an obsession it can be both mentally and physically damaging. Many women with eating disorders also become exercise addicts (every gym in the country has a few). When you push yourself to work out despite injury or ill health, your exercise programme has become a form of self-abuse and you need help.

ARE YOU ADDICTED TO FITNESS? On a scale of 1 to 10, with 10 being the strongest, weight each of the following statements as they apply to you. Then total your numbers and check the interpretations at the end of the test.

1. Working out is extremely important to me. I'll be doing it for the rest of my life.
2. I need to do at least two hours a day to feel I have pushed myself.
3. If I cannot get my workouts in today, I will double up tomorrow.
4. If I don't get a workout in I can't function.
5. A little pain indicates that I am making progress.
6. If I have an injury, I will just take a couple of aspirin/ibuprofen and keep going.
7. More is always better.
8. My string of work out days must remain unbroken.
9. I stick very carefully to my routines and it upsets me if I can't follow them.
10. Many exercise-related pains can be got rid of by working through them.

SCORE • 80–100: You need to get some help. Talk to your GP • 50–80: You are leaning towards addiction, go easy on yourself • 0–10: Addiction is really not a problem • 0: Get yourself to the gym

ANABOLIC STEROIDS Last year the British Medical Association estimated that steroid use was up 13% in some gyms around the UK and some needle exchanges in the UK report that 60% of the patients using their services are not heroin addicts but intravenous steroid users. An increasing number of women are taking anabolic steroids in an effort to achieve a toned, muscular look without having to put in the hours at the gym. Tablets such as Clenbuterol or Winstrol are generally bought over the Internet or distributed around gyms. Derived from the male hormone testosterone, anabolic steroids cause increased muscle mass, though not necessarily bulk. They also reduce body fat, boost libido, cause enlargement of the clitoris and apparently, enhanced orgasm.

Sounds great? Read about the side effects. Anabolic steroids also cause hair loss, voice deepening, extra body hair, shrunken breasts, irritability, insomnia, panic attacks and a higher risk of heart disease, liver disease and cancer. And when you stop taking them, you suffer chronic withdrawal symptoms and pile on the weight.

There is a girl at the gym where I teach who is clearly an exercise addict. She goes running on the treadmill, then does one and a half hours of Ashtanga yoga and then runs into a one-hour aerobics class. Everyone realizes that she is sick but I don't think she does. I do feel that some of the staff should say something to her but they just give each other knowing looks when she comes in to the gym.
Boo, 24, UK

I have been taking Clenbuterol for a year now. I do six weeks on and six weeks off and I feel fantastic. My body is in great shape and I am having more sex than ever. However, I have noticed a fine down of hair on my face. It is blonde so it is not very noticeable but if it gets any worse I guess I will quit for a while. I sort of don't think about the fact that I am taking drugs but if I think about it, I am only 22 so I can't go on taking them for the rest of my life but I am worried that when I stop I will lose my shape.
Annie, 22, UK

Exercise addiction? In my dreams. I have been trying to catch anorexia unsuccessfully for years too.
Monica, 29, US

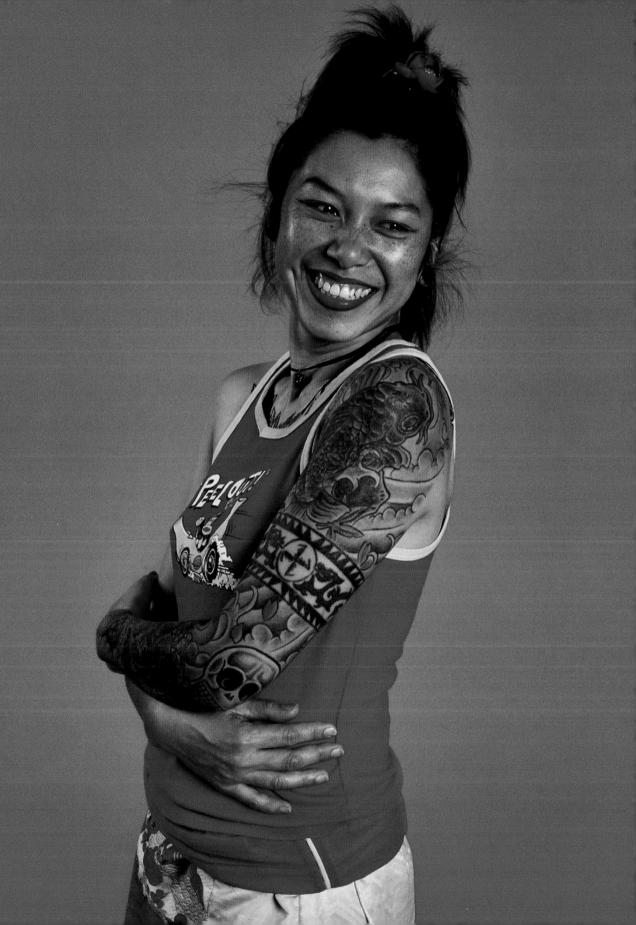

THE
Beauty
CHAPTER

From science to science fiction

Bad skin has never been a good look, but at least it is no longer seen as a sign of moral failure. We now know that acne is linked to hormones, but 200 years ago spots were thought to be, at best, a symptom of TB or smallpox, at worst, an indication of syphilis, excessive masturbation or sexual promiscuity. In the 1800s, dermatology and the study of venereal diseases were considered to be joint fields and medical journals such as *The Archives of Dermatology* and *Syphilology* advised doctors that if spots did not respond to treatment, immorality should be considered the root cause. Faced with the embarrassment of medical, religious and social disapproval, spotty 19th-century teenagers were often forced into early marriage – the only acceptable outlet for sexual expression – as a cure.

Since, at that point in time, marrying well was about the most important thing a girl could hope to achieve in life, good skin became a passport 19th-century parents were prepared to pay for. Naturally, the doctors who helped to treat skin conditions had a financial interest in nurturing parental concerns about the negative implications of pimples, and manufacturers soon learned to exploit adolescent anxieties too. Advertising copylines such as, 'When a man marries, nine times out of ten he chooses a girl with a pretty complexion', reinforced the social significance of perfect skin and set the precedent for an industry that has been relentlessly hammering away at female self-esteem ever since.

With the arrival of affordable domestic mirrors at the turn of the century, self-consciousness escalated. Having previously studied themselves in shiny shop windows or public department stores, women were suddenly able to examine their flaws in the privacy of their own bathroom. Sales of face creams and acne treatments escalated and, as commercial photography, movies, women's magazines and mass market advertising subjected the female face and figure to further scrutiny, women began experimenting with cosmetics such as face powders, rouge, lipstick, and eyebrow pencils and eyelash curlers. Many of these products contained irritants that exacerbated skin conditions, boosting sales of creams and treatments even further, but by the 1950s, medical advances and a better understanding of the causes of acne had led to the introduction of prescription antibiotics, and the first generation of prescription drying lotions such as Clearasil.

With the arrival of the pill in the 1960s young girls acquired simultaneous protection from pimples and pregnancy (acne is triggered by an excess of the male sex hormone testosterone which is balanced by the oestrogen in the pill). But the annihilation of teenage zits forced the beauty industry to look elsewhere for business. As the first wave of baby boomers waddled out of nappies, ageing was not an obvious angle, but within forty years, manufacturers and advertising agencies had managed to convince women that the ageing process was something that needed to be 'fought'. As a continual media assault heightened awareness about 'signs of ageing', for women over the age of thirty maintaining a youthful complexion became an obligation rather than an aspiration. Junk science and rehashed press releases posing as medical research medicalised ageing, effectively turning it into a 'treatable condition. And, given that this was a 'condition' that affected 100% of the population at some stage, cosmetics manufacturers couldn't lose.

For the beauty business, the shift of emphasis from something attainable – clear, blemish-free skin, to something unattainable – youthful skin with no fine lines or wrinkles, has been an ingenious move. But the anti-ageing market is now so saturated and competitive that it has weakened its own credibility. Advertising campaigns featuring airbrushed 25-year-olds claiming to be in their 40s irritate their target audience - media savvy middle aged women who are well aware of the limitations of 'miracle creams'

Though the beauty business continues to thrive, when questioned, most women say that they know the promises preached on packaging are not worth the paper they are printed on, however they continue to buy beauty products because they provide a great deal of pleasure. The anointing rituals of cleansing, toning, purifying and moisturizing are seen a much needed opportunity for personal nurturing and as long as women view this process as 'indulgent', sales will continue to grow.

Although the hunt for an 'active' anti-ageing ingredient appears to be a triumph of hope over experience to date, 'hope' in any form is still hope. Current skincare technologies may not have managed to turn the clock back yet, but what women want now drives research and development in the cosmetic and beauty industries and, since an anti-ageing cream that really works would create a cash cow most manufacturers can only dream of, the GDP of several small nations is currently being invested in turning that hope into a reality.

At present, it is impossible for any beauty product to definitively state that a specific ingredient repairs skin, but advertising and packaging employ an arsenal of visual and editorial ammunition to force us to think otherwise. It can be incredibly difficult for anyone to remain objective in the face of such convincing pseudo-science so this chapter aims to translate the persuasive mumbo jumbo into a reassuringly simple 'does it work, or doesn't it'. By demystifying product ingredients and labelling it will help you to differentiate between cosmetics that have the potential to do good, those that have the potential to harm, and those that almost certainly do nothing at all.

Packaging and advertising influence what I buy, but for me, part of the pleasure of beauty products is the way they look and smell. I would rather have beautiful things on my bathroom shelf.
Josie, 38, US

I have been paranoid about ageing since I was about twenty-five. Now that I am 40 I realize how stupid it was for me to worry about wrinkles because at that stage I didn't even have any.
Lilla, 42, France

My husband is the mirror in which I view my attractiveness. If I look at myself I judge every wrinkle harshly but he sees the years on my face as a calendar of our relationship together.
Barbara, 62, UK

Skin care seems to be changing so rapidly that it is difficult to keep up with new products and innovations. If a woman was to take it all seriously, her skincare routine would take hours, not minutes, and she would need to build an extension to house her products.
Lisa, 29, US

Basically, I don't have time to be beautiful.
India, 35, US

The skin

Skin types

To determine your skin type, wash your face, wait 30 minutes, then put a single piece of tissue paper against each area of your face: forehead, nose, chin, cheeks. The areas that leave oil on the tissue paper should be exfoliated and cleaned more thoroughly and don't need moisturizer.

Normal skin

Medium-sized pores. When you pull the skin away from the bone, it quickly springs back to normal position. Needs regular cleansing, exfoli-ation and occasional moisturizer. Avoid using moisturizer at night.

Oily skin

Overactive oil glands lead to larger pores. Oil retains dead skin cells in the hair follicles, which can darken and form blackheads. May be acne prone and may develop larger pores later in life. Exfoliate regularly and avoid heavy moisturizers.

Dry skin

Rough texture and a tendency to become flaky. Pores tend to be smaller because less oil is produced. More likely to wrinkle as it ages. Feed the skin with hydrating facial oils. Use moisturizers containing liposomes, which disperse moisture into the epidermis.

THE EPIDERMIS Skin is made up of three different layers all of which have varied functions. The epidermis is the protective outer barrier of the skin and is made up of millions of dead skin protein cells known as keratinocytes, which are constantly shed and replaced with new layers from below (90% of household dust is dead skin cells). Keratinocytes are produced in the lower layers of the epidermis and over the course of about two weeks they become progressively flattened and advance towards the surface of the skin. In a young woman, the average keratinocyte takes 28 days to get to the surface of the skin but in women over 50, it can take an additional week and a half. If you leave dead skin cells to accumulate they can make your skin look dull and flaky so they should be sloughed off regularly with an appropriate exfoliant.

The lower layers of the epidermis are stimulated by sunlight to produce melanin (p.176), the pigment that protects the skin from UV radiation. The darker your skin the more melanin your skin contains and the less likely you are to age quickly. Though too much sun damages our skin, a certain amount of sunlight needs to penetrate the epidermal cells to stimulate the production of vitamin D, which keeps your bones strong. Skin colour is also determined by haemoglobin, the pigment that gives blood its colour. When haemoglobin combines with oxygen, blood has a bright red colour and this produces a rosy complexion. Anaemic women tend to have pale skin because they have reduced levels of haemoglobin but any woman who takes regular exercise can boost the oxygen levels in her blood.

THE DERMIS The middle layer of connective support tissue contains tiny blood vessels that allow the skin to breathe and feed the outermost layers of the skin. It also contains hair follicles and sweat glands, surrounded by fibrous supporting tissue and collagen. Collagen, a fibrous protein produced by fibroblast cells, is responsible for most of the skin's mechanical strength and elasticity. Age and exposure to the sun's rays (p.176) gradually break down these proteins and it is the declining production of collagen and elastin that gives mature skin a thin, papery, wrinkled look. At the base of each hair follicle are the sebaceous glands, which secrete sebum, an oily substance that lubricates the skin. These glands provide the 'acid mantle', a natural film that protects the skin from outside attack. Over-functioning sebaceous glands can lead to blackheads and pimples (p.149).

THE HYPODERMIS This is the base layer of fatty tissue. It provides nourishment to the dermis and upper layers of skin, controls body temperature, cushions internal organs against trauma and contains the sweat glands that excrete waste through perspiration and control temperature by evaporation on the skin's surface. If the muscles in the hypodermis contract, we get 'gooseflesh'.

Free radicals and antioxidants

The words 'free radical' are plugged as 'the science bit' in adverts for cosmetics and shampoos all the time, but most women haven't got a clue what they mean, which is hardly surprising, because free radical theory is actually very complicated and very scientific. It was first put forward over 40 years ago as a cause of ageing and cellular degeneration and is based on the fact that all the atoms or molecules that make up our bodies contain one or more pairs of electrons. Free radicals are atoms or molecules that are missing one of their electrons, a state that makes them highly reactive. To find a partner for their single electron, free radicals go around stealing electrons and destabilizing other molecules. With their structure disturbed, in turn, these molecules fail to function, and continue the damaging process by seeking partners for their newly divorced electron.

It doesn't exactly make the most obvious angle for a shampoo ad but, over the years, scientists have linked pretty much every chronic degenerative disease – cancer, arthritis, Parkinson's disease, multiple sclerosis and diabetes – to free radicals. With regard to ageing of the skin, it is thought that free radical damage causes the production of chemicals that eat collagen, the stuff that keeps our skin plump and bouncy, and this obviously leads to wrinkles. But free radical damage is hard to avoid. It is exacerbated by exposure to environmental pollutants, exhaust fumes, cigarette smoke, pesticides, herbicides, industrial chemicals, margarines, partially hydrogenated oils, sugars and processed foods, chlorine in our water, household cleaners, paint and petrochemical fumes, ozone, mobile phone radiation and ultra-violet light from the sun.

That's the bad news. The good news is that the body has created a mechanism for coping with free radical damage. This mechanism kicks in courtesy of antioxidants, enzymes that terminate the chain reaction before vital molecules are damaged. However, the key antioxidants – vitamins C and E, beta carotene, selenium and zinc – cannot be manufactured in the body, so they must be supplied in your diet (p.43). Because the link between skin damage and antioxidants is one of the few scientifically proven aspects of skincare, antioxidants such as vitamins A, C and E, amino acids, enzymes, alphalipoic acid and co-enzyme Q10 are now added to almost every cosmetic product on the market, but it is unlikely that applying them topically is as effective as including them in your diet. None has been clinically tested to evaluate their effect on wrinkling and since free radical damage is ongoing and omnipresent in the body, it is impossible to establish how much of these particular ingredients might be needed, how long they should be on the skin or how long any effects might last. Though major investigations are underway, at the moment the only way you can be sure of getting the maximum benefit is by eating them. It's a lot cheaper, tastes better and is, without doubt, more effective.

Combination skin
Usually the T-zone – the forehead, nose and chin – are prone to oiliness, whereas the cheeks and neck tend to be dry. Exfoliate oily areas and feed neck and cheeks with a light moisturizer.

Dehydrated skin
Taut, scaly and lacks elasticity because it isn't making enough natural sebum (oil). Extremely sensitive to sun, wind and cold and more likely to show spider veins and broken capillaries. Drink six to eight glasses of water every day. Eat enough oily fish, e.g. mackerel or wild salmon. Lubricate the skin with vaseline, aqueous cream, liposome moisturizers and facial oils.

Sensitive skin
More common in people with dermatitis and eczema. Irritates easily, has a blotchy, red colouring and is very sensitive. Can be an allergic reaction. Avoid new products and stick to brands with a limited number of recognizable ingredients. Use aqueous cream, E45 or Emulave as a cleanser/moisturizer. Oilatum products are specifically designed for sensitive skin and feel as luxurious as any skincare range. Vaseline is often very effective at reducing redness, but don't use it all the time.

Dermatologists' top tips

DIY skincare

Commercial products make a big deal about containing 'natural ingredients' but the quantities used in commercial products are so minuscule and so heavily processed that making your own is far more effective. Women with sensitive skin or egg allergies should avoid recipes containing egg whites or egg yolk. Cleanse your skin before applying face masks to avoid sealing in the dirt and use a facial oil or soothing moisturizer afterwards.

Papaya facial peel

Papaya contains the exfoliant and antioxidant papain. Dissolve a small packet of gelatin in boiled water. Peel, de-seed and chop a small papaya. Then juice or blend it and strain off the liquid. Mix the juice with the gelatin and refrigerate it for 20 minutes until it begins to set. Apply the facial to your face and neck avoiding your eyes and leave on for 15 minutes. Peel off and rinse well.

Moisturizing facial

Mash one avocado with 1 tsp of lemon and 2 tsp of wheatgerm to form a paste. Smooth on skin, leave on for five minutes and rinse.

In the US, it is common for a woman with normal skin to consult a qualified dermatologist to establish her skin type or condition and work out a personal skincare routine. In the UK it is considerably more difficult for women to get this kind of objective advice. There are only 400 dermatology consultants in the whole country and, naturally, most of their time is taken up treating serious skin problems. So, many women end up getting skincare directives from magazines, beauticians or sales girls, most of whom have a vested interest in selling a specific product, whether it is right for a customer's skin or not. Though most women believe they need to spend a small fortune on skincare, dermatologists suggest a simple routine of regular exfoliation with a cheap moisturizer is all you need. If you follow the basic guidelines below, within one month you will see an improvement in your skin.

EXFOLIATE Though dermatologists pooh pooh a lot of commercial skincare products, most of them believe that regular facial exfoliation with fruit acids such as glycolic acid or salicylic acid is the key to maintaining wrinkle-free skin and promoting the development of new collagen (p.138). Exfoliants work by taking away the top layer of dead skin, which stimulates the layers below to produce new skin cells. They can be quite abrasive and can cause irritation in some women, but if used correctly, they make a noticeable difference to the skin. They are usually used twice a day but because they make your skin more sensitive to the sun you have to wear a sun protection factor (SPF) 15 moisturizer or sunblock whenever you are outside. Milder cleansers such as Eve Lom Cleansing Cream, which comes with a soft muslin cloth, provide more gentle exfoliation without acids.

USE A CHEAP MOISTURIZER Dermatologists say that as long as you use a good exfoliant and a sunblock, you are wasting your money buying costly moisturizing creams. Inexpensive pharmacy products like aqueous cream, which have been designed for sensitive skins, are just as good at temporarily plumping out fine lines and wrinkles. Dermatologists also believe that many women over-moisturize and, in doing so, destroy their skin's natural balance. Night time is when the skin rests, breathes and eliminates toxins through your pores. Going to bed with a heavy layer of moisturizer all over your face prevents your skin from excreting waste matter and effectively seals in the dirt.

WEAR SUNSCREEN Dermatologists estimate that up to 80% of skin ageing is photo damage, so anyone who wants to maintain good skin should use a day cream with a high UVA (the rays that wrinkle) and a high UVB (the rays that burn) and steer clear of the midday sun (p.177). Facial tanners such as Clarins Auto Bronzant or Benetint YouRebel tinted moisturizer incorporate an SPF 15 sunscreen and give you a healthy glow at the same time.

QUIT SMOKING Smoking reduces collagen production and is a major cause of premature skin ageing, particularly around the lips. Wrinkles are five times more likely in smokers (p.268).

EAT WELL Antioxidant foods repair free radical damage (p.137). New research indicates that highly processed foods may increase testosterone which encourages spots. Spots are virtually unknown in places like Papua New Guinea where refined foods are not eaten, but the Inuit of Alaska have seen an escalation in adolescent acne since doughnuts, bread and waffles appeared on their once fish-based menu.

DRINK PLENTY OF WATER Moist skin is stronger and more resilient than dry skin. Remember to drink six 225ml (8fl oz) glasses of water every day. Still water at room temperature is easiest for your body to absorb.

GET ENOUGH SLEEP AND EXERCISE Sleep gives your skin an opportunity to repair daily damage. Stress or burning the candle at both ends eventually leads to less oxygenated and more exhausted skin, which loses elasticity and wrinkles faster. Exercise helps tired skin by improving circulation and increasing the amount of oxygen in the blood, which feeds your skin and so you look rosy.

LESS IS MORE Stick to a limited number of beauty products and don't wear make-up when you can get away without it. The fewer products you put on your face, the better, because over the years rubbing, scrubbing and pulling at your skin take their toll. When applying anything to your face always use a gentle upwards stroke from collarbone to chin and chin to forehead and try not to rub downwards.

MAKE LIKE A MOVIE STAR The skin around your eyes is the most sensitive area of your face. Wearing sunglasses protects it from the sun and prevents you from squinting in bright light, which contributes to fine lines and wrinkling.

CLEANLINESS IS NEXT TO GODLINESS Clean your skin morning and night with a warm wet muslin and a gentle cleanser (or a facial wipe if is 2am and you are seeing double).

DON'T STEAM Traditionally, steaming has been used as a way of opening pores before cleansing. However, dermatologists don't think this is a very good idea because the moisture swells blockages in skin pores and can make spots worse.

DON'T SQUEEZE Tempting though it is, if you press hard enough to make a mark, you can burst tiny blood vessels, causing spider veins and scarring.

Skin smoother
Whisk one egg yolk, 1 tbsp of honey and 1 tbsp of olive oil to form a paste. Apply mixture with a soft pastry or make-up brush over the face, avoiding the eyes. Leave on for 15 minutes then rinse off.

Depuffer
Yogurt contains lactic acid, which is an antioxidant. Straight from the fridge it will reduce redness and puffiness. Apply 2 tbsp of yogurt to the face and neck, avoiding the eyes. Relax for ten minutes and rinse well. Then sweep cotton pads dipped into chilled green tea over face and rinse.

Skin tightener
Albumin in egg white can leave a light film over the skin, which temporarily constricts and tightens it, making it look smoother. Beat two egg whites with ten drops of fresh lemon juice. Smooth over clean, dry skin, avoiding the eyes. Let set for five minutes then rinse. Finish with facial oil.

Exfoliator
Combine a couple of handfuls of coarse sea salt, with olive or avocado oil. Scent it by grating in the rind of an orange or a lime. Use the scrub over your whole body and the soles of your feet and then shower.

Moisturizers

Moisturizers, particularly the ones with a built-in SPF, are an important part of a skincare routine. They protect your skin from the sun and form a barrier that helps to keep your skin cells intact and keeps bacteria and dirt out. Though many products would like you to believe they can, by law, no moisturizer can permanently affect or change the structure of your skin (p.152). At best, moisturizers will temporarily plump up your skin by hydrating it. At worst, they can block pores and cause spots or sensitivity. Moisturizers contain an enormous range of chemical ingredients that mimic our skin's efforts to moisturize itself: ceramides, hyaluronic acid, cholesterol, fatty acids, triglycerides, phospholipids, glycosphingolipids, amino acids, linoleic acid, glycosaminoglycans, glycerin and sodium PCA, to name but a few. But there are plenty of natural ingredients that work just as well: apricot oil, canola oil, olive oil, coconut oil, corn oil, jojoba oil, jojoba wax, lanolin, lecithin, olive oil, safflower oil, sesame oil, shea butter, soybean oil, rose moqueta oil, squalane and almond oil. Women who suffer from spots should not moisturize and should avoid any products containing lanolin, isopropyl myristate, mineral oil or liquid paraffin, ethanol or alcohol denat or D&C red.

CHEAP AND EFFECTIVE Aqueous cream is a great all-round, moderate-strength moisturizer that suits many people because it is non-greasy, very cheap and available in bulk without a prescription. Because it contains an emulsifier, aqueous cream can mix with sweat and it can be washed off. It can also be used as a cleanser and, because it is cheap, you can use it on your whole body. It is also very good for sensitive skin and unlikely to cause irritation. If your skin is very dry, you may want to use an oil such as olive or almond oil or even glycerine, all of which can be bought very cheaply. Vaseline is also a very effective moisturizer if your skin is very dry or red, but it shouldn't be used consistently on inflamed skin.

ADDED INGREDIENTS Many moisturizers contain built-in sun block, which is a real advantage and worth paying more for. Clarins Hydration plus moisture effect lotion has an SPF 15 and is a very effective moisturizer. Many moisturizers also contain antioxidant ingredients (p.139) such as vitamins A, E, C and beta carotene. The Paula's Choice range of products from Paula Begoum contain both sun block and antioxidants, as does Olay Total Effects Time Resist moisturizer.

LIPOSOMES These are not ingredients, but a delivery system for 'active ingredients'. Liposomes are microscopic hollow spheres manufactured from fatty substances called phospholipids. When mixed with water, phospholipids will 'trap' any substance that can dissolve in water or oil. In cosmetics they are used to trap anti-ageing or moisturizing ingredients. The liposomes are then absorbed by the skin where they melt and deliver their ingredients directly into the epidermis. Liposomes

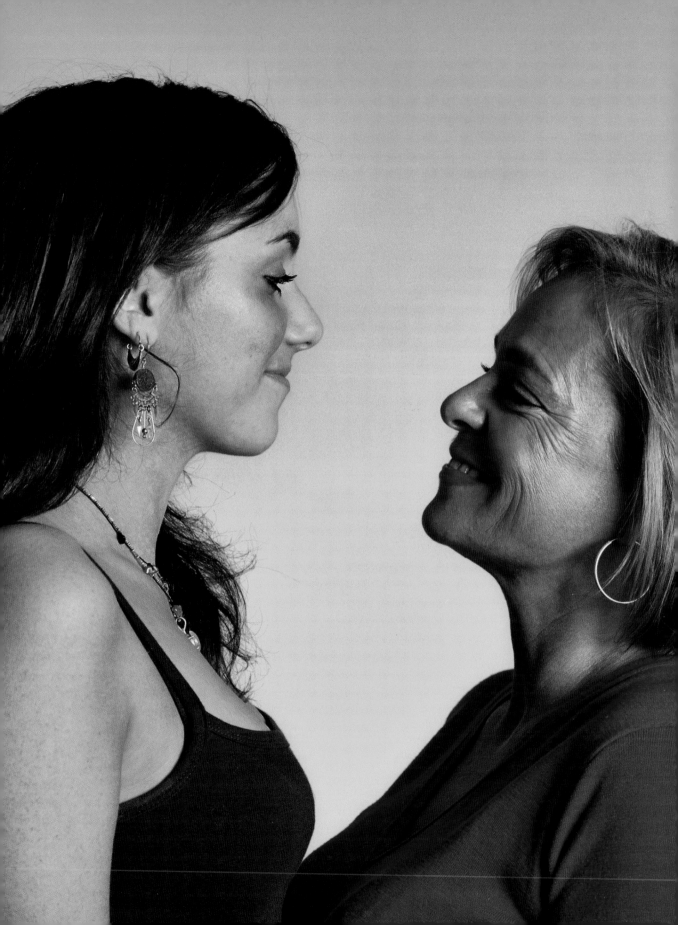

are being investigated as a method of targeted drug delivery, which suggests that they do work, but whether the ingredients they carry do what they are supposed to is another matter entirely. Try Christian Dior Capture Anti-Ageing Complex for the face or Nivea Liposome Cream as a cheaper option.

HYALURONIC ACID (HA) HA is naturally found in the skin and is the key substance involved in skin moisture (p.194). With ageing, the HA content of the outer skin layer (the epidermis) decreases. It is estimated that 50-year-olds have less than half the hyaluronic acid they had in their youth. Products containing 0.025–0.05% HA act as moisturizers by forming a hydrated film on the skin surface that lasts for a considerable period of time. Murads Perfecting Day Cream contains hyaluronic acid, antioxidants, oat protein and has a built-in SPF 15.

SILICONE AND CERAMIDES Silicone provides silky emollience and it helps to smooth out your skin. Paula's Choice Super Antioxidant Concentrate is a silicone-based product that also contains high concentrations of antioxidants and anti-irritants. Women with sensitive skin may like to try Triceram Cream. It was developed as a non-steroid-based treatment for eczema and atopic dermatitis and dermatologists have been impressed with the results. Its ceramide base allows the skin to repair and heal and makes it an effective and reasonably priced moisturizer.

CRÈME DE LA MER Unless you have been hiding under a rock for the last ten years you will have heard about Crème de la Mer, one of the world's most expensive face creams. Now manufactured by Estée Lauder, Crème de la Mer was apparently developed as an emollient to treat scars in 1953 when NASA scientist Max Huber suffered severe burns in a rocket fuel explosion. The cream is apparently made from a special seaweed plucked from the Pacific at moonlight and, in a manufacturing process unlikely to be copied by competitors, the weed is then fermented to the pre-recorded sounds of previous batches being made.

Dermatologists and burns specialists are cynical about the product, pointing out, quite sensibly, that any cream that was so great at healing burns would be used in hospitals all the time. It's not. And when CBS conducted an investigation into the legend of Max Huber, they couldn't find any record of him being employed by NASA. Ever. In 2000, *Time* magazine commissioned Chemir/Polytech Laboratories in the US to do a chemical analysis of Crème de la Mer. When the results revealed that levels of the active ingredient, Vitamin E ester were barely detectable, Estée Lauders responsded by saying that the fermentation process makes it hard to detect the active agent. Most people who use it say Crème de la Mer is a nice moisturizer, but at £135 for a 60ml (2oz) pot, is that enough of an endorsement?

I have been using Crème de la Mer for about two years now. It suits my skin and it seems to work well as a moisturizer. Some people might find it very heavy but I have quite dry skin. I only use it at night, but it doesn't leave my skin feeling oily or greasy. I suppose I bought it because of all the hype and I have probably been using it for too long to notice any difference now. I do believe in changing products every so often because I think if you use something for too long, it doesn't work any more. I have reasonably good skin and I think I could probably just use a cheap Pond's moisturizer and it would be as good. I don't know if there is any truth to Crème de la Mer. I don't think I saw much difference but to be honest I can't really remember what kind of condition my skin was in before I started using it, so I can't really tell if it works or not. I'd have to live life again and not use it to be able to tell you whether it works or not.
Julie, 51, Ireland

The secret to good skin is good diet, fresh air, exercise and lots of water. Creams don't matter a damn.
Betty, 52, UK

Common problems

BRUISING Bruises are the result of tissue damage and bleeding beneath the skin. Women with thinner skin bruise more easily, particularly asthmatics, diabetics or those on medication. Immediately applying ice (or chilled steak) will reduce swelling and minimize bruising by slowing blood flow and preventing coagulation. Arnica tablets may aid healing and arnica cream massaged into the area will stimulate circulation. Use toothpaste, concealer or foundation to disguise bruises.

CELLULITE Cells in the lower part of a woman's body store six times more fat than cells in the upper body. Originally, nature's way of ensuring women had an emergency store of energy (very few of us have required this facility since the arrival of Häagen Dazs and Starbucks) cellulite is caused by a honeycomb network of supportive fibres under the skin, which accumulate fat and bulge out forming the distinctive cottage cheese/orange rind on the bum, hips and thighs. Nine out of ten women are affected by cellulite, but no matter how expensive they are, anti-cellulite creams simply don't work and the best you can hope for is a pleasant smelling rear end. Salon treatments such as mesotherapy, vitamin B1 injections, or lymph massage don't work either though massage may temporarily increase blood flow. Ultimately, the only way to boost circulation and get rid of fat is through exercise and diet.

DARK CIRCLES Dark circles can be hereditary, but if you don't get enough sleep, the toxins that should be dispersed during the night reduce the oxygen in your blood, making it appear darker and more visible under the eye where the skin is the thinnest. Exercise, good diet and fresh air help but you can remove some of the dark colour by placing cold compresses. e.g. ice cubes in a soft cloth, chilled cucumber slices or chilled damp green teabags (keep a stack in the fridge) over your eyes for 15 minutes. This will help to contract the blood vessels and brings down puffiness and redness. If all else fails, use a good concealer.

ENLARGED PORES These are more common in people who have oily skin, but pore elasticity decreases in everyone as they age. Products such as Dr Hauschka cleansing clay mask with witch hazel contain a high concentration of tannins that help the skin to regain some strength and contract pores. Alternatively, you can buy bottles of witch hazel cheaply in any pharmacy to use as a daily toner.

COLD SORES Cold sores are a very infectious form of oral herpes. Over 45% of people have had a cold sore by the time they are 18. If someone who has a cold sore performs oral sex on their partner, the herpes virus can be passed on, and can cause genital herpes (p.255). The virus lives in a nerve near the cheekbone and can be triggered by emotional trauma, illness, accidents and over-exposure to the sun. There are plenty of effective over-the-counter cold sore treatments.

I suffer very badly from mysterious bruising. I have so many bruises on my legs sometimes that it looks as if I have been attacked. I really don't know how I get them and I have to wear jeans in the summer.
Jackie, 26, UK

I can't help squeezing my blackheads and spots. In fact it is something of an obsession and I want to squeeze my boyfriend's as well. I do it mostly when I am bored but I can not stop. Really can not stop.
Donna, 30, UK

I have recently started using a Salicylic acid exfoliant and I am hoping that it will help me to even out my skin tones and get rid of my blackheads. In the past I have been lazy about skincare and I may be shutting the stable door after the horse has bolted but I am giving it a go.
Marcy, 56, US

Using a facial tanner gave me the worst blackheads I have ever had. I scrubbed and scrubbed but in the end the only thing that seemed to get rid of them was swimming. I don't know what happened but they went white straight away. Weird.
Ella, 27, UK

Common skin conditions

Skin conditions may not be life threatening but in many ways they have a more immediate and more damaging effect on people than other illnesses because they affect self-confidence so hugely. When my psoriasis is really bad I can hardly move and I feel like a leper. People don't mean to be hurtful but when I go out, I am stared at, and children are the worst. It has really made me hate children and I know that is not something a woman should ever say. I think I would rather have anything else than this.
Diana, 35, US

My 11-year-old daughter got impetigo last year. I didn't have a clue what it was at first. I thought it was something to do with her ear piercing so I got her to clean it with antiseptic, but it kept getting worse. In the end it spread all the way down the side of her face and I took her to the doctor who diagnosed impetigo and put her on antibiotics. She could not go to school because it is highly contagious, which I didn't know. By the time I found out what it was she had given it to half her class. Terribly embarrassing!
Sandra, 40, UK

CELLULITIS Cellulitis is a bacterial infection of the tissues under the skin, which usually manifests itself as red streaks up the arm. The skin becomes intensely inflamed, swollen, tender and warm to the touch, and the streaks have spreading, indistinct margins. It should be treated with antibiotics as soon as possible because in certain people it is potentially life threatening.

DERMATITIS There are several different kinds of dermatitis. *Contact dermatitis* occurs when you touch something you are allergic to, e.g. poison ivy, washing powder, soap, rubber, metals, jewellery, perfume, cosmetics and weeds. Since the reaction happens almost immediately, it is usually quite easy to identify the culprit. The allergen causes skin inflamation and itchiness and, in severe cases, you get blisters and weeping sores. Repeated scratching brings on neurodermatitis, which appears as small, flat, raised areas with definite margins. *Stasis dermatitis* often occurs with varicose veins and can make the skin at your ankles and over your shins thick, itchy and a reddy brown colour. *Seborrheic dermatitis* can be caused by stress or by conditions such as Parkinson's disease. It manifests as greasy, scaling areas at the sides of your nose, between your eyebrows, behind your ears or over your breastbone and can also appear as a stubborn, itchy dandruff that is cleared up by using a tar shampoo containing zinc pyrithione on the head, neck and shoulders. Dermatitis can be treated by topical steroids to relieve inflammation and itchiness.

ECZEMA In the UK, about one in 12 of the adult population suffers from eczema. In mild forms, the skin is dry, hot and itchy, whilst in more severe forms the skin can become broken, raw and bleeding. Although it looks unpleasant, it is not contagious. It can be caused by allergies, genetic factors, physical and mental stress, and chemical irritants. It most commonly appears on the elbows, hands, face, inner arms and the back of the knees and can be made worse by cold, dry weather. Warm weather often improves it, as does keeping it dry. Treatment with oral antihistamines relieves itching, and topical steroids with hydrocortisone relieve inflammation though they are not a great long-term option as they can eventually thin the skin. Use specific eczema moisturizers such as Emulave or Oilatum products.

HIVES Hives are an allergic reaction, usually to something you have eaten, but they can be brought on by stress too. The pink, itchy swellings are caused by the release of histamine, a natural chemical produced by the body in reaction to a particular substance. Eggs, chocolate, seafood, nuts, milk and medications are common triggers of hives. Less commonly, exposure to cold temperatures or water can cause them. Hives generally fade in 24 hours or less, but may occasionally take several weeks. Very occasionally, hives develop in the throat, making breathing difficult. This requires urgent treatment with antihistamines and steroids.

IMPETIGO Sometimes, the open sores and fissures that occur with eczema or dermatitis become infected. This usually happens when a weeping sore is touched and the infection is transferred to another part of the body, often the face. The infection is caused by staphylococci bacteria and is highly contagious, so it needs to be treated with a course of antibiotics as soon as possible.

PSORIASIS This chronic disease causes skin to become inflamed with patches of red thickened skin, covered with flaky, silvery scales. Experts think psoriasis is a genetic abnormality that encourages excess skin production. Normal cells replenish themselves about every 28 days, but psoriasis causes the skin cells to multiply so quickly that they replenish themselves every two to four days. This new skin grows so fast that the cells don't have a chance to separate. It typically appears on elbows, knees and scalp, but it can also arise on your lower back, buttocks, palms, soles and genital region. Lesions are often triggered by stress, infection, climate changes and medications. There is no cure for psoriasis, but topical steroid medications are the most popular help. UVB light therapy is now being used and remission rates can last several months or longer. Several studies demonstrate that Dead Sea minerals have a positive and cumulative effect on psoriatic skin.

VITILIGO People suffering from vitiligo begin to lose the melanin or pigment that gives their skin its colour. This results in white patches all over their body, face, lips, hands, arms, legs and genital areas. It affects one or two in every 100 people and experts suspect that it is either genetic, related to a compromised immune system or due to abnormally functioning nerve cells. There is no single cure. PUVA is a form of re-pigmentation therapy involving a drug called psoralen, which has a 50–70% chance of returning colour to the face, trunk and upper arms and upper legs, but hands and feet respond very poorly.

Vitiligo patches can be disguised with make-up, and stains that dye the skin can be used to make the white patches match your normal skin colour. Self-tanning compounds work on vitiligo patches because they contain a chemical called dihydroxyacetone that does not need melanocytes to make the skin a tan colour, and micropigmentation or tattooing can be used to add colour to a white patch. None of these techniques treat the disease or provide permanent cover, but they can improve appearance. For patients with severe vitiligo the most practical treatment may be to remove all the remaining pigment from their normal skin and make the whole body an even, white colour. The treatment is done with a chemical called monobenzylether of hydroquinone. It takes about a year to complete and is permanent. For people with darker skin, like Michael Jackson, the transformation can be fairly radical.

I've had vitiligo since I was about 12 but it wasn't diagnosed until much later. I was teased about it as a child because I looked different and my hair lost its pigment early so I looked like a badger. Both my parents went grey quite young but I don't know if that is related. The vitiligo now covers most of my arms and legs and I have patches on my back, neck, sides and chest too, with spots of it on my face. I have tried pretty much everything and I have had a little success using herbal treatments. The de-pigmentation was so aggressive at first but it seems to have stalled in the last few years. I am now thinking about complete de-pigmentation. I know it is not very nice but if I get rid of all the pigment then basically I don't have to wake up every morning wondering whether I have a new patch or whether I have any more pigment. It is the not knowing that drives me mad and I would rather just lose it all. I suppose it wouldn't look as bad on me because I have fair skin to begin with. I imagine if I was darker, it might be a lot more difficult.
Jo, 30, UK

Acne

It is estimated that 85% of people have acne at some point in their lives and studies show that no amount of cleansing the skin can get rid of the problem. Acne can be exacerbated by stress, which is a vicious circle because most people with acne are stressed by their spots. Studies of people with acne have revealed that three out of four sufferers felt depressed, almost half felt anxious and almost all would prefer to have a cure for the skin condition rather than £5000 in cash. Some 15% felt suicidal and more than a third felt they would have a better job if they didn't have acne. Among the women questioned, 37% spent £120 a year on skincare products and 27% spent the same amount on make-up. Most non-prescription products are only effective for treating mild acne. For more severe cases, the best treatments are available through dermatologists and doctors.

ACCUTANE®/ROACCUTANE/ISOTRETONIN Accutane is a controversial drug treatment licensed for the treatment of severe cystic acne in 1982. Although the Federal Drug Administration (FDA) has linked the drug to foetal malformation and miscarriage, about 5 million people in the US and 12 million worldwide have been treated with it – half of them women in their child-bearing years. Revised labelling now makes it clear that women should not take Accutane if they are, or may become, pregnant, and doctors cannot prescribe it without a full health assessment and informing patients of the risks. In the US and the UK it is broadly acknowledged that this drug should only be used as a 'last resort'. However, a study by UK dermatologists has shown that Accutane was prescribed to some 74% of patients with just mild or moderate acne. Because this product actually works, it is immensely popular with adolescent girls who are the most desperate to have clear skin and the least experienced when it comes to controlling fertility. Though the manufacturers have dealt with the issue of birth defects, they are more reluctant to tackle the relationship between Accutane and psychiatric illness. The link remains unproven, but from 1982 to May 2000, the FDA received reports of 37 Accutane patients who committed suicide and 110 Accutane users hospitalized for depression. The FDA recommends that any doctor who prescribes this drug should act as if Accutane has psychiatric effects until there is more information. Treatment lasts four to six months and besides the side effects noted above, it causes severe flakiness and dryness around the eyes, lips and inside the nose. It can also cause severe dehydration. Taking the tablets straight after food in the evening can help minimize side effects. Alcohol should be avoided.

COMEDOLYTICS A comedolytic is a substance that loosens the plugs in clogged pores and lets the pores open. Salicylic acid, azelic acid, combinations of sulfur and resorcinol are common comedolytics. The vitamin A derivative tretinoin, or Retin-A (p.154), works by expelling acne plugs and preventing new ones from forming. Pregnant women should not use Retin-A as studies have linked it to foetal damage. Topical isotretonin and adapalene are more potent than Retin-A and work by normalizing the growth of skin cells. Always use with a sunblock.

HORMONE THERAPY/THE PILL While other acne medications reduce the amount of oil produced by the skin, anti-androgen medications counter the effects of the male hormones or androgens, which contribute to enlarged skin pores and oil production. Oral contraceptives containing oestrogen can improve acne by balancing hormone levels but progesterone-only birth control pills are very bad for acne, as are contraceptive injections, mini pills and IUDs that contain progesterone. Acne friendly pills must be 'third generation' pills, which contain a different form of synthetic progesterone, but there is a slightly increased risk of blood clots with these pills.

N-LITE LASER TREATMENTS Developed to remove birthmarks and wrinkles, this treatment is now being used with tremendous success on acne. The laser heats small blood vessels, which provokes a natural healing response and stimulates the production of collagen. In tests at the Hammersmith Hospital, London, 41 patients were given one treatment and monitored for 12 weeks. Some 81% of the patients showed significant improvement and, in 58% of patients, spots were reduced by 50 per cent. A single treatment lasts about three months.

ORAL ANTIBIOTICS Ten years ago, oral antibiotics were routinely prescribed for the treatment of acne, but rising drug resistance in bacteria has made doctors increasingly reluctant to dish them out unless it is absolutely necessary. Although more effective than topical applications, 40% of acne bacteria are insensitive to oral antibiotics and you need to take the medicine for at least three months before you see a real improvement. Sometimes symptoms get even worse before they begin to subside and, since improvement is often very gradual, permanent scarring may occur before the antibiotics actually work. There are three main groups of oral antibiotics: tetracycline (oxytetracycline, lymecycline, minocycline and doxycycline) and erythromycin and trimethoprim. Tetracycline antibiotics should not be taken if you intend to get pregnant, or are pregnant or breastfeeding. Erythromycin is thought to be safe to take during pregnancy.

TOPICAL ANTI-MICROBIALS Benzoyl peroxide is available both in prescription (combined with antibiotics) and over-the-counter products. It will loosen blackheads but it has no effect on cell build-up and so is a less successful treatment than comedolytics. Can cause blotchiness, allergy and photosensitivity.

Having bad skin affects everything, your posture (you hunch so people don't notice you), your hairstyle (curtains so it covers your face), you avoid eye contact when talking, and wear clothes that cover as far up as possible, and choose outfits on the basis of where your spots are that day. Hell – spotty people are seen to be untrustworthy so it can even do you out of a job! In the winter my spots show worse, and in the summer their scars show up against a tan –you can't win!
Izzy, 25, US

Having acne affects my confidence and self-image. I always feel dirty, scabby and messy. I also feel that people are looking at my skin and find it repulsive. I don't go out as often and when I do I don't feel confident talking to members of the opposite sex.
Vio , 28, UK

When talking to people I avoid eye contact because I am so conscious that they are staring at my skin. I am obsessed with washing my face and I believe that even the slightest bit of dirt will make it worse. Doctors are sympathetic but useless.
Nina, 22, UK

How to read cosmetics' labels

When I was younger I would see my mum putting on Nivea cream and Oil of Olay and I started to copy her. I use an exfoliator from Synergie on my face every morning and I use moisturizer from Clinique though I don't think the brand of product is important. I exfoliate and moisturize my body too. I don't really wear make-up. I think using foundation dries out your skin and some girls just cake it on and it doesn't look natural. My mum is a bit obsessed with beauty. She takes every supplement under the sun and she has special creams for her neck, her cheeks, her eyes – you name it. Whenever any new anti-ageing product comes out she buys it, even though I tell her it won't do anything. I do sometimes use a moisturizer that has an SPF in it but sometimes I don't use sunblock on holiday, which is probably bad because I know the sun is ageing and they say that you should start thinking about wrinkles in your twenties. I do think it's a ploy to sell more products though. They always use models that are 20 in their ads and they don't have any wrinkles anyway.
Laura, 21, Iran/UK

You would need a PhD in Latin to understand most skincare and cosmetics labels but most of the big words are simply chemical names for the stuff that holds a product together or adds the necessary slip and slide. When buying cosmetics, the most important thing to look at is the 'active' ingredient, which should be listed first on the label, after water. This is the 'X' factor that will, or won't, as the case may be, eliminate your wrinkles or get rid of the bags under your eyes. Few manufacturers actually list the percentage of 'X' in a product, mainly because they contain such tiny amounts. For example L'Oréal's Plenitude contains one of the highest over-the-counter percentages of vitamin A derivative, but at 0.1% per pot, divided by the number of applications, eating a mango is likely to be far more effective.

Cosmetics manufacturers rely on 'X' factor additives to differentiate their product from others. But cosmetic ingredients go in and out of fashion very quickly, so as soon as a manufacturer's original research has been copied, adapted, repackaged and reproduced for the cheaper end of the market, they lose interest and move on to try to find the next big thing. What this means is that the stuff that makes this year's miracle repair cream miraculously expensive will appear on the label of a cheaper brand in six months' time. But in the meantime a new 'X' factor will be claiming to do all the great things that last year's 'X' factor failed to do.

ACTIVE INGREDIENTS Active ingredients must be listed first on an ingredient label and, since active ingredients are considered to have a pharmacological altering effect on skin, the amount and exact function of each active ingredient must adhere to specific regulations. These effects must be documented by scientific evaluation and approved by the FDA. Active ingredients include sunscreens, retinoids, skin-lightening agents and acne treatments (p.148).

INACTIVE INGREDIENTS Inactive ingredients are listed by quantity. The main ingredient in most skincare products is water and this usually comes first, but thousands of inactive ingredients are then added so that creams can be applied and absorbed more easily. Since many have not been tested for long-term effects, naturally enough, a lot of dermatologists question the wisdom of women plastering their skin with untested chemicals twice a day.

NATURAL COSMETICS Concerns about chemicals and animal testing have led to an exponential growth in the natural skincare market. It is possible to take a natural approach and companies like Aveda, Jurlique and Espa pride themselves on adhering to natural ingredients. But although the term "all-natural" has considerable promotional value, a closer look at the ingredients label often reveals that plant extracts make up only a small percentage of the product. When it comes to cosmetic products it is virtually impossible to tell whether a product is 100% natural or not because when natural raw materials, such as fruit or nuts, are processed, preserved, stabilized and added to a cosmetic with other ingredients, they lose their natural qualities. The base ingredients are often the same as other non-natural cosmetics and naturally occurring preservatives such as vitamins E and C can produce both delayed allergic contact dermatitis and immediate allergic hives. Natural doesn't mean pure or clean or perfect either. All plants, including those used in cosmetics, can be contaminated with bacteria, pesticides and chemical fertilizers, which can produce skin irritation in sensitive individuals.

VITAMINS The US FDA insists that products that contain vitamins must list the ingredients by their chemical names, e.g. vitamin E must be listed as d-alpha Tocopherol, because listing it as a vitamin gives consumers the misleading impression that the vitamin E in the product offers nutrient or health benefits. In actual fact vitamin E is usually added as a preservative to prevent chemical deterioration of the product. However, manufacturers have been able to exploit this regulation by acquainting consumers with the chemical names of vitamins through advertising and then marketing them as 'scientific' ingredients which imply improved efficacy.

HYPOALLERGENIC This term is routinely used by the cosmetics industry to suggest that using a product will not cause allergic reactions. However, the word 'hypoallergenic' is not regulated and there is not a single cosmetic or skincare product on the market that can guarantee that no one will be allergic to it. If you have sensitive skin or allergies always try before you buy.

ANIMAL TESTING Within the last ten years, test tube experiments, synthetic skin and computer models have become a cheaper alternative to animal testing. The EU believes that animal testing is now largely unnecessary and plans to ban most new cosmetics tested on animals from 2009, though some tests will continue to be used to check for dangers such as cancer or allergic reaction. The US is less keen to legislate but approximately 550 companies have voluntarily signed a pledge with the Coalition for Consumer Information on Cosmetics stating to, 'neither commission nor conduct animal testing for their ingredients, product formulations or finished products'.

pH BALANCE When 'pH balanced' appears on a label it makes the product sound carefully formulated, but it actually means very little. Anything with a pH above 7 is alkaline and anything with a pH below 7 is acid (water has a pH of 7). Since skin has an average pH of 5.5 and products with a pH of 8 or above can cause skin irritation, most products are formulated to have a neutral pH.

I need moisturizer now, which I never did before. I started a couple of years ago, when I was 25, and my need for it seems to have grown since then. Of course, maybe it's like lipsalve – I never needed it until I started using it …
Liz, 28, UK

I have very dry skin, which I take care of by smothering myself regularly with Clarins thirst quenching masks. I cleanse, tone and moisturize twice a day using Clarins products.
Carra, 31, La Réunion

Moisturizers and anti-ageing creams don't work. Good skin is down to genetics, staying out of the sun and not smoking.
Judith, 26, UK

I make my own intensive moisturizer by snipping the tops off a fish oil and a vitamin E oil capsule and mixing the two together. Then I dab the sticky mixture over my face and let it sink in while I take a long bath.
Maggie, 49, Ireland

I have a clear olive complexion and I don't use any skin products at all! just water!!
Catherine, 18, UK

Cosmeceuticals

THE POLITICS OF COSMETICS Cosmetics are defined by the FDA as 'inert substances that cleanse or enhance the skin but don't affect or alter the structure or function of the human body in any way'. What this means is that the majority of beauty products on the market cannot, by law, actually change your skin in any way, because if they do, they have to be classified as drugs rather than cosmetics. Cosmetics are not approved by the FDA prior to sale. However, if a cosmetic product claims to have therapeutic properties, it is subject to the same approval procedures as a drug and must be proven both safe and effective before it can go on sale. Because the clinical trials and medical research cost so much money, many cosmetics firms try to violate the law by marketing a cosmetic and implying that it has active properties, or by marketing a drug as if it were a cosmetic without providing the necessary research and safety information to the FDA.

Aromatherapy is a good example of an industry trying to navigate through these issues. Most essential oils don't say what their intended use is so they can be sold as fragrances or cosmetics. However, an oil that is marketed with 'aromatherapy' claims, such as 'aids sleep', meets the definition of a drug because of its intended therapeutic use and so has to go through more rigorous approval procedures. Examples of products that are both cosmetics and drugs are dandruff shampoos, acne medications, antiperspirant deodorants and foundations or tanning preparations that contain sunscreen. All of these will list their 'active ingredient' first on the label.

COSMECEUTICALS In the last five years, scientific developments have pushed cosmetics into a grey area between cosmetics and pharmaceuticals. Though the term 'cosmeceutical' is not recognized by law, these products are not traditional cosmetics because they do have a physical impact on the skin. As such, they do not conform to current 'cosmetic' definitions, but most cosmeceuticals still try to pass themselves off as cosmetics to avoid having to go through regulatory drug testing. Though all manufacturers are obliged to test for safety, whether a product actually works or not is rarely investigated. This makes it incredibly difficult for consumers to determine whether scientific claims of efficacy are actually valid.

Carefully worded labels allude to therapeutic benefits but, much of the time, products marketed as cosmeceuticals contain such tiny concentrations of any active ingredients that the products are completely ineffective. Since labelling does not generally list the percentage of the ingredient, it is virtually impossible for consumers to work out how efficiently they are being ripped off. At the moment, cosmeceuticals are both confusing and unreliable, but there is no doubt that over the next ten years these products will take over the skincare market and become more effective, more popular and more heavily regulated.

Active ingredients that work

ALPHA-HYDROXY ACIDS (AHAs) AHAs were originally derived from fruit acids, though 99% of the AHAs now used in cosmetic products are synthetic. The most effective and well-researched AHAs are glycolic acid (sugar cane) and lactic acid (sour milk). Malic acid (apples), citric acid (citrus fruits), and tartaric acid are considered less stable and less skin friendly. AHAs are labelled with a variety of beneficial claims such as exfoliating, moisturizing, cleansing, wrinkle reducing, texture improvement, increased firmness and elasticity, improvement of photodamage, skin protection, scar reduction, anti-ageing, anti-acne, skin tone evening, skin lightening and skin conditioning. And, unusually, most of it is true.

At concentrations of over 4% and in a base with an acid pH of 3 to 4, AHAs exfoliate skin cells by breaking down the substance that holds skin cells together and 'burning off' the outer layer of skin. When the top layer of cells are removed, healthier cells come to the surface, improving skin texture and colour, and allowing moisturizers to be better absorbed. AHAs make your skin feel and appear smoother and visibly reduce stretch marks, but if you stop using AHAs, your skin will return to its normal state since cell regeneration is no longer occurring. Typically, products sold over the counter have an AHA concentration of approximately 10% though US brand Aqua Glycolic, which is relatively cheap, contains concentrations of 12% and Paula's Choice contains 8%.

The products are used twice daily and initially they can make the skin feel quite dry and flaky. Many women develop redness and irritation when they first start using them, but most find that using an AHA on a regular basis for six to eight weeks improves the condition of their skin. If you intend to start using AHAs you might want to kick start your treatment with a stronger treatment. AHA products used by trained cosmetologists run at between 20% and 30%. Those used by doctors in glycolic peels can range from 50% to 70% but they literally burn the top layer of skin off on contact and it can take weeks to recover (p.197).

Dermatologists agree that AHAs are effective but because they seem to be capable of penetrating the skin's barrier, they have been the subject of a great deal of investigation by the FDA. The concern about AHAs is less to do with their immediate impact on skin and more to do with the fact that studies continually indicate that long-term use of AHA products increases sun sensitivity causing photoageing and increasing the risk of skin cancer. One study that looked at the effects of glycolic acid found that people who had AHA product treatments and were then exposed to sunlight experienced twice the cell damage in areas where the AHA had been applied. Manufacturers now have to put a sunburn alert on all AHA products and anyone using them should take the warning seriously and always use a sunscreen.

Though I am a make-up artist, I tend to buy very basic creams. I look for food based ingredients. If I don't recognize the ingredients, it doesn't go on my face. I believe that oil- and beeswax-based creams help seal in your own moisture and help to keep skin soft and supple. They are also effective as barrier creams against the elements. I do not believe that they reverse the signs of ageing or stop the ageing process. My favourite brands are Kathleen Lewis Good Plain Cream and Weleda creams.
Regina, 40, US

I realize that the beauty industry manipulates women into buying things they don't need and I seem to be a prime target because I have lots of half-used cosmetics and skincare products in my bathroom, but I keep hoping I will find 'the one' that works.
Tracey, 35, Canada

I am against animal testing so I tend to make my own cleansers and moisturizers from food products and yogurt and oils. I believe they work just as well.
Lois, 48, US

BETA-HYDROXY ACIDS (BHAs) The only cosmetic BHA is salicylic acid, found in willow bark, sweet birch and wintergreen leaves. It is a fat-soluble acid that can penetrate into the pores, thereby exfoliating inside as well as outside the pore. Because it also has anti-microbial properties it has been used at high concentrations for many years for the treatment of spots, blackheads and whiteheads and for the removal of dry, scaly skin and warts. Salicylic acid is one of the only products that has been studied for safety and effectiveness and approved by FDA for treating signs of sun-damaged or ageing skin and it has been demonstrated to improve skin thickness, barrier functions and collagen production. Its effect is less potent than that of AHAs though it can also cause some skin irritation. Salicylic acid in skin-care products works best in a concentration of 1–2% and at a pH of 3 to 4. Unlike AHAs, which must be listed in the top three ingredients to indicate the appropriate concentration, salicylic acid can be listed in the middle or even towards the bottom of the ingredient list because it is effective at lower concentrations. The Paula's Choice range includes a choice of either 1–2% salicylic acid exfoliants. Anyone using salicylic acid product must use an SPF 15 sunscreen.

POLY-HYDROXY ACID (PHAs) PHA products are the next generation of AHAs. They are less irritating and more easily tolerated by sensitive skin and contain antioxidant benefits not found in other fruit acids. Since PHAs have larger molecular structures, they don't penetrate into the skin as deeply which means they tend to have less irritating side effects. However, reduced absorption doesn't seem to hamper their effectiveness. In fact, research on PHAs shows that there is only a '6% decrease in dermal penetration compared to glycolic acid'. The US brand Lubriderm, originally produced for dermatologists, now produces several relatively inexpensive products containing PHAs. Always use a sunblock with PHAs.

PRESCRIPTION RETINOIDS Retinoids (chemicals that are related to vitamin A) such as retinoic acid or Retin-A became available in cream, gel and liquid form in the early 70s, but overexcited consumers used so much of them that they burned their skin, so these products are now only available on prescription. Under the trademark name of Retinova, retinoids were the first drug to be given a licence for treating sun-damaged skin and to obtain their licence the manufacturers had to show beyond doubt that the product worked in the majority of people with limited side effects.

In a study of 251 people aged 29–50 with sun-damaged skin, Retinova cream used once a day for six months produced some type of improvement in 79%, made the skin 29.3% less rough and faded age spots by 37 per cent. By taking before and after silicone impressions of the skin, the researchers were also able to prove that it improved wrinkles by 27.1 per cent. However, 48% of people who used only sunscreen and moisturizers also showed improvement, too, which just goes to show how much a regular skin-care routine and sunblock really helps.

Retinoids are FDA-approved for reducing the appearance of fine wrinkles, mottled darkened spots and rough skin. They don't have any effect on very noticeable wrinkles, such as the deep lines that appear between the nose and mouth. Retinoids work in much the same way as acids. By removing the top layer of skin, they force the skin below to compensate by making new cells. The skin produces more collagen and plumps out wrinkles after about four months. Retinoids inhibit the production of skin pigment, which means that over time, treated areas become lighter in colour and age spots begin to fade after six to eight weeks.

A pea-sized dab of cream is used to cover the entire face every night and, although the results are not immediate and not miraculous, it does work. Eventually, with regular usage your skin continues to improve for about six months. After that there is no further change, but you keep using the cream between two and three times per week to prevent your skin going back to the way it was. In other words, once you start, you have to continue using retinoids for the rest of your life. This could be a problem because the safety of daily retinoid use has not been established for longer than 48 weeks and, ironically, since retinoids are a product that would appeal to older women, their effects have not been studied on women over 50 years old.

Although no serious medical problems have been associated with retinoids, they do irritate the skin and can cause dryness and flakiness, sometimes with itching, soreness, redness and a tight feeling. If the products cause severe irritation, you may need to stop using them or get a milder formula from your doctor. Because retinoids are drying to the skin and make it more sun sensitive, you will need to apply an SPF 15 sunblock or moisturizer twice a day and retinoids should not be used in conjunction with fruit acids or products containing alcohol and benzoyl peroxide as these products can increase the effects of the cream and cause severe skin irritation. Retinoids are available on prescription from cosmetic surgeons, dermatologists or GPs but should not be used by women who are pregnant or planning to conceive in the next six months.

RETINOL Retinol is an over-the-counter relative of the prescription retinoid. Theoretically, retinol can be absorbed into the skin but retinol is a very unstable ingredient. Any container that allows the product to be exposed to sunlight or air will render the active ingredient completely useless within a couple of days. Retinol can cause skin irritation, but there is some evidence showing that it can increase

When I was 21 years old I worked at a national newspaper. I was the assistant to the beauty editor but I basically wrote the beauty column for her. Every week I would be sent loads of stuff to try out for the tried-and-tested section. One week it would be eight different anti-ageing creams, the next week it would be the ten best leg waxes and I had to give them all marks out of ten. Well, I never actually tried any of them. I would decide which PR girl had been nice to me or which one smelt nice or which one had the nicest packaging and I would write a review of them pretending that I had done a scrupulous analysis. I did feel a bit guilty about it but no one at the paper, particularly not my boss, seemed to care. Naturally I never trust any of those tried-and-tested things in papers. Well I might trust them if I was buying a toaster, but I certainly don't trust them for beauty products because I know what goes on. When they say Elle McPherson uses this cream or Kate Moss uses that cream —do they bugger.
Sally, 35, UK

epidermal thickness, so you might want to give it a try anyway. Neutrogena's Healthy Skin Anti-Wrinkle Cream comes in an opaque pump-action bottle and contains both retinol and an SPF 15 sunblock. And, unlike some retinol products, it won't break the bank.

PALMITOYL Palmitoyl pentapeptide (Pal-KTTKS) is the new retinol. In two studies it has proved as effective as retinol in improving the effects of photoageing but it doesn't seem to cause the inflammatory reactions frequently associated with retinol treatment. In studies on both retinol and palmitoyl, both products increased skin thickness by an average of 9% after four months. However, the two-month data suggested that palmitoyl pentapeptide thickened the skin about one and a half times faster than retinol. As with many new ingredients, the research on palmitoyl was carried out by doctors sponsored by the product's manufacturer. However, the results are encouraging and anything that causes less irritation is a step in the right direction. Olay Regenerist Daily Regenerating Serum contains palmitoyl but no sunscreen, so use it with an SPF 15 sunscreen.

SKIN WHITENERS Three skin whiteners are prescribed to inhibit melanin production and remove age spots – brown patches caused by ageing and over exposure to the sun. *Hydroquinone* is used to get rid of age spots, freckles and general brown patching. It works by inhibiting the production of melanin, though it has to be used for a long time to be effective. Hydroquinone in 1–2% concentrations is available in over-the-counter products while 4% concentrations are available by prescription. Occasionally, sunlight reverses the effect of hydroquinone by increasing melanin production and, at higher concentrations, people with darker skin can experience increased pigmentation. However, this is relatively rare and the most common side effects are mild skin irritation and the possibility of an allergic reaction. There is concern that hydroquinone is potentially carcinogenic. Tests on animals led to tumours and DNA damage but monitoring of people who work with hydroquinone on a daily basis revealed a lower than average death rate. *Arbutin* is a melanin inhibitor often used in de-pigmentation. It is combined with retinol to fade brown spots caused by ageing or sun exposure. It needs to be used for at least 30 days to take effect. *Kojic acid* is an effective skin lightener that inhibits melanin production. It is produced from a fungus and was discovered in Japan in 1989 and there is plenty of evidence that it works, but since the product loses its active properties when exposed to air, it is not available in many products. Many cosmetics companies use kojic dipalmitate as an alternative because it is more stable in formulations but there is no research showing that it is as effective as kojic acid. Look for kojic acid in airtight dispensers. Always use an SPF 15 sunblock with skin whiteners.

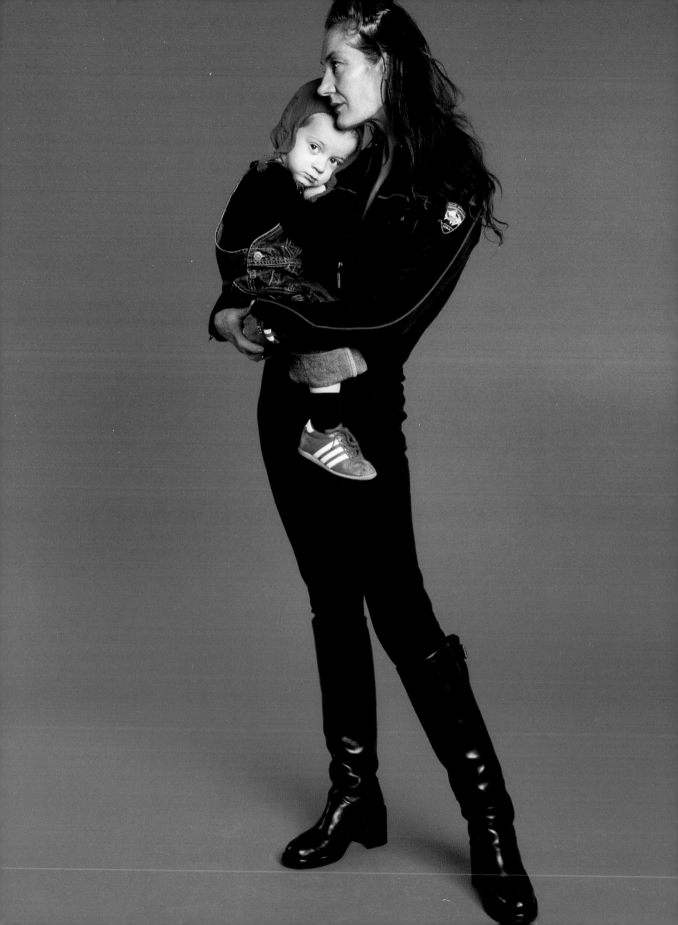

Active ingredients that don't work

COLLAGEN We all wish we had more collagen but, sadly, using a collagen cream is not the way to get it. Collagen creams make decent moisturizers but the collagen molecule is actually too large to penetrate the skin so it simply sits on the surface. The only way to increase the amount of collagen in your skin is to have collagen injections (p.191).

ENZYMES Pure enzymes from fruits such as papaya (papain) and pineapple (bromelain) make great exfoliants but the minute quantities added to commercial skincare products make no difference at all because isolated enzymes are the skincare equivalent to a single piece of a jigsaw puzzle. If a gazillion others are not present, one on its own is totally useless.

HUMAN GROWTH HORMONE (HGH) Though a glut of convincing 'medical' websites promote the miraculaous benefits of HGH pills and injections (all of which are available at a price), it is not a magic anti-ageing bullet. HGH is produced naturally in the body and affects protein, glucose, fat and carbohydrate metabolism and regulates the division and reproduction of cells. As with all hormones, levels of HGH decline as we age and, as a result, lean muscle mass decreases and our skin becomes thinner and more wrinkled. HGH is used medically to correct pituitary growth hormone deficiency and Turner's syndrome in girls, but its use by people with levels that are normal for their age is untested.

The hormone's potential as an anti-aging cure-all first came to light in 1990 when a study of 12 healthy men, aged 61–81 years of age, showed that growth hormone injections over a period of six months resulted in less fat, more muscle mass and a slight increase in lumbar-spine density. The study attracted a lot of attention, but the injections were carried out by professionals over a short space of time and there is no information on whether long-term administration of HGH is potentially harmful. Anything that interferes with cell division can influence the growth of cancers, and in another study of 152 healthy men, the development of prostate cancer was increased by a factor of 4.3 among men who had high doses of HGH. HGH did not cause the cancer but it raises concern about the use of this product for cosmetic reasons. HGH levels can be boosted naturally by eating less, taking exercise and getting enough sleep, and in tests of men on HGH versus men on a programme of resistance training and regular exercise, the men who worked out both looked better and felt better.

HUMAN PLACENTA Products containing processed embryonic tissue claim to provide hormones that stimulate tissue growth and remove wrinkles. When they first appeared, the FDA took these claims seriously and tested the products as drugs, but they found them to be completely ineffective so the manufacturers then decided to re-market the products as protein-rich cosmetics. There is absolutely no evidence that they work.

KINETIN Though there has been a lot of hype about kinetin (N6-furfuryladenine), at the moment there is no objective research to support claims that it reduces signs of ageing or improves sun damage. Two positive clinical studies were sponsored by the manufacturers so they should be taken with a giant pinch of salt.

OESTROGEN AND PROGESTERONE Hormone replacement therapy (HRT) was originally designed to boost declining hormone levels in menopausal women, but the treatment proved to have some interesting side effects, one of which was a significant improvement in skin tone and elasticity. Oestrogen deficient women tend to develop more pronounced lines between the nose and the mouth and these seem to improve once oestrogen levels are balanced out. However, despite its cosmetic benefits, hormone treatment is not an option for pre menopausal women because HRT has a significant relationship with breast cancer in later life (p.278). Unfortunately, in the quest for short-term benefits to physical appearance some women are willing to overlook long-term health implications. HRT type creams containing active hormones should only be used if prescribed by a doctor for symptoms of menopause. Natural alternatives such as wild yam based creams are a waste of money because research shows that have absolutly no effect on skin quality when applied topically.

OXYGEN The therapeutic use of oxygen under pressure is known as hyperbaric oxygen therapy (HBO2). The treatment was originally developed to recompress divers and involves sitting in a huge tank that uses pressure to provide tissue with 11 times more oxygen than normal. Science supports the idea that oxygen encourages the production of collagen but the teensy percentage delivered by a jar of cream will have absolutely no impact on your skin. The only way to boost oxygen levels in your skin is to exercise and increase your aerobic capacity (p.113).

ROYAL JELLY Secreted by worker bees as food for queen bees, royal jelly has been afforded all sorts of beneficial qualities but the buzz about royal jelly's ability to prevent wrinkles or cure acne is not supported by any research.

VITAMIN K Vitamin K is a known blood coagulant and, as such, is marketed as a miracle cure for spider veins. However, tiny concentrations in a topical application will have absolutely no effect on anything other than your wallet. Vitamin K is readily available in dark green vegetables and oils, so eat more broccoli and use less lotion.

I'm fortunate that I've found a massage therapist that visits at home. I've not had a facial for a long time but I regularly go to my friend who's a wonderful beauty therapist for manicures, pedicures and waxing – and a laugh! Aromatherapy works for me. It always has for me and I was fortunate enough to start my aromatherapy journey with Lyn Harris in her early days as a massage therapist before she became famous! My body has always responded well to the oils.
Ruth, 43, UK

When you think of the number of chemicals women consume or put on our skin or hair as part of our cleansing/ beauty regime every day it is pretty frightening really. Toothpaste, cleansers, soaps, shampoo, bubble bath make-up, moisturizer, antiperspirant – they are all chemicals. It's really a miracle that more of us don't develop terrible allergies as a result of relentless exposure to unnatural substances.
Nanette, 44, UK

The whole beauty business stinks. If I see another girl with vagina lips pouting at me, I think I will be sick.
Louise, 34, UK

And active ingredients that might be of benefit

Antioxidants are best absorbed through food (p.43) and there is no concrete evidence that topical applications can penetrate the skins layers. However, they are routinely added to cosmetics and *may* provide additional protection for your skin. Promoted as preventing sun damage and photoageing, lessening redness and neutralizing existing free-radical damage (p.139), there are lots of antioxidant products on the market. The N.V. Perricone, Environ and Paula's Choice ranges contain the broadest range and highest percentage of ingredients. You should always use an SPF 15 sunblock with antioxidant products as they make the skin more sensitive to UVA and UVB rays. There is no single best antioxidant and none of the following ingredients will prevent or cure wrinkles.

ALPHA LIPOIC ACID Studies of its effects on human skin are limited. Most of the research has been done on human skin cells in test tubes and it is not known whether the promising results will ever translate to human skin. There is research showing that when taken orally, this enzyme can have a positive impact on cellular damage. As a cream or a serum it will protect the skin, but take wrinkle reduction claims with a pinch of salt.

BETA CAROTENE Beta carotene is converted to vitamin A (retinol) in the body and is a member of the carotenoid family. Beta carotene is a potentially good antioxidant and can reduce the effects of sun damage, though obviously this depends on the quantity of beta carotene in the product and whether it actually penetrates or adheres to the skin.

CO-ENZYME 10 (Q10) Co-enzyme Q10 is found in most of the body tissues but levels decrease as people get older. In cultured human cells, Q10 has been shown to decrease photodamage and limit the activity of enzymes that degrade collagen, but whether that translates into fewer human wrinkles is not something that has yet been established. There is a great deal of research currently being done to investigate the rejuvenating properties of Q10 but at present it is used for its antioxidant properties. Eucerin Q10 Anti-Wrinkle Sensitive Skin Creme may be worth trying.

GINGKO BILOBA The leaves of the gingko biloba tree are thought to increase blood flow and circulation. The leaves are now used in skincare products because they have both antioxidant and anti-inflammatory properties (P. 49).

GRAPE SEED EXTRACT Grape seed extract contains powerful antioxidants known as oligomeric proanthocyanidins (OPCs). They won't prevent wrinkles but have been shown to have wound healing properties.

European studies have indicated that OPCs inhibit enzymes (collagenase, elastase and hyaluronidase) that are involved in the breakdown of structural components of the skin, but these effects nevertheless need to be proven by clinical trials. There is no difference in the antioxidant potential between different types of grapes.

GREEN TEA Polyphenols, the active ingredients in green and white tea, possess powerful antioxidant, anti-inflammatory and anti-carcinogenic properties, but studies have not established whether these benefits would translate into a topical preparation. In one 3% preparation, green tea cream was shown to have a beneficial effect on acne lesions, but the minute percentages added to commercial cosmetic products are unlikely to have any impact.

TOCOTRIENOLS Super-potent forms of vitamin E that are considered to be stable and powerful antioxidants. Research on animals shows tocotrienols to be more potent antioxidants than other forms of vitamin E, but studies on humans are limited and are based on very large oral doses.

VITAMIN C Vitamin C is a very fragile vitamin that is unlikely to cope with heavy processing. Although topical preparations may be able to deliver a higher dosage to specific areas and several animal studies have suggested topical vitamin C provides protection against ultra-violet radiation, this may not be the case with humans, and C certainly won't get rid of existing wrinkles. In creams, vitamin C usually comes in a modified form, as an ester, but it must be converted back to the native form to have any effect. Studies suggest it is more effective if combined with vitamin E, but further research would help.

VITAMIN E (D-alpha tocopherol) Vitamin E is a fat-soluble vitamin that is known to be an excellent antioxidant when applied topically to skin. Many scientific studies that have been conducted on animals have shown that a topical application of vitamin E reduces redness, swelling and wrinkling caused by ultra-violet radiation. However, although vitamin E is often used to heal scars, there is no clinical proof that it works. In people with very sensitive skin, vitamin E can actually impede the healing process.

WITCH HAZEL Witch hazel contains high concentrations of tannin, which is a known antioxidant that soothes the skin and reduces inflammation from burns. It is relatively cheap and can be bought in any pharmacy but check the alcohol content, which can irritate skin if used too often.

I have worked in the same office for about five years now and in that time most of the people who used to smoke outside on the fire escape have quit. One very pretty girl who joined the company when she was 26 is now 31 years old. She hasn't quit smoking and, of course, I can't say if it is cigarettes for sure, but her skin seems to have aged a lot more than it should have in that time. I try not to stare, but I have become increasingly fascinated by it.
Theresa, 35, US

I stick to very plain, simple products, a light exfoliating wash and gentle cleanser with moisturizer when I need it. It seems to work! I do try new products if I think they might be a new development but I don't think I ever have very high expectations. Based on past experience, nothing works as well as not drinking and getting an early night.
Auriel, 28, UK

Though I am as cynical as the next person about their effectiveness, beauty products are my addiction. My bathroom is full of every brand under the sun and I take great pleasure in all of them, whether they work or not.
Elizabeth, 32, US

Top beauty tips

GO SHOPPING NAKED If you are going to buy make-up products don't go wearing foundation. Test products on your clean skin so that you can really see whether you are buying the right shade.

DON'T SHARE MAKE-UP Sharing cosmetics means sharing germs. Avoid using tester products in-store, which are often contaminated with bacteria. If you need to check a lipstick colour, put it on the back of your hand, not your mouth.

TRY BEFORE YOU BUY Preservatives and fragrances are the number-one cause of skin irritation and the words 'natural' or 'hypoallergenic' on the packet are no guarantee that you won't have a reaction.

MAKE SURE YOU BUY THE RIGHT COLOUR Unlike other products, if you buy something like a mascara and it turns out to be the wrong colour, most pharmacies will not exchange it, even if it is unopened.

DON'T STICK TO A SINGLE SKINCARE BRAND Although sales people and advertising suggest that to get the maximum benefit from a skincare product you have to buy and use a single range (the one they are trying to sell you), that is not true. You can, and should, mix and match your skincare products in the same way that you mix and match your clothes.

DON'T USE MAKE-UP THAT IS OUT OF DATE Cull the crusty old mascaras and lipsticks that have been knocking around your bathroom cabinet for years. Every time you open a bottle of foundation or case of eye shadow, micro-organisms in the air have an opportunity to rush in. Over the years, products can become contaminated with moulds, fungi and pathogenic organisms, which may not be visible. Foundation lasts about a year, moisturizer lasts about a year and a half, lipstick lasts about a year, but mascara should be renewed every six months, whether it is used up or not.

FOUNDATION You can get away with cheap blusher, eyeshadow and mascara, but foundation needs to be colour matched. Prescriptives custom blending is available at most big stores and, although it is more expensive, you can at least be sure that you have got your foundation colour spot on. Foundations that contain light-reflecting pigments, which bounce light off the face, tend to look more flawless than regular foundations, and the older or drier your skin, the more important it is to use a creamy, more moisturizing foundation.

CONCEALER The best is the Yves Saint Laurent Touche Eclat applicator pen.

MAKE-UP FOR DAY TIME For daytime don't overdo the colour. Use a tinted moisturizer instead of a foundation and use a concealer to even out areas of redness around the nose or eyes. Stick to more neutral colours and use a tint like Benetint blush to give yourself a healthy, natural-looking glow and a slick of clear gloss on your lips. Carrot oil will bring out the yellow in your skin tones and facial bronzers such as Lancôme flash bronzer or Clarins Anti Ride Visage will give you a sun-kissed look.

MAKE-UP FOR NIGHT TIME Lighting at night is usually softer, so you can compensate by wearing a light-reflective foundation and concealer to even out your complexion and go for stronger coloured lipstick, smoky eyes and shimmer shadows. Don't forget to smooth foundation up from your neck so you don't get a line around the base of your jaw.

CONCEALING SPOTS First dab the spot with tea tree oil which has disinfecting properties that are effective against the bacteria that cause blemishes. Use the actual oil rather than tea tree preparations, which only contain about 1% concentrations rather than the 5–10% that is recommended. Then conceal the blemish with your usual foundation, paint over the top of the spot with concealer and gently blend it with your finger. Then take a small amount of translucent powder on a puff and pat it over the top to keep the concealer in place.

TO EXFOLIATE CHAPPED LIPS To exfoliate flaky or chapped lips, moisten your lips then apply a strip of Sellotape across your lips and when you remove the tape you will also remove the unwanted skin flakes. After exfoliating apply lip balm and leave your lips lipstick-free for half an hour.

NATURAL LIPSTICK INGREDIENTS Women who wear lipstick eat the equivalent of four tubes of lipstick in a lifetime. Hardly surprising that there has been an increasing demand for more natural products then. Dr Hauschka, Jurlique, Aveda and Origins avoid the use of nasty petrochemicals in favour of natural base products such as beeswax, shea butter, vitamin E and jojoba oil. The downside of natural lipsticks is the fact that their range of colours is not as extensive. Fewer pigments mean they generally have a more neutral palette which is fine if you like lots of muted seventies browns and plums, but not so good for brights.

For those women who would rather eat four tubes of lipstick than go through life without a bright red smile, then MAC lipsticks are just about the best in terms of colour range and they are really very long lasting. The Channel and Sephora own-brand ranges are also very good.

When Nigella Lawson wrote her Times beauty column I used to buy things she recommended. I trusted her judgement and I knew that there wasn't an advertising department breathing down her neck.
Rose, 38, UK

If you say women are manipulated into buying things they don't need that makes it sound as if all women are easily manipulated – if you say women are not manipulated into buying things they don't need, well that's ignoring the fact that it happens. I think everyone can be manipulated if they have insecurities and want to believe what they hear.
Sue, 35, UK

Inside every overweight, overtired, overwhelmed woman is a beautiful, rested and calm woman who is trying to get out.
Tonya, 42, UK

I can't see how women are meant to be able to differentiate between the different products on the market. There is nothing to tell you definitively what works and what is useless and what is even bad for you. I will never know if there is a magic product will I?
Angela, 32, UK

TO KEEP YOUR LIPSTICK ON ALL DAY To maintain your lipstick, use a matching lip liner to outline your lips, then colour in your entire upper and lower lip with liner. Apply a heavy coat of lipstick on top and then press your lips against a dry tissue. Repeat this process three times to build up an intense layer of lipstick. Then apply either a coat of gloss or a sealing lipcoat.

TO STOP YOUR LIPSTICK BLEEDING Apply Touche Eclat concealer all around the outside of your lips, then outline your lips with a lip liner, taking care to work within the lip and not go over the edges. Apply your lipstick as usual and then seal it with a lipcoat.

PERMANENT MAKE-UP Permanent make-up is a form of tattooing that needs to be carried out by a trained beautician. The treatments most commonly requested are eyebrows, eyeliner and lips. Eyebrows can be given better definition from filling in small areas to total brow recreation. Eyeliner can be applied in any colour for a soft, natural enhancement or a more defined line. Lipliner can outline the lips, correct uneven lip shape or deepen lip colour, which tends to get paler with age. Full lip colour can give the impression of fuller lips. The technique involves using a hand tool (which is about the size of a fountain pen) containing tiny needles to implant pigment just under the surface of the skin. It can be quite painful if you are a bit of a wimp and the result can look a bit scabby for the first day or two. Pigments fade over time, though the rate depends on how well they react with your skin and beauticians recommend that you come back to have the colour checked within ten months of your treatment so they can see how rapidly colour fades on your particular skin type. The pigment colour can be changed and adjusted at any time.

TRICK OF THE LIGHT Lighter eyeshadow colours (pinks, blues, whites, silvers) highlight your eyes and make them appear larger whereas darker colours (smoky browns, blacks, greys) make your eyes recede. A dot of white eyeliner in the corner of your eyelid near the bridge of your nose and along the lower rim will make the whites of your eyes look clearer though women with pale skin may feel that lighter liners make them look a little anaemic. If you don't wear eye shadow, a pale concealer like Touche Eclat on the upper lid and below the eyebrow will brighten your eyes and give a natural looking all-over tone and smooth out any blotchiness or broken veins.

EYELASH CURLERS Using an eyelash curler before you apply your mascara makes eyelashes look more dramatic. After your lashes are curled, you're ready to apply mascara. Clean eyelash curlers with eye make-up remover.

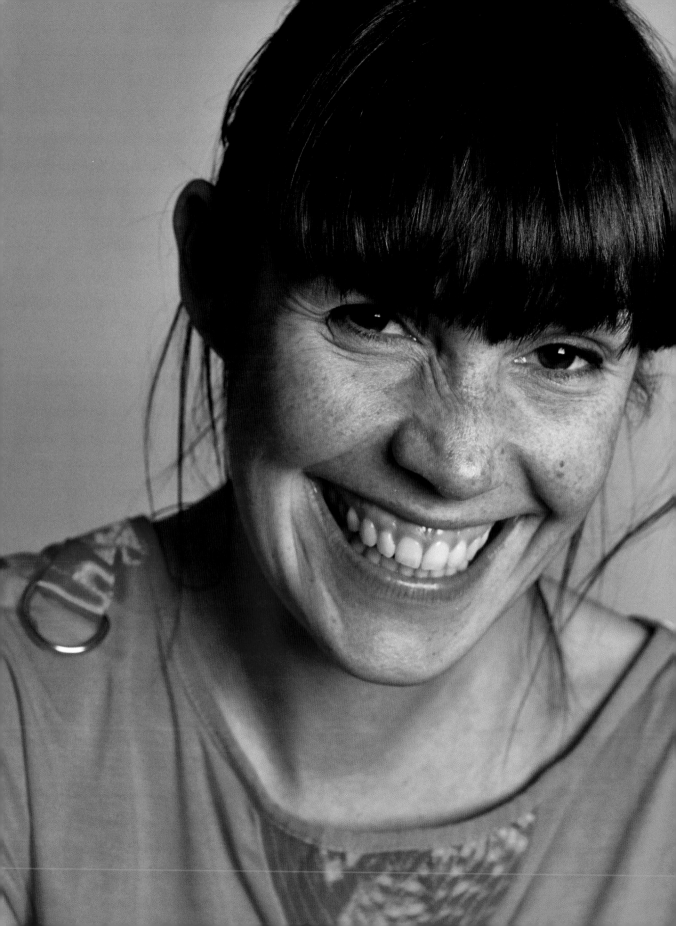

APPLYING MASCARA Swirl the brush within the tube rather than pumping it in and out. Anything that lets air into your mascara causes the product to age and spreads bacteria. When you put the brush to the base of your lashes, wiggle it slightly so that the lashes don't clump together and then extend the wand outward. Always apply two coats, but allow the first to dry completely before applying the second. For a natural look, don't use either liner or mascara on lower lashes. Remove smudgy mascara with a cotton bud and cleanser or liquid filled beauty tips. Clean mascara brushes once a month with eye make-up remover. If you run out of mascara Vaseline on your lashes will make them look longer and thicker.

FALSE EYELASHES False eyelashes are an inexpensive way of making yourself stand out in the crowd. Make sure you buy a reputable brand and test the glue on the back of your hand to make sure you are not allergic to it.

EYELASH AND EYEBROW TINTING Tinting is great for women who have very pale lashes or brows, sportswomen, swimmers or even just those that can't be bothered with applying mascara and brow pencil every day. It lasts between four and six weeks, depending on the tint, and colours can be matched to your natural colouring if desired. A patch test should be done in advance to make sure you are not allergic to the tint.

BRIGHT EYES Using a blue tinted eye drop will make the whites of your eyes appear brighter and cleaner and give you a dewy sparkle. Try Optrex Eye Dew Blue Eye Drops.

EMERGENCY EYEBAG REPAIR Supermodels favour the use of a thin layer of haemorrhoid cream such as Anusol under the eyes to shrink puffy bags. To make eyes look brighter they apply a little matt pink eyeshadow beneath their eyes then cover the entire area with a powder that is a couple of shades lighter than their natural skin tone.

EYEBROW SHAPING Professional eyebrow shaping is probably the quickest, cheapest, most immediate beauty fix there is. It is best to get it done at a salon first and then pluck at home to keep the shape. Shavata Singh's eyebrow stencil kit contains four eyebrow stencils that you can use at home. The Liz Hurley, The Kylie Minogue, the Grace Kelly and the Brooke Shields stencils are pasted over your existing brow and you then pluck around them.

GREASY HAIR If you have greasy hair but your scalp is dry, then you are probably using a shampoo or conditioner that is too heavy for your hair. Stop using conditioner and use a tea tree oil shampoo. If your scalp is greasy, you may need to wash your hair less often. Frequent shampooing stimulates the oil glands in your scalp and aggravates the problem. Wash twice a week, don't brush your hair repeatedly and avoid rubbing your fingers through your scalp.

DRY, DAMAGED HAIR Too many chemical processes, colour changes, perms and relaxing treatments can damage your hair and dry it out. Invest in a good leave-in conditioner, use an intensive conditioning treatment once a week, avoid blow drying and heat treatments and make sure to get your hair trimmed regularly. Kerastase products are great for dry, damaged hair.

HEAT Blow-drying, curling tongs and straightening irons make your hair look great, but they are terribly hard on hair condition. GHD straightening irons are a great investment for women wanting dead straight hair but use a thermal protector lotion such as GHD Iron Oil before heat treatments to protect your hair.

DANDRUFF Though dandruff is not harmful, it is certainly unsightly. There are a range of products on the market, such as TGel or Head and Shoulders, which are specifically designed to combat dandruff. A tar-based medicated shampoo is more likely to be effective if you are suffering from seborrheic dermatitis (p.146). Massaging olive oil into your scalp before you go to bed can help stop flaking.

GREY HAIR As we age, the amount of hair pigment (melanin) that we produce lessens, turning the hair 'grey', though when and how much this happens is mainly genetic. Though stories abound of women going grey overnight, this never really happens because the colour molecules in the hair are formed below the scalp and then proceed to grow down through the hair, eventually becoming noticeable. Occasionally, shock or illness can cause people to lose a lot of hair and, if the hair left behind is predominantly grey, it can appear as if they have literally gone grey. Fewer and fewer women opt to go grey now that hair dyes and tints have become so realistic. In fact, a head of grey hair is now so rare that you can expect to see more women opting to return to their roots in the near future. Grey hair tends to suffer from yellowing, particularly in smokers, but it is mainly due to pollution. A purifying shampoo will remove build-up and shampoos with a blue/ash or silver tone help to naturalize any yellow and enhance white or grey hairs.

HAIR COLOUR Sadly, when it comes to hair colour, 'permanent' does not mean forever. Roots and colour have to be touched up every four to eight weeks and this can become incredibly expensive. Many women make the mistake of having a go at home but it is not advisable, particularly if you intend to completely change

If you want great looking shimmery lips, apply a little sparkling eye shadow over the top of your lipstick to create a new, shiny shade, absolutely free.
Zoe, 25, US

I was going to a big party and I decided to wear false eyelashes. I bought a pair which came with a little tube of glue, which you had to squirt over the base of the lashes. Unfortunately, I was rather too liberal with the glue and it squelched all over the lashes. I cleaned it off and tried again and then put them on with tweezers. They looked really good and I put some eyeliner over the join so they looked more natural. I was a big hit at the party but after about an hour my eyelids got really itchy and I had to go and take the lashes off. When I removed them, my eyelids were red, itchy and swollen so I suppose I had a reaction to the glue. Although they do look good I would advise anyone thinking of using them to test the glue on its own on their eyelid before they go to a big event. I looked really rough for a few days afterwards.
Natasha, 26, UK

colour. Most hairdressers insist on an allergy patch test before colouring and are better at working out whether a particular colour will suit you. After colouring, the condition of your hair changes. Permanent colours and bleaches leave the hair slightly swollen so, if you already have very thick hair, you may need to get a hairdresser to thin it out.

LOWLIGHTS AND HIGHLIGHTS If you don't want to change your colour completely, lowlights or highlights can break up your existing colour. Lowlights make sections of hair darker and highlights make sections of hair lighter. For women with grey hair, lights can be chosen to match their natural colour and blend out some of their grey. Because this type of colouring will only be on 30–50% of the hair, the re-growth will not be as strong and will only require touch-ups every eight weeks plus. The more contrasting the colour you choose, the more often it will need to be done.

SEMI-PERMANENTS These gradually fade out over a period of weeks or washes, although a slight re-growth will be visible as they fade more slowly than your hair grows. If your hair is very fine or if you repeat too often (before the last one fades out), you will, however, get a re-growth. Nicky Clarke Colour is a relatively inexpensive option for home colour, gives high shine and lasts for about 20 washes.

HAIR IN PREGNANCY During late pregnancy, hair grows around 10% more than normal and shedding reduces by a third. Following childbirth, shedding increases and, by nine weeks after the birth, shedding, in percentage terms, has gone from an all-time low in the late weeks of pregnancy (around 5%) to a high of 30–35 per cent. Typically, the shedding lasts less than six months and the majority of women return to normal hair density within a year. If you can get away without having your hair coloured while you are pregnant, do. Though the risk is unproven, some scientists suspect that chemical dyes on the hair are capable of passing through the skin and into the bloodstream. Foil lowlights or highlights are more acceptable as they are not in direct contact with the scalp.

HOME IMPROVEMENTS To bring out the natural colour of darker hair soak dry hair with cooled strong coffee and leave it in for 30 minutes. Rinse, dry and style. For lighter hair, soak hair in cooled camomile and lemon tea and leave in for 20 minutes. rinse, dry and style.

WAXING Brazilian waxing was pioneered in Brazil, home of the itsy-bitsy, teeny-weeny bikini. But it really hit the big time when the J Sisters (seven Brazilian sisters whose names all begin with J) perfected the method at their New York salon and built up a huge celebrity client list. There are four basic kinds: the bikini wax simply removes hair from outside the panty line; the Brazilian leaves an inch-wide vertical stripe of hair up the front; the Playboy removes all hair leaving only a very narrow strip in the front, and the Hollywood, which takes everything off everywhere, Kojak style. Professional waxing has obvious benefits. Women say it makes them feel really clean and groomed. And re-growth is often softer and easier to remove, so the more you do it, the less it hurts. But most of all, women say it's worth the money because it drives men wild.

LASER HAIR REMOVAL. Up to six treatments are required to remove facial or body hair using a laser beam, which destroys the follicles of the hair. It's expensive but results last about a year.

DYEING PUBIC HAIR Dyeing pubic hair has mixed results. Bleaching tends to turn pubic hair orange and can also cause severe irritation and burning on sensitive skin. Black dye tends to look the most convincing, but use dye made for beards because it is better for stronger hair.

STRONG NAILS Nails, like hair, are made of keratin. To keep them strong and flexible, rub hand cream or oil into the cuticles and base of the nails daily.

FIXING A BROKEN NAIL When nails crack or split, using nail glue or mending tape is your best solution. Dab a bit of nail glue onto a small piece of a tea bag or coffee filter paper, then cover the nail where it is torn. File the nail smooth, and cover it with polish.

BRITTLE NAILS Brittle nails can be caused by over-exposure to the sun, a poor diet or using hardeners or varnishes that contain formaldehyde, which has a drying effect on nails. Rub the nails with a waxy lip balm and cover with a transparent waterproof coating to seal in the moisture.

RIDGES Ridges on the nail are, unfortunately, mostly down to genetic causes, though they can be caused by illness or extreme pressure on the nail. You can smooth the ridged nail surface with a buffer and buffing cream. However, if you have only recently developed ridges on your nails, this could be a sign of anaemia, and you may want to consult your doctor.

WHITE SPOTS Occasionally these are caused by a zinc deficiency but more usually they are a result of damage to the nail, general wear and tear or prodding beneath the cuticles and you just need to let them grow out.

I only had my eyebrows shaped for the first time when I was 34 and it made a huge difference to my face. I can't imagine why I waited so long to do it.
Bunty, 39, UK

I've always been very self-conscious of my hair as it's thick and quite wavy – there's loads of it! Getting all my hair cut off when I was 15 and then again at 25 made a big difference to my life – it was literally like I felt lighter. I once got my hair 'layered' when I was 13. Unfortunately, it wasn't the look I was aiming for and, with loads of short layers at the front, was effectively a mullet. What a nightmare!
Lorraine, 29, UK

I haven't seen my natural hair colour for about 20 years. I get my roots done every three weeks come rain or shine and I hope I will never see any grey because I don't intend to change my routine. The only thing is that it is incredibly expensive. It costs £78 for roots and a further £70 if I need a haircut. I have never worked it out before but I think I spend several thousand pounds a year on my hair. Better not tell my husband.
June, 47, UK

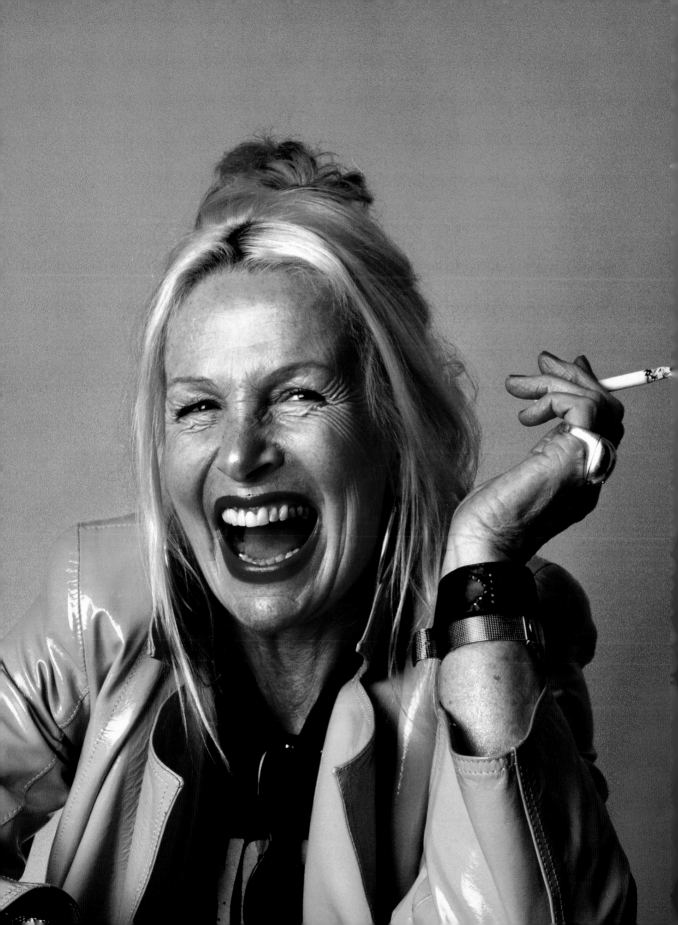

THE Ageing CHAPTER

From fertility to invisibility

Ageing as we know it is a relatively recent phenomenon. Life expectancy has doubled in the last 100 years, and over the next 50, the proportion of people aged 60-plus around the world is predicted to grow by a further 250 per cent. By 2050, for the first time in human history, old people will outnumber children on the planet. Better health care and greater independence means most women can plan on longer, healthier, more fulfilling lives. However, as confidence in longevity has increased, so too has paranoia about the negative implications of looking older in a society obsessed with youth.

Because women are governed by their biological function to a much greater degree than men are, increased longevity has made the transition from fertility to infertility much more significant. Men simply continue to get older, but after menopause, women lose something that has traditionally defined, or even justified, their existence. Theoretically, men can carry on reproducing until they die, but women now lose their ability to reproduce when they still have half their life to live. This forces them to renegotiate their position in a society that still prefers to see the female menopause as notice of imminent redundancy, rather than a promotion to greater physical freedom. Crow's-feet and grey hair make a man look 'distinguished', but for women, the same features symbolize dwindling opportunities in the community, in the workplace and in the bedroom and, as such, ageing has become synonymous with a process of gradual disqualification.

The unspoken perception that women over the age of 50 are less 'useful' than men of the same age is reinforced by their complete invisibility in the media. Nowhere is society's hypocritical approach to ageing more apparent than it is in Hollywood where an actress's working life ends at 35. At that point she finds herself stranded in the 'babes and grannies gap' - too old to be young and too young to be old. If she is lucky she may, in later life, get cast in character parts, but it must be galling for the very many redundant 40-something actresses to watch men like Harrison Ford, Mel Gibson and Jack Nicholson continue to play lead roles opposite women who are young enough to be their daughters.

This movie industry double standard is not a recent phenomenon. Fred Astaire was dancing into his 70s but Ginger Rogers was out to pasture at 34. Even parts that actually required 'older' women have not been given to them in the past. In Hitchcock's *North by Northwest* Cary Grant was 11 months *older* than his mother, played by Jesse Royce Landis and in *The Graduate*, student Dustin Hoffman was only six years younger than Anne Bancroft, the mother figure he was sleeping with. Sadly, until the movie industry stops peddling fantasy and starts acknowledging reality, older women will continue to be overlooked.

Obviously, because actresses have a short shelf life and are, in effect, paid to look good, many begin investing in maintenance and anti-ageing treatments a lot sooner than ordinary mortals. But the average 50-year-old woman hitting menopause may well have had little time or money to invest in her appearance as she raised her kids or ran her home. For her, the triple whammy of menopause, an empty nest and time to look in the mirror can bring the sudden and somewhat shocking realization that she has been so busy caring for everyone else in her life that she has completely forgotten to care for herself.

The feminist argument that fear of ageing is just a crisis of the imagination - one that will only be resolved when women decide to tell the truth and let their faces show the lives they have lived - is all very well. In theory. In practice, accepting grey hair, wrinkles and an expanding waistline goes against the culture of self improvement that this generation has grown up on. We have been under instruction to improve our health, our homes, our careers, our relationships, and our looks for decades now. And we are programmed to start fighting 'the seven signs of ageing' before they even appear. As such, one would think that the decision to add botox or collagen shots to an existing beauty programme would be a no brainer. But it isn't. It's not just that non surgical anti ageing treatments are expensive. Even women who can afford them find the negative connotations associated with any form of intervention terribly offputting.

It is fair to say that more women would probably explore ways to counter ageing if vanity didn't generate such a froth of cynicism from both sexes. Women who choose to paralyze signs of ageing are generally viewed as narcissistic at best, and dysfunctional at worst. But the perception that women who seek to improve the way they look and, in turn, feel about themselves are somehow cheating, implies that, although help is out there, there is something wrong with a woman who chooses to take it. Damned if she does and damned if she doesn't, an ageing woman is hung by her desire to conform to a standard that starts strangling her as soon as she turns thirty.

Though climbing a mountain or getting a law degree are a far more effective way of boosting self-esteem, non surgical anti-ageing treatments can provide instant, if temporary, benefit to a woman who is bothered by her wrinkles. Although the cost is still prohibitive, they are a more affordable and more acceptable alternative to surgery because they don't involve anaesthetics, incisions, stitches and long recovery times. So, as well as examining preventative measures, this chapter outlines the latest and safest non surgical anti-ageing treatments for those who would like to limit the damage of a misspent youth.

After the age of about 45, ageing is like falling off a cliff. It happens really fast and you feel out of control. Your body weight creeps up overnight and every morning brings a new imperfection. The only way to cope is to keep yourself active and try not to get paranoid about it all. Oh, and date older men who will tell you how young you look.
Margaret, 54, UK

My husband left me for his 30-year-old secretary on my 50th birthday. Menopausal and depressed, for my self-esteem it was the final twist of the knife. In February I took an overdose but luckily, though I did not think so at the time, my son found me and I recovered. Over the past five years I have rebuilt my life. I lost weight (15lb [6.8kg]), partly in recovery, partly by diet, and when I felt I was looking better I had Botox and an eye lift. I now look better than I did at 45 and I am more physicaly active than I have been for most of my adult life. I now feel in control of my life and, ironically, my ex-husband is now suffering from depression.
Ellen, 55, Aus

Signs of ageing

I started to go grey when I was about forty. I had ordinary brown hair which started to change colour quite gradually and I just let it grow through. It has taken 20 years for my hair to go this colour but it's still not completely grey and my hairdresser refuses to let me dye it. I have so many friends who look like rather old foxes. They've all dyed their hair and gone slightly gingery and they all look the same. I like to look different. My background was in the theatre. I was a dancer and I did classical ballet and I still believe it is terribly important to keep fit. I swim every day to keep myself flexible because I have arthritis in my hand. You never think you will inherit things, but you do. I got it from my mum who had it and my grandmother was in a wheel chair at the age of 36 years. I got it when I first had children because I didn't have extra calcium but doctors are much more vigilant now about welfare. I have had three operations on my hand and I have had the bone taken out of my thumb because it was so painful.
Penny, 60, U.K.
(Pictured right)

THE SKIN The skin of a 20-year-old is plump with collagen and elastin (p.138) and the outer skin cells renew every 28 days. By the time a woman hits 35, the first signs of ageing – tiny wrinkles or crow's-feet at the corners of the eyes and frown lines on the forehead – are noticeable. Because women have thinner, less oily skin than men, signs of ageing appear up to five years faster.

The sun is the major cause of wrinkles and your lifetime exposure to it largely determines how lined your skin will get. Exposed areas such as the face, neck, forearms and hands age more quickly than the rest of your body because they are in the sun more. They also develop small brown or black patches, known as liver spots or sun spots. They are not cancerous, nor do they lead to cancer, but any blemish that appears to change should be evaluated by a doctor.

People who smoke tend to have more wrinkles than nonsmokers of the same age, complexion, and history of sun exposure. The reason for this difference is not clear but it may be that smoking plays a role in damaging elastin. Facial wrinkling increases in direct proportion to the number of cigarettes a person has smoked throughout their lifetime.

By the age of 50, skin takes up to six weeks to renew itself. Lines become more pronounced and grooves appear running between the nose to the mouth, particularly in smokers. During menopause, women produce less oestrogen and skin becomes thinner and less flexible. It starts to sag at the cheeks as the elastin fibres and collagen in the middle layer of skin dries and shrinks and fat deposits concentrate under the eyes, chin and earlobes. As muscle tone is lost, the face can take on a droopy appearance and the jowls may sag, creating a double chin.

Collagen also supports the tiny blood vessels in the skin, but because your skin is thinner and blood flow is decreased, small injuries cause bleeding which forms tiny bruises and mottled discolorations, and since cell repair is so slow, healing takes much longer. Thread veins and varicose veins can appear on the face, hands and legs and as melanin production decreases and oil-producing glands become less active, the skin on the hands and feet becomes thinner and more transparent, making these veins more visible.

Facial hair increases as a woman ages. Pubic and axillary hair decreases and head hair begins to lose its pigment at the roots and gradually goes grey. Eyebrows also go grey and eyelashes begin to disappear. The outer surface of the eye (cornea) may develop a gray-white ring while the colored portion of the eye (iris) loses pigment, giving very elderly people grayish or light blue eyes.

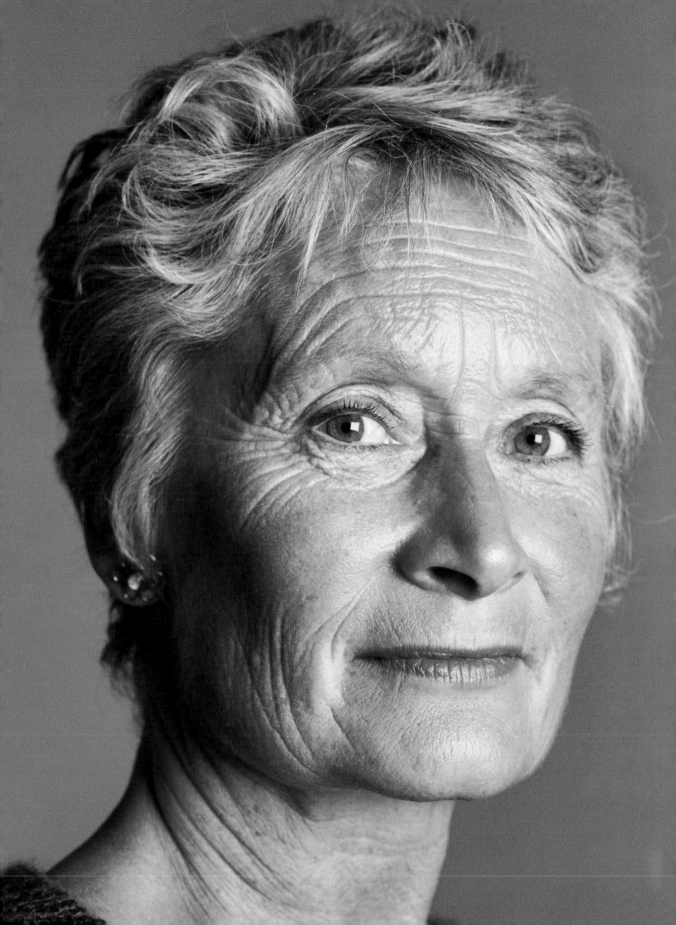

Photoageing

DEAD FASHIONABLE Though a golden tan has been considered a fundamental fashion accessory since the 1920s, the sun's impact on the skin hasn't always been appreciated. In ancient Greece and Rome, a tan indicated a life of poverty and outdoor labour so ladies preserved their pale complexions by staying indoors and whitening their faces with a deadly cocktail of carbonate hydroxide and lead oxide. By the mid-10th century, arsenic was the preferred, though equally deadly, skin whitener and, during the reign of Queen Elizabeth 1, women began painting thin blue lines on their whitened foreheads to give their skin a translucent look (unfortunately if they sat too close to the fire they quickly 'lost face' as their make-up melted). In France, fake beauty spots emphasized pale skin and in 19th-century America no young lady would venture outside without a parasol. All this changed when Josephine Baker and Coco Chanel made skin colour cool. As fashions through the 20s and 30s became more revealing and sunbathing and swimming became acceptable pastimes for women, darker complexions became *de rigueur*. In an extraordinary about turn, tanned skin, once a sign of poverty, was transformed into a symbol of wealth and leisure, because only the rich could afford to holiday, while the working class slaved away inside factories.

EARLY WARNING SYSTEMS Growing awareness that burning damaged the skin led to the introduction of the sun protection factor (SPF) sunscreen system in 1979. By 1985, the American Academy of Dermatology (AAD) had begun an educational campaign to warn the public about the dangers of sun exposure; and in 1988, the AAD held a major conference on photoageing and photo damage. Their conclusion was that, 'there is no safe way to tan'. Dermatologists now say that, bar smoking, most of the visible signs of ageing, such as wrinkles and thin, dry skin, are a direct result of largely preventable sun damage, 80% of which occurs before the age of 18 years.

SUNBURN Tanning is caused when UV rays in sunlight trigger melanocyte cells in the skin to produce melanin, a dark pigment that builds up a protective barrier against the sun in the surface of the skin by turning it brown over a period of about five to seven days. Sunburn occurs when UV rays burn the skin. The effect is similar to burning yourself with steam or very hot oil. The blood vessels swell and, as cells are damaged, your skin cracks or forms small blisters, which then burst and layers of skin peel off. Every time your skin becomes burnt, you damage your skin cells and your DNA. Some cells die and some repair themselves by getting rid of the damaged DNA, but UV light lowers the body's immune system and makes it less capable of destroying defective cells. In some cases, defective cells grow into cancerous tumours or melanomas, a formation of dark-pigmented malignant moles or tumours, which can appear suddenly, with no warning. Melanomas can develop from or around moles and can occur anywhere on the body but are most frequently found on the upper back and legs. You should be aware of unusual changes in size or colour of moles or birthmarks, dark or irregular growths or spots, bleeding around birthmarks, the spread of pigment into the surrounding skin, itchiness, tenderness or pain in the surrounding area.

SKIN CANCER Warnings about the sun's dangers have been no match for the lure of cheap package holidays to hot destinations and the number of people chasing a two-week tan continues to escalate. Because skin cancer takes 10–30 years to develop, the conditions doctors are currently treating probably date back to the 1970s and since the fashion for tanning hasn't let up since the invention of the bikini, the situation is likely to get a lot worse.

65% of melanomas and 90% of basal and squamous cell skin cancers are attributed to UV exposure and the rate at which skin cancer is being diagnosed doubles every ten years. There are over 69,000 new cases of skin cancer each year in the UK. Of these, 6000 are malignant melanomas and 1,500 will result in death. The problem is obviously more severe in hotter climates, however half of all Australians develop skin cancer at some point, and one of every three cancers now diagnosed in the US is an entirely preventable form of skin cancer. Darker skinned people have a more even spread of melanin in their skin which gives them more protection and, consequently, they have a much lower incidence of skin cancer but even in relatively sun-free countries like Britain, it can take as little as half an hour to get sunburnt. Although surveys show that 90% of the population are aware of the risks associated with sunbathing, three-quarters of young women still actively seek a suntan every year. And the other quarter probably would if they could afford it.

UVA AND UVB RAYS Physicists classify UV light acccording to wavelengths: UVA, UVB and UVC. The shorter the wavelength, the greater the energy level of the light and the more damage it can do. UVC, which has a very short wavelength, is completely absorbed by the ozone layer before it reaches the ground, but the longer wavelengths of UVB and UVA pass right through the atmosphere, even on cloudy days, causing sunburn. UVB rays are the main cause of sunburn and skin cancer but they cannot pass through glass and the molecules in sunscreens are very effective at protecting the skin from them. In the past, UVA rays were thought to be less harmful than UVB rays, which is why sunbeds – which produce 99% UVA and 1% UVB rays – were once promoted as a safe tanning method. However, UVA is now known to be just as damaging as UVB because, although the rays are milder than UVB, they penetrate deeper through the skin's layers, pass through glass and, unknown to most consumers, the majority of SPF

I don't feel I have to look extremely tanned, although my husband wants me to look tanned! I have fair skin, so I have always tried to protect my skin, but I have experienced sunburn, and it is very painful. Sometimes I use facial tanners because I think it is a brilliant way to look fresh. Over the last few years I have used a Dior product, which I think works very well.
Line, 33, Norway

As a small child at a Brownie picnic in Australia I got so sunburnt and I had blisters on my shoulders, but I have not sunbathed since I was 13. In Australia those were the days of using baby oil instead of sunblock. Now whenever I am out in the sun. I never use less than Factor 20.
Joy, 39, Aus

Living in Ireland where the sun doesn't shine much and the winters drag on makes using a sunbed a necessity sometimes. When it is dull and grey and cold I feel that I need a blast of heat. There is no doubt that a ten-minute sunbed session lifts my spirits.
Ellen, 28, Ireland

sunscreens offer no protection against them. Dermalogica Full Spectrum Block SPF 15 protects against UVA, UVB and infrared rays, and contains soothing herbal extracts and skin-conditioning Vitamins A, C and E. Dermalogica Full Spectrum Wipes SPF 15 protect against UVA, UVB and infrared rays. Individually wrapped towels come in packs of 15 so you can slip them in your handbag.

SUNBEDS Studies now show that the artificial UVA rays in tanning booths may be as much as 20 times stronger than natural sunlight. In fact, just ten trips to a sunbed per year increases your likelihood of developing skin cancer by 700%. Unprotected exposure to UVA rays creates inflammation, abnormal cell production, skin thinning and the deterioration of elastin. Furthermore, because people with a base tan from a sunbed believe that they won't burn when they go in the sun they are statistically less likely to wear a sunblock. Though various bodies have tried to publicize the dangers of sunbed use, the message just doesn't seem to be getting through. In the UK about 800,000 people had at least one sunbed session in the last year and most of them were women aged 16–24 years. The sunbed industry is still relatively young but there are already several known cases of early skin cancer in sunbed users and health experts believe that this is just the tip of the iceberg. As a result, they are now debating whether sunbeds should simply be banned completely.

SUNSCREENS To be effective, sunscreens must protect skin from both the sun's UVA and UVB radiation. There are only three approved ingredients that protect across the full UV range: titanium dioxide, zinc oxide and avobenzone (also called parsol 1789 and butyl methoxydibenzoylmethane). Outside of the US, mexoryl SX is also used.

Sunscreens that protect against both kinds of rays are often labelled as 'broad spectrum' sunscreens, but unless a sun lotion contains one of the ingredients listed above, the SPF number on sunscreens relates only to UVB exposure. And although an SPF of 30 might suggest that it provides double the protection of an SPF 15, this isn't the case. Sunscreens with SPFs above 15 only provide 2–3% more protection than those with lower SPFs and, since they are likely to contain high concentrations of active ingredients, they can cause rashes in people with sensitive skin. People with sensitive skin are better off applying a lower SPF more frequently than using a very high factor. Studies show that the public under-applies sunscreens by as much as half of the recommended amount and recent research suggests that overall, sunscreen use is actually dropping rather than increasing. All sunscreens are only active for two hours from application and should never be used to prolong the time you spend in the sun. Re-apply after swimming, sweating or towel drying.

The future is bright, the future is orange'ish'

YOU'VE BEEN MELANOTANGO'D Researchers at the University of Arizona have developed a drug that boosts tanning by speeding up the rate at which skin darkens when exposed to sunlight. In tests, subjects who were injected with Melanotan-1, a synthetic version of the hormone that stimulates the the release of melanin in skin cells, needed half as much tanning time to go brown. Though a commercial product is a long way off and experts acknowledge that it is unlikely to stop people spending the day at the beach, it is hoped that a tan accelerator might at least discourage sun bed users from over exposure.

TANNERS' LIB Five years ago just 28% of women aged 18–24 and 9% of women aged 25+ used fake tan on a regular basis. Since then there has been a dramatic improvement in products for home and salon use. Easier application and faster drying times mean that fake tans now provide a realistic, accessible and affordable alternative to the real thing and sales reflect this. Around the globe a bottle of San Tropez fake tan sells every 10 seconds and in a 2003 study of 2000 British women aged between 16-65 three quarters said having a tan made them feel better and over half admitted to using fake tan.

ACTIVE INGREDIENTS Most self tanners (and tan extenders) contain dihydroxyacetone (DHA), a chemical that is refined from sugar cane. It was discovered to be an effective temporary skin-colouring agent back in the 1920s and has been in use ever since. It works by reacting with the protein keratin to produce a brown colouring in the top layer of your skin. Erythrulose, a natural keto-sugar, is used in combination with dihydroxyacetone (DHA) to prevent streaking and create a deeper, more uniform and natural tan. Since the outer layers of skin are continually being replaced, fake tans only last about a week but unlike true tanning, it is a completely safe process. New and better products continually appear on the market but it is always a good idea to do a patch test before you buy tanners because people with sensitive skin can find that they react to certain ingredients.

TAN ACCELERATORS Available as tanning pills or lotions. These preparations contain the chemicals psoralens and tyrosine. There is no evidence that they have any effect and, when applied to the skin, tan accelerator products can cause painful conditions, including blistering. When taken by mouth, possible side effects include nausea, headaches and itchy skin. Using tan accelerators over a long period of time has also been associated with an increased risk of skin cancer.

GOOD BODY TANNERS St Tropez Whipped Bronze Self Tanning Gel or mousse gives the longest lasting and deepest tan. The gel is less drying on your skin than the mousse, though both contain aloe leaf juice and AHA ingredients. The

I love lying in the sun. It makes me feel charged. I am aware of the risks so I always use sunblock, even in winter, but I just need it. In winter I use sunbeds though I don't use sunblock when I use them. Maybe I should.
Lucy, 34, England

If I use fake tan, I end up looking like Tango man. I just don't have the knack and end up looking particularly orange and streaky!
Kellie, 30, UK

When I was younger I bought a bottle of tan tablets because I thought that it would be a good way of getting a tan but then someone told me that they dye your insides and that if you are taking them and you are pregnant, you give birth to an orange baby.
Sophie, 31, UK

I try and avoid sun exposure where possible. It's a combination of pure vanity and a skin condition called vitiligo, which I think may have been triggered by getting terribly sunburnt when I was 12 years old. I am also pretty good at applying fake tan and use factor 30 on my face and hands when in the sun. The rest of me stays covered up.
Lucy, 34, UK

product range includes extras like barrier creams, but moisturizer or vaseline works just as well. It can be used on the face and body and because it is chocolate coloured you can see where you are applying it though you need to use latex gloves to ensure that it doesn't stain your hands.

APPLYING FAKE TAN TO THE BODY Use a body scrub over your whole body to exfoliate your skin. Then rinse, dry and moisturize your skin. It is best not to apply tanner to warm skin so give your body time to cool down. Sweating can alter the chemical composition of the tanning agent and ruin the colour so apply the tan in a cool rather than steamy room. Before application, lightly cover any areas of drier, more absorbent or whiter skin such as knees, toes, ankles, heels, inner arms and elbows, with an additional layer of moisturizer. Once you have done this, put a surgical glove on each hand and rub a large squirt of tanning cream between your two hands to warm it up slightly.

Apply the tanner in regular movements making sure you achieve an even coverage and try to avoid tide marks. Don't forget to do the sides and back of your neck, up behind the backs of your ears, the sides of your waist, your underarms, inner thighs and backs of your knees and, if possible, get someone else to do your back. If some areas, like elbows, look slightly dark, wipe them with a little damp cotton wool or rub in some additional moisturizer to dilute the product.

If you want a darker tan, it is best to do two coats of a medium colour rather than one coat of a deep tan. Wait at least four hours after the first application, then wash off the first coat and apply the second coat. The longer you leave the tan on before showering, the better the result will be. If you can, put the tan on at night and then sleep in old pyjamas and wash it off the next morning. If you find you have streaks after your self-tan is absorbed, rub them with half a lemon or scrub them with an exfoliating brush. Keeping your skin moisturized will prolong your fake tan, but shaving your legs or exfoliating may cause streaking. Most fake tans will last between four and seven days, though if you swim or bathe more frequently, they will fade more quickly.

GOOD FACIAL TANNERS Dermalogica's Protective Self Tan delivers a natural, golden colour and also contains SPF 15 and antioxidant vitamins to protect against UV rays. Essential fruit oils and extracts provide a pleasant, light scent. Because Dermalogica is not coloured it is not as easy to see where you have applied it, but on the plus side it does not block your pores in the same way that coloured tanners do. Lancôme Flash Bronzer contains tinted pigment, which gives an instant sun-kissed look and is designed for darker skins. The colour then builds up gradually underneath so that by the time you wash your face you have a natural tan. Again, it can make your face look a bit dirty if you over apply it, and you need to make sure you exfoliate at night. Clarins Facial Self Tanners are very effective and, unlike most fake tan products, they contain an SPF 15. However, although the facial tanner says it is non-comedogenic, i.e. it doesn't block pores, all facial tanners have a tendency to collect in pores. You can overcome this by using an exfoliant once the colour has developed. It means you have to use the tanner more often.

APPLYING FACIAL TANNERS Keep your hair off your face and remove jewellery. Exfoliate your face, apply a thin layer of moisturizer and wait about half an hour till you cool down. Brush vaseline or moisturizer over your eyebrows to stop the tanner discolouring the brows and the skin underneath. Use latex gloves to protect your hands and dot the tanner around your face, neck and upper chest. Don't forget to do the back of your neck and behind your ears. Rub the tanner in circular movements and be careful when you do your eyelids and below your eyes. If you add a little moisturizer, the tanner will blend more easily. Afterwards, use a damp cottonbud to remove the tanner and vaseline from your eyebrows. Take a 'less is more' approach to facial tanner. You can always apply a second coat if you don't feel the colour is dark enough.

SALON TANS Most salons offer professional fake tan application which include a great full body exfoliation, followed by a shower and a tan application. You look like you have fallen in a puddle of mud afterwards so if you have a hot date out, ask the beautician to use a non-tinted tanner such as Dermalogica on your face. Make sure that your beautician does your whole bottom, including the crack of your cheeks.

SPRAY-ON TANS A hot favourite with celebs like Jennifer Aniston, the latest tanning methods involve standing in a booth and getting sprayed with either an airbrush or moving jets of tan. The entire procedure takes between sixty seconds and five minutes and the results are absolutely fantastic. As with any fake tan the results will only last about a week. If you are being airbrushed your beautician should add some extra spray to your cheekbones to make that area a little darker and more defined.

A WORD OF CAUTION Statistically, women who use fake tans are twice as likely to get sunburnt because they wrongly assume that a fake tan serves as a base tan and protects them from UV rays. They also suffer from the misapprehension that if they apply a tanner containing an SPF, the protection will last as long as the tan is applied. It wont. An SPF is only active for two hours after a tan is applied.

I got burnt when I was younger and now suffer the consequences but I have discovered fake tan and beach umbrellas! Ella Bache – thank you. I wear factor 30+ every day but I worry about skin cancer. Living in Oz I just keep my fingers crossed.
Kirsty, 35, Aus

I don't lie in the sun a lot. I am very aware of the risks – especially when I see what years of sun worshipping have done to women from older generations. However, I still like a healthy glow so I use fake tan in the summer and when I go on holiday. I got badly burnt on holiday even though I had a high factor on. It's so easy to overdo it – by the time you realise you are going pink, it's already too late and the damage is done. Then I spend days worrying about the consequences. I have fair skin so after I've peeled I just go white again – it's pointless really.
Kari, 27, UK

My top tip for fake tanning is apply it every three days so that you build up a base colour. Then, when you overlay the next layer, you don't get any streaks.
Lois, 36, UK

Facial exercises

PREVENTION IS CHEAPER THAN CURE Fans of facial exercises claim that they prevent wrinkles forming by toning up the muscles in the face. Others argue that overuse of the muscles in the face is precisely what causes wrinkles in the first place. Though normal daily expressions put our faces through a range of movements, facial exercises concentrate on working the muscles that are ignored in normal day-to-day facial use. There is no scientific evidence that they work, they take a long time to show any results and doing them for ten minutes every day requires a degree of discipline that eludes most of us. However women who are concerned about specific features, e.g. a double chin, would obviously be well advised to take facial exercises seriously before resorting to the pain and expense of surgery (p.229). Though you will look pretty goofy, doing these exercises in front of a mirror will help you too see which muscles you are working.

FOR FACE AND NECK Touch the corners of your mouth with your index and middle fingers. Holding your back teeth lightly together, part your lips and smile as wide as you can. Try and feel the muscle lifting, hold for a count of six and don't squint. Repeat five times.

FOR SAGGY JOWLS Pull your bottom lip up over your top lip. Press your tongue against the back of your lower teeth. Your mouth turns down and you will feel a tightening in your lower jaw and throat. Hold for five seconds, release and repeat five times. Next, tilt your head back, looking at the ceiling, lips closed and relaxed. Stick your tongue out as if you were trying to touch your chin with the tip of your tongue. Hold for ten counts.

CRÊPE NECK AND DOUBLE CHIN Put your bottom teeth in front of your top teeth as far as you can. Smile and chew for 60 bites. Then tilt your head back, looking at the ceiling, lips closed and relaxed. Pucker your lips together in a kiss and stretch, as if you were trying to kiss the ceiling. Keep your lips puckered for ten counts, then relax and bring your head back to normal. Repeat five times.

LOWER JAW AND CHEEK MUSCLES Keep your teeth and lips closed and puff air into the side of your mouth, inflating your left cheek side and hold for ten, then puff air into your right cheek and hold for ten; puff air under your lower lip and hold for ten; puff air under your top lip and hold for ten. Repeat five times.

FOREHEAD Lie on a bed with your head hanging over the edge. Lift your eyebrows as high as possible, with your eyes opening very wide. Relax and repeat ten times. Place your thumb and index finger above your eyebrows and stretch the skin away from your eyes. Close your eyes, relax your face and hold for 30 seconds.

LIPS Sit upright, lips closed and teeth together. Smile as broadly as possible, without opening your lips and hold for five counts. Then relax. Pucker your lips into a pointed kiss. Hold for five counts and relax – repeat ten times. Sit relaxed with lips hardly opened and curl your lips outwards. While your lips are in the outward position, move your curled top lip towards your nose. Hold in this position for ten counts and repeat five times.

FOR THE UPPER EYELIDS Looking in the mirror, curve your index finger over your eyebrow holding it against the bone. Raise your eyebrows slightly over the bone and close your eyelids, feeling a gentle stretch. Repeat six times on each side.

FOR THE LOWER EYELIDS Stand with your eyes closed and without opening them, look upwards as far as you can and then downwards. Repeat ten times. Stand looking ahead with eyes open. Look up and then down, while keeping your head still. Repeat ten times. Then repeat the sequence with your eyes both closed and open, but look left and right.

EXERCISES TO IMPROVE VISION Your eyesight gets worse as you age because the muscles in the eye lose strength and your lenses lose elasticity. As focusing becomes more difficult, your eyes can get tired more easily and this can lead to headaches and eye strain. The following excercises help to maintain vision and strengthen focus. They may also delay the onset of near-sightedness, a condition that commonly affects women in their mid- to late 40s making it difficult to read small print without reading glasses. Before beginning, put two chamomile teabags in a cup of hot, not boiling, water

AROUND THE CLOCK Stand in front of a mirror with your back straight. Stare straight ahead and slowly rotate your eyes clockwise around a complete circle two or three times. Then repeat the process in the opposite direction. Next, look from north to south three times, and east to west three times. Then repeat the sequence starting from south and west.

EXERCISES TO IMPROVE FOCUS Stand about 180cm (6ft) away from the mirror. Hold one finger out in front of you pointing towards the ceiling. Focus on your actual finger, then focus on your finger in the mirror. Alternate your gaze between the two fields of vision for a minute or more.

RELAXING THE EYES After doing the exercises, wring out the teabags, lie down and cover your eyes with the warm chamomile infusion.

When my mother was 40 I thought she was over the hill. Now I am 40 myself and I feel like I am only just starting to become an adult. I think it is terrifying that I and so many of my friends seem to be so juvenile in comparison to how our parents were at the same age. At 40 my mother had an 18-year-old and a 16-year-old. I had my first child a year ago and may now have left it too late to have another. I was too busy with my career and having fun to settle down, and having kids was something I kept putting off. I just felt I was too young, and I believe I look young too, at least younger than my mother did at my age. However, that may also be to do with fashion and the fact that I have more time and more money to spend on my appearance than she did.
Ros, 40, UK

I have been doing facial exercises for about two years now and I do think that my face has better muscle tone than it had before I started though the difference is not terribly dramatic. I do my routine at my desk in work so I don't usually miss it.
Angela, 46, UK

The wrinkle diet

Dr Nicholas Perricone, MD, author of *The Wrinkle Cure* and *The Perricone Prescription*, believes that diet and supplements are the key to great skin and good health. Perricone says sugar is responsible for up to 50% of ageing and suggests that the rapid increase in blood sugar that occurs after eating starch triggers the inflammation that makes skin look puffy. According to Perricone, sugar also creates chemicals in the body that attach to collagen in the skin, reducing elasticity and causing sagging and wrinkling.

The Perricone diet essentially follows the glycaemic index principles (p.38). The diet avoids foods that are high in sugar (such as cereals with processed sugar, corn, fruit juices and raw sugar), and since pasta, white rice, white bread, and potatoes are also rapidly converted from carbohydrates into sugar in the body, they are off the list of acceptable foods too. Instead, Perricone suggests that women concentrate on low-sugar foods such as asparagus, beans, broccoli, citrus fruits, leafy greens, peaches, plums and spinach.

Perricone also believes that in a mistaken attempt to control weight, women eat too little protein and that this is one of the primary reasons that their skin ages faster. Protein provides cells with amino acids, the building blocks needed to repair damage by free radicals, so Perricone concludes that a diet high in protein and omega-3 and omega-6 fatty acids will repair skin cells, make your skin clearer and less puffy, and increase your skin tone. Perricone strongly recommends that women should up their protein intake to 60g (2¼oz)/day, but although the diet does include low fat dairy products, beans, peas and poultry, it concentrates on cold-water fish such as salmon, mackerel, bass and trout, which are all excellent sources of both omega-3 and omega-6, both of which are anti-inflammatory agents.

Perricone's fish of choice is salmon, which contains a chemical called dimethylaminoethanol (DMAE). Perricone says that increasing DMAE intake strengthens the connection between nerves and muscles, automatically improving skin tone. As salmon is now a comparatively cheap and widely available source of protein, this diet doesn't have to be expensive, but in light of recent reports about the level of toxins in farmed salmon it is wiser to base this diet on wild or organic varieties, though this substantially increases the cost.

Women who can't afford, or can't stand fish, are advised to take a daily fish oil supplement to provide the omega-3 and omega-6 essential oils. However, a supplement will not give you the protein benefits, or co-enzyme Q-10 (a powerful antioxidant) (p.160), or any of the other nutrients which are contained in fresh fish.

The diet is relatively simple to follow and like all diet doctors, Perricone turns chef and provides a list of recipes. To be fair, his culinary offerings are simple to prepare and don't rely on ridiculous ingredients, so they are actually very manageable. The diet is mostly based on raw and fresh foods and there is very little planning or cooking required, which is a distinct advantage in any diet plan. The portions are small but because the same foods appear several times in the same day you won't waste much either. Perricone is keen that women drink plenty of water. This provides the double benefit of keeping you hydrated and making you feel full.

Arguably anyone who is eating a diet rich in fish, seeds and leafy green vegetables doesn't really require expensive pills on top. But Perricone is keen on supplements of antioxidants and anti-inflammatories, so he manufactures and sells Perricone-branded alpha lipoic, vitamins such as C ester and E, DMAE, conjugated linoleic acid (CLA), co-enzyme Q-10, borage oil (GLA), L-carnitine fumarate, L-tryosine, omega-3 and selenium. Perricone's books also provide lists of recommended beauty brands and cosmetic products.

According to Perricone, people of all ages and skin types can expect to see improvement in just three days on the diet. There is no doubt that eating plenty of fish will benefit your skin and, since it is also low in calories, chances are, anyone who sticks to it is likely to lose a few pounds too. (And losing a few pounds makes everyone look and feel younger, fitter and more attractive). Though Perricone's books are a touch too fond of pseudo-science, the wrinkle diet is generally a sensible and healthy programme that works on several levels, and testimonials suggest that it is a more successful method of improving skin and general health than other 'miracle' anti-ageing treatments.

A SAMPLE DIET DAY A typical day's diet might include: *On waking*: Drink 225ml (8fl oz) water and a further seven glasses during the course of the day. *Breakfast*: An egg-white omelette, a piece of grilled salmon, some oatmeal, cantaloupe melon and a handful of blueberries. *Lunch*: Grilled salmon or low sodium canned tuna in water or sardines in oil or broiled chicken with romaine lettuce dressed with lemon and extra virgin olive oil. Cantaloupe melon and blueberries for pudding. *Afternoon snack*: Small piece of grilled chicken breast with a tablespoon of unsalted hazelnuts and half a green apple. *Dinner*: Broiled salmon fillet with steamed asparagus, broccoli or spinach and a salad of romaine lettuce dressed with lemon juice and olive oil. Fresh cantaloupe and honeydew melon with a handful of blueberries for dessert. *Before bed*: A small amount of chicken or turkey breast with a dessertspoonful of almonds or olives and half a green pear or green apple.

I would like to try the wrinkle diet because it is quick. I think anyone can do a three-day diet and then, if they feel better, they can carry on. It is a good idea.
Bonnie, 25, UK

When I eat fish I literally feel it making me healthier. I don't know if it is my perception of it as health giving that makes me feel like that, but if I feel low or down or tired or toxic a big plate of sushi and sashimi makes me feel heaps better.
Andrea, 29, Aus

In my view, seeds are underestimated in our diet. If you think about it in evolutionary terms, seeds and nuts must have been a primary food source for early man and, in terms of growth, the seed is packed full of nutrition because it is designed to grow into a shoot. I snack on pumpkin and sunflower seeds during the day, sprinkle them on salads and put them in soups too.
Tara, 44, UK

My wrinkles always seem to look better the morning after I have been drunk. Don't ask me why. Maybe it is just that my eyesight is worse.
Dianne, 34, UK

Non-surgical, anti-ageing treatments

As little as ten years ago, women who wanted to turn back the clock, or at least stop it ticking for a while, had only one option. And it wasn't a particularly pleasant one. Surgical procedures have always been dangerous but, historically, cosmetic surgery results have been very disappointing too. Generations of women who opted for a full face lift at 50 found that after the procedure, they didn't look any younger, they just looked like they had had cosmetic surgery.

Although surgical techniques have improved considerably, the future of anti-ageing lies in the myriad of non-surgical treatments that aim to emulate the plump bouncy skin of Scarlet Johannson, rather than the scarily stretched paper thin skin of Anna Wintour or Joan Rivers. Most dermatologists and cosmetic surgeons agree that staying out of the sun and avoiding smoking are the best ways of maintaining good skin. But, failing that, they suggest that women who want to delay ageing are better off opting for earlier use of non-surgical, anti-ageing procedures than waiting for a full face lift at fifty. The new procedures are less invasive, they don't require general anaesthetics and they can be carried out quickly and safely in a doctor's office. As with any medical treatment, who carries out the procedure is of paramount importance. Make sure to check your surgeon's qualifications and don't get non-surgical, anti-ageing procedures anywhere other than a reputable treatment office. At the moment, a lot of injectables are given by nurses, but it is often safer if a doctor administers them.

The problem with the treatments is that they are currently very expensive and since most of the effects only last between three and six months, repeat injections can add up to several thousand pounds a year. This prohibitive and ongoing cost creates a divide between women who can afford to avoid ageing and those that can't, but in the future, drugs that can reproduce collagen or elastin fibres or creams such as Dimericine (which contains an enzyme that helps to repair DNA) will probably make current anti-ageing treatments look prehistoric and the market will become much more affordable and accessible.

For women who can currently afford them, anti-ageing treatments boost self-confidence. Women know that they are judged by their looks and as they have to present some physical self to the world, it might as well be a self that they feel comfortable and confident about. Every time a woman looks in a mirror she sees herself as she is, and feeling confident about her reflection is a critical part of her positive self-image. In a sense, anti-ageing treatments are really about preserving identity for the older woman who feels her face no longer fits her sense of self. It is not about trying to look 25-years-old, but a gesture of goodwill to the face she plans to inhabit for another 40 years.

Botox

FROM CHEMICAL WEAPON TO SECRET AGENT Botox is a poison (Botulinum toxin A), which acts specifically on nervous tissue. It is related to botulism, a severe form of food poisoning that can cause paralysis and is sometimes fatal. Botulinum toxins work by attaching themselves to nerve endings and blocking the signals that would normally tell your muscles to contract. In the early 80s, doctors began to experiment with very low doses of the toxin to treat muscle disorders such as uncontrollable eyelid spasms and misaligned eyes. The results were immediate and much more effective than medication so, in 1989, Botox received FDA approval to treat a limited number of medical conditions.

It was a Canadian eye surgeon who first noted that patients receiving treatment for eyelid spasms seemed to have fewer wrinkles and frown lines between their eyebrows and around their eyes. One can only hope that he was smart enough to buy shares in the manufacturer, Allergan Inc., because his discovery led to the development of the fastest growing and most hyped cosmetic treatment in the world. Allergan's sales increased from $25m in 1993 to $310m in 2001 and global sales of Botox totalled $200.8 million in the first six months of 2002.

The use of Botox to combat facial lines has increased by 1500% in the US over the past four years and although it is only approved to treat frown lines between the eyebrows, doctors routinely use the product on other areas of the face, such as the forehead, around the eyes, on the neck, on vertical lip lines and on chin dimpling. Doctors continue to explore the 'off-label' possibilities of Botox and many are successfully treating symptoms of Parkinson's disease, multiple sclerosis, cerebral palsy, urinary incontinence, stuttering, migraine headaches, back pain, excessive sweating and chest wrinkles. Botox has not been tested for use during pregnancy.

HOW IT WORKS Botox works on the face by paralysing the muscles involved in frowning and raising the eyebrows. Small doses of the toxin are injected directly into the target muscles and the toxin then travels to the junction between the nerve ending and the muscle and binds to the nerve ending. This stops the nerve releasing the chemical acetylcholine, which triggers muscle movement and contraction, and as the muscle can no longer contract, wrinkles gradually smooth out. When, for example, Botox is injected into the forehead the muscles cannot 'scrunch up' when you frown so the lines along your forehead temporarily disappear. Injections take effect about three days after treatment and last for 10–12 weeks, at which point the nerve ending breaks through the Botox binding to release acetylcholine and muscle action returns. With repeated treatments, atrophy or thinning of the muscles occurs, which produces longer lasting results, but this may prove to have negative implications in the future.

THE PROCEDURE Treatment usually takes less than ten minutes. Your doctor will ask you to frown and smile and will mark points on your face with a pen to indicate which muscles need to be injected. A thin needle is then used to inject the Botox. It stings slightly and some patients temporarily experience slight bruising, bleeding at the injection site or a burning sensation. You see initial results from the injection within three days, though full results appear within two weeks. A set of Botox injections costs about £250 and you need follow-up injections every three or four months or your wrinkles will return. Certain vitamins and medications can make you more prone to bruising if you are getting any form of injections, so avoid vitamin E and aspirin for ten days before treatment. Remain upright for a minimum of two hours following treatment to make sure that the Botox doesn't migrate to a different part of the face. Excessive smiling and frowning should be avoided for a few hours.

SIDE EFFECTS Though Botox has relatively few known side effects, when treatments are overdone they can leave the face devoid of expression (Hollywood directors and casting agents can't remember the last time they saw a woman frown). There is also concern that repeated use of Botox makes other muscles in the face overcompensate for lack of movement, giving rise to a whole different set of wrinkles. Some people have an adverse reaction to Botox though patch testing is not normally offered before treatment. The most common complaints are headache, respiratory infection, flu, droopy eyelids or eyebrows and nausea. Less frequent reactions (less than 3% of patients) include pain in the face, redness and muscle weakness. These reactions are generally temporary, but can last up to 12 weeks or as long as the effects of the Botox last.

FDA SCRUTINY Though scientists, doctors and the FDA stress that Botox is completely safe, there is little doubt that many people are apprehensive about the long-term effects of the Botox explosion. Because the product has been available as a cosmetic treatment for less than five years, there is concern that the Botox generation will arrive at 50, at best looking worse than they would have had they let time take its natural toll, at worst having permanently damaged their facial muscles. Last year, in an effort to reassure the public about the safety of Botox, Ella L. Toombs, MD, a former FDA director who helped to approve Botox in the US, emphasized the fact that drugs such as Botox, which are considered to be 'lifestyle enhancers' rather than 'lifesavers', actually fall under more intense FDA scrutiny than proposed treatments for serious conditions. It's an important point. Every product is examined for a benefit to risk ratio and while authorities might be willing to settle for some side effects with a drug that keeps people alive, they wouldn't approve products with side effects if the goal was purely cosmetic.

Botox is a treatment that has suffered more than its fair share of bad press but for me it has been a very positive experience. I have had a real thing about the way my mouth and chin drooped from the age of about 35 onwards. My chin was dimpled and I had lines all around my lower jaw that looked out of place really because the rest of my face didn't seem to have aged as badly. Anyway, Botox every three months has corrected the problem. My doctor simply gives me one botox injection in the middle of my chin along with the usual ones around my eyes and the combination seems to have completely altered the shape of my face. My chin does not dimple or sag anymore. My eyes still crinkle when I smile so no one really notices, but it makes a huge difference to the way I feel about myself.
Aqifa, 35, UK

I started doing Botox about three years ago and I have noticed that my skin seems thinner now. It is hard to say whether that is a natural sign of ageing, but I worry that it is Botox related.
Tamsin, 39, UK

BOTOX PARTIES Though Botox has an immaculate safety record to date, to maintain that record it is important that it continues to be administered by experienced and well-trained doctors or nurses. Though medical treatments can require higher doses, Botox for cosmetic purposes is used at the lowest dosage. Only one-tenth of a teaspoon of the toxin is injected into a muscle and a full treatment might only use half a syringe. Allergan packages Botox in 50mm vials for one-time use only and as it doesn't contain any preservatives, if the same vial is used to treat two or more patients it is impossible to guarantee that it is still sterile. Needless to say, the practice of sharing vials to avoid waste is already rife and the company is concerned that as more and more people demand the treatment, it will become increasingly difficult to monitor who is giving the injections, and how. The popularity of Botox parties, where groups of women club together to get discounted Botox injections while sipping champagne, is an accident waiting to happen. Not only is there a high risk of cross-contamination, but booze intensifies bruising and it can wash the toxin away from the target muscle, which renders the treatment ineffective at best, dangerous at worst.

DOSAGE REGULATIONS Because Botox is potentially lethal, appropriate dosage is critical. At the moment, scientists know how much Botox will kill a mouse but they have no parallel figures for humans. They are aware that sensitivity varies from person to person, but admit they don't fully understand the response curve in humans. Regulations require that the lowest effective dose should always be used and injections must be given no more frequently than 12 weeks apart, but unfortunately, wealthy women who are paranoid about their looks and used to getting their own way, often decide that three months is too long. In Mayfair, Manhattan and Melbourne it's not unusual for ladies who lunch to have two hairdressers, two fitness trainers and two Botox doctors. The fact that they are receiving twice the recommended amount of Botox will only concern them when someone comes up with a good reason as to why it's a bad idea

It is highly unlikely that Allergan, are ever going to do that. In September 2002, the US FDA ordered them to withdraw misleading advertisements that failed to mention that Botox is only a temporary cosmetic fix and cannot be used to treat all sorts of wrinkles. More crucially, they also forgot to mention that Botox is only approved for people aged between 18 and 65 years. Doubtless the manufacturers of Botox, and all those who pay for it, will also choose to ignore a recent study which found that 23% of all the patients who were seeking treatment with Botox at a dermatology clinic were suffering from body dysmorphic disorder (p.206) and psychotherapy was considered to be a more appropriate treatment for them. If you can frown, do it now.

Fillers that work

Fillers are used to plump up and contour wrinkles, smile lines, frown lines and sunken cheeks as well as to improve depressions resulting from injury, surgery, or certain types of scarring. Fillers last longer in larger areas that don't move much, so they can also be used to provide definition to the cheeks and the chin. If you are planning to have any injectable fillers, you should not take aspirin, blood thinners, anti-inflammatory drugs, vitamin E or alcohol in the week prior to your treatment as they may cause a reaction or slow the healing process.

BOVINE COLLAGEN Bovine collagen is a liquid gel made from the connective tissue of cows. It was approved as a cosmetic treatment by the FDA in 1981 and because it has been around for so long and has a much longer safety record than any of the newer fillers, it remains the standard against which all other dermal fillers are measured. Though BSE made many patients concerned about bovine collagen, the product is derived from the hides of isolated herds of domestic cattle so there is no risk of contamination. Around 3% of people are allergic to collagen that comes from cattle, so doctors perform a skin test two weeks before beginning the injection procedure. Any sign of redness, itching, swelling or illness should be reported to the doctor. If you display a reaction to bovine collagen, you won't be able to receive the injections because in rare cases it triggers anaphylactic shock, which can be fatal.

Injected collagen smooths out wrinkles and fills in furrows, such as those around your nose and mouth and between your eyebrows. The collagen gradually degrades and is absorbed into the body over a period of three to four months when treatment needs to be repeated. However, because the treatments trigger your body to increase your own collagen production, over time you may need fewer treatments. Collagen injections usually take about 20 minutes. After cleaning the skin and administering a local anaesthetic, the doctor will inject a mixture of collagen and lidocaine, a topical anaesthetic, into each wrinkle. Pain is minimal, as are side effects, though you will probably look red and swollen around the site of the injection and it can take 24 hours to look normal.

Any injection will cause redness and bruising but applying an ice pack to the area before and after the injection will compress the blood vessels. In particularly fair-skinned patients, this redness may persist for a week or more. Tiny scabs may also form over the needle-stick areas, though these generally heal quickly. No bandaging is needed and you are free to eat, drink and wear make-up with sunblock protection shortly thereafter. Because the anaesthetic agent lidocaine is mixed in with collagen, additional anaesthetic is usually not used. If you are especially sensitive, your doctor may use a topical anaesthetic or spray to numb the injected area.

I finally plucked up the courage to have collagen when I was about thirty. First I had to do a test to check that I didn't react badly and then I went back a few weeks later for the treatment. I didn't really think it would be a big deal because it was just in a beauty salon and it seemed a bit like having a facial, but when I saw the syringe I began to feel a bit nervous. I didn't expect it to hurt but it really did and I had tears in my eyes, particularly when she did delicate soft areas. They had told me that I would be able to go back to work afterwards but I had needle marks which were swollen into lumps all over my cheeks. I knew there was no way that I could go back to work so I had to pretend I was sick and go home.
Jo, 32, UK

About 18 months ago I noticed that every time I wore lipstick it bled into the fine lines around my lips. I had Perlane I think, and it worked incredibly well. I did look like I had two tyres around my mouth for a couple of days but once the swelling went down it looked great. I would give it a complete thumbs up.
Jill, 42, UK

There are three forms of collagen, Zyderm I, Zyderm I I· and Zyplast. *Zyderm I* is used for very fine or superficial lines but because the body absorbs so much of the product the doctor injects twice as much as is necessary to compensate for the absorption. *Zyderm II* is used for coarse lines, acne scars and lip augmentation. It has a higher concentration of collagen and is slower to re-absorb so there is less over-correction. *Zyplast* works on deeper furrows and contour defects, such as droopy nasolabial folds, heavy lipstick lines and significant lip augmentation. No over-correction is required.

FAT TRANSFER Fat transfer involves extracting fat cells from the patient's abdomen, thighs, buttocks or elsewhere and reinjecting them beneath the facial skin. In many ways it is safer than other filler options because there is little risk of your body rejecting its own fat cells but, as one patient who had her lips enlarged so elegantly put it, 'you do end up talking out of your ass'. The procedure differs from collagen injections in that much smaller amounts of fat are injected. If the procedure is carried out in conjunction with a liposuction operation, the patient will be sedated throughout. During liposuction your surgeon can harvest a much larger amount of fat, then freeze and store your fat for future injections when they become necessary.

Fat transfer is performed on an outpatient basis and can take up to two hours. Both the area from which the fat is taken and the treatment site are anaesthetized with a local anaesthetic. The doctor chooses a donor site where your fat is most tightly packed, such as your abdomen or your buttocks and withdraws fat with a syringe attached to a suction pump. Sometimes an adhesive bandage is applied over the injection site. Once removed, your fat is processed to remove excess fluids and then reinjected using another needle, which is placed just under your skin. This process may be repeated until the desired correction has been achieved.

Because fat needs to be injected with a larger needle it can be more painful than having collagen or hyaluronic injections. As with collagen, some 'overfilling' is necessary to allow for fat absorption in the weeks following treatment. When fat is used to fill sunken cheeks or to correct areas on the face other than lines, this over-correction of newly injected fat may temporarily make the face appear abnormally puffed out or swollen. There will be some swelling, bruising or redness in both the donor and recipient sites, though the severity of these symptoms depends upon the size and location of the area being treated.

After the injections you should stay out of the sun until the redness and bruising subsides – usually about 48 hours. In the meantime, you can use make-up with

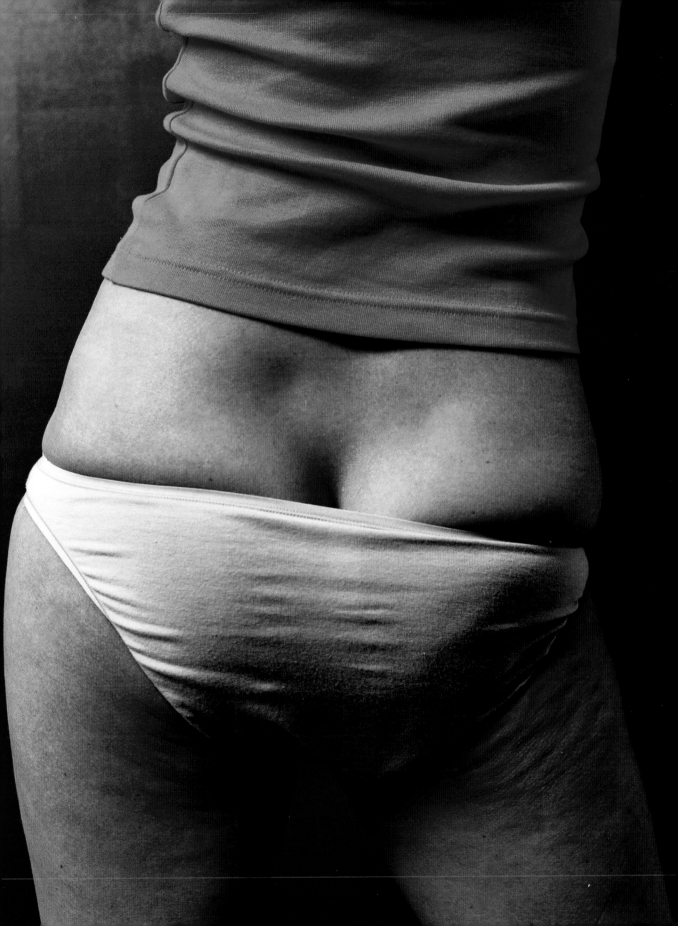

sunblock protection to help conceal your condition. The swelling and puffiness in the recipient site may last several weeks, especially if a large area was filled. Occasionally, the swelling never goes down and requires surgery and further treatments to rectify a 'trout pout'.

Your initial injection should last up to six months. Over the first few months, about 65% of the fat will be absorbed by your body. The remaining 35% will usually stay in place for years. For best results, fat transfer injections should be repeated every two to three months for the first year.

FIBRIL This is a relatively new technique. The filler is made from your own blood plasma, which is then mixed with a freeze-dried gelatin derived from connective pig tissue and a chemical to encourage the formation of new collagen. Although allergic reactions are fairly uncommon, skin testing before treatment is still necessary. The procedure usually lasts about 30 minutes. A thin needle is used to inject Fibril at several points along the site that's being treated. A local anaesthetic may be used, as the injections can be painful. After the procedure, you may experience moderate pain, swelling, redness and bruising. These side effects usually subside in a few days. The benefits of Fibril injections can last anywhere from eight months to two years. No allergy tests are need.

HYLAFORM GEL Hyaluronic acid is a polysaccharide found in the skin of all mammals, which can be refined and used as a cosmetic filler. Hylaform gel is a form of this acid, which is derived from the rooster combs of domestic fowl. It has become popular as a filler because it is reported to cause fewer allergic reactions and lasts longer than bovine collagen. Another significant advantage is that it is less likely to clump up under the skin and goes in more smoothly. Also, unlike other fillers, over-correction is not needed. Although Hylaform gel is widely used throughout the world for wrinkles, scars and lip augmentation, it only received FDA approval for use in the US in November 2003.

NEW-FILL This product has been available in Europe since 1999 but was only given FDA approval for use in the US in August 2004. New-fill is a polymer derived from naturally occurring lactic acid, which has been used for decades by the medical profession to form re-absorbable sutures inside the body and to carry out ligament repair. It is also completely inert, so it will not produce an adverse allergic reaction. It is distributed freeze-dried, can be stored at room temperature, and is reconstituted with sterile water. New-fill is injected either into the superficial dermis for treatment of wrinkles and acne scars or subdermally to treat sunken cheeks and hands, liposuction contour deformities and lip atrophy. The procedure takes about

20 minutes and has to be done twice for maximum effect but the results can last up to two years. Side effects may include the delayed appearance of small bumps under the skin in the treated area and some redness, bruising, or swelling.

NON-ANIMAL HYALURONIC ACIDS (NAHA) Most dermatologists believe that Restylane and Perlane are now the best fillers for women, particularly those who suffer from allergies. Although they have been used in Europe for some time, Restylane was only given FDA approval in the US in December 2003. Being hyaluronic acid derivatives, similar to Hylaform gel, Restylane and Perlane have less risk of clumping and go in more smoothly.

PERLANE Perlane is a more robust hyaluronic acid used to fill deep wrinkles or for shaping facial contours, such as the cheeks or chin or for increasing lip volume. Over-correction is not needed. Treatment lasts 6–12 months.

RESTYLANE This filler is not derived from an animal source and lasts longer than collagen. It is used to treat deeper wrinkles, scars and in lip augmentation. In a study involving 285 wrinkles treated in 113 patients, Restylane correction was noted to be 82% at three months and 33% at one year. Restylane Fine Line is a lighter product designed for thin, superficial lines around the eyes, mouth, forehead and smile lines. Treatments last between four to eight months.

FILLER SAFETY Fillers are generally pretty safe as long as you know you are not allergic to the substance being injected. It is important that the person who administers your injection is fully qualified and experienced and that all syringes and equipment are fully sterilized. Occasionally, superficial beading or lumping of skin occurs when fillers are used. It usually resolves by itself but, in serious cases, lancing the skin will express the excess material and correct the problem.

Though it is very unlikely, it is possible for the needle to be accidentally placed through a blood vessel during injection. This can affect blood circulation leading to temporary discoloration of the treated area, or in tissue death, which can lead to a scab or scar forming. Very occasionally, this can block blood flow and in one instance in 1981, a blood flow blockage caused loss of vision in a patient. As a result, injectable fillers such as collagen should be avoided close to the eyes.

Any discomfort should go within 24 hours, but if it doesn't, you should consult your doctor. Pain, redness or inflammation starting 24–72 hours after treatment may be a sign of allergy or bacterial infection and you may need to be put on a course of steroids or antibiotics.

I don't need to bother with anti-ageing treatments because apparently I have a special gene which slows down the rate at which I am ageing. I had cancer 12 years ago and during the course of my treatment I had a lot of complicated blood tests. Some time afterwards, when the results came back, my doctor said that on the tests to see how fast I was ageing he would have been happy to see a score of 12 given my medical history. He said 15 was generally an excellent score but I had actually scored 32. It didn't surprise me really because most of my family look very young for their age. My grandfather died at 94 and looked 60 and my father always looked very young too. My brother looks about 15 years younger than he really is and my aunt in Alaska is 85, still works a 40-hour week, has had nine children and only looks about 45 years old. It has made me feel much better. Despite the cancer, those results helped me to make lots of long-range plans about work. I went on a diet and did a TV series last year – not bad for a gal of 57 years.
Meredith, 57, UK

Fillers to avoid for now

ISOLAGEN Isolagen injections may be the fillers of the future but right now, the procedure is too complicated and the results are not significantly more effective than non-animal hyaluronic acids so the £2500 cost just isn't worth it. Dubbed 'grow-your-own facelift', by the media, Isolagen borrows techniques used in stem-cell (cells that have the unique ability to transform themselves into every type of body cell) research to provide patients with a long-lasting supply of their own collagen-producing fibroblast cells. The method does not yet have FDA approval in the US but it is available in Australia and the UK and has sparked controversy about a future where cells are harvested at birth from babies' umbilical cords and stored for cosmetic or therapeutic use later in life.

Isolagen requires taking a very tiny piece of your skin from behind the ear. The skin cells are placed in a tissue culture to stimulate them. Processing takes about eight weeks and then a test dose is sent back to the physician, which must be administered within 24 hours. Once the sample has been given, if there is no reaction after two weeks, the stimulated collagen cells will be reinjected into your wrinkles to create more collagen. A skin sample and the first three injections have been shown to give improvement for up to 22 months but it can take four to six months for the results to be noticeable.

SILICONE Silicone is not approved for use in the US though it is used in the UK. Because it has a history of migrating from the site of injection and ulcerating, it isn't particularly stable and it is unclear whether injectable silicone poses the same autoimmune problems as silicone implants. Used correctly, it is an effective filler but the product has to be injected very very slowly. Tiny droplets have to be injected once a month over a period of six months. Although silicone injections will fix the injected wrinkles permanently, no one ever stops ageing and by the time you get the big ones sorted out, others have replaced them anyway.

HUMAN COLLAGEN Cosmoderm and Cosmoplast are similar to bovine collagen and last the same amount of time. They contain natural human collagen harvested from the cells of infant foreskins. Yes, that's right, infant foreskins. Say no more.

HUMAN INJECTABLE TISSUE Cymetra is an injectable mixture of donated cadaver skin. Yes, that's right. Dead human skin. A small plus is that because it comes from dead humans no allergy testing is required. A big minus is that the material is lumpy and viscous so a larger needle is required for injection, which means local or regional anaesthesia is required and it can be very painful. Also, results don't last any longer than collagen.

Chemical peels and dermabrasion

CHEMICAL PEELS Chemical peels have been used for the last 50 years to treat signs of skin ageing, such as discoloration, wrinkling, liver spots, scarring or acne. The chemicals burn the skin, which makes the outer layer peel off, revealing a fresher-looking layer of skin. Though wrinkles can be reduced or even eliminated, sags, bulges or more severe wrinkles do not respond well. Generally, fair-skinned patients are the best candidates for chemical peels. Anyone who has a chemical peel has to stay out of the sun and wear heavy sunblock constantly.

SAFETY Your doctor needs to know if you have any past history of unusual scarring tendencies, extensive x-rays on the face or recurring cold sores. In certain skin types, there is a risk of developing temporary or permanent colour change in the skin. Taking birth control pills, pregnancy or a family history of facial discoloration may increase the possibility of abnormal pigmentation. Although low, there is a risk of scarring in certain areas of the face and there is a small incidence of the reactivation of cold sores or herpes infection in patients with herpes. There are three different peel strengths.

SUPERFICIAL PEELS These need to be carried out once every couple of weeks over a period of months. The peel is usually made from either glycolic acid at 30–59% or Jessner's solution, which contains a mixture of acids used at 10–15 per cent. Superficial peeling usually involves redness, followed by scaling, which lasts between three and seven days.

MEDIUM PEELS These can be carried out once a year and involve glycolic acid used at 70% or trichloroacetic acid (TCA) at 35%. You should expect to look like a burns victim for about two weeks following a medium depth peel. On days one and two, your skin will be pink. On days three and four, your skin will darken, your face will be swollen and you will develop water blisters that will break, crust, turn brown and peel off over a period of 7–14 days. On day five, your skin begins to peel off and carries on peeling for up to five days.

DEEP PEELS These can only be done once in a lifetime and have pretty much been replaced by laser resurfacing because they take so long to recover from. They involve the use of powerful acids, phenol or TCA, and should only be carried out by very experienced surgeons because full sedation is required and patients have to be hooked up to a heart monitor. Your face will be bandaged for several days and it takes two to three weeks to recuperate. The skin looks red and raw for about three months and ends up looking much lighter in colour than the rest of the body. Peeling can cause skin thinning, enlarged pores, permanent sun sensitivity, discoloration and a bleached-out complexion. The new paleness may get rid of hard

My sister has exactly the same lines as me and she is 45, so we are going to look into doing something about it together. I am curious about non-invasive, anti-ageing treatments and I may investigate Botox, but I wouldn't have full plastic surgery. I have seen too many women who start to look alike. My hairdresser fills me in on which of my friends have had surgery but I can't tell by looking at them, which makes me think it is completely pointless. There is a certain type of New York socialite in her 60s or 70s that seems to look identical to every other New York socialite of the same age – skinny, frightened to smile in case their knees go up. I don't think I know enough about the options, but I am unlikely to go under the knife.
Annabel, 51, UK

I have been thinking of having Botox recently. Two friends of mine have been 'done' and I must admit it looks good. I would also like to try fillers as I have some deep lines around my mouth. I am a bit worried that if I start I won't stop and the cost is ok once or twice but not four times a year.
Tessa 51, UK

shadows under your eyes, but it may also mean you will need to wear tinted foundation every day. Peeling also creates a visible tide mark around the edge of the face so you will need to blend your make-up into the treated skin. A peel that is too deep can cause permanent skin damage.

DERMABRASION When dermabrasion was first developed, it was used predominantly to improve acne scars, chickenpox marks and scars resulting from accidents or disease. Today, it is also used to treat other skin conditions, such as pigmentation, wrinkles, sun damage, tattoos, age (liver) spots and certain types of skin lesions. Although this process is done with a local anaesthetic, it takes a long time to recover and should only be undertaken once every two years at most.

During dermabrasion, or surgical skin planing, the surgeon anaesthetizes the patient's skin, then a high-speed rotary instrument with an abrasive wheel studded with diamond particles mechanically removes, or 'sands', the surface to encourage the growth of new skin. Afterwards, the skin bleeds and crusts over, which is pretty disgusting but, generally, most people can resume normal activities within two weeks. Make-up can be used as a cover-up as soon as the crust is off but the pinkness takes 8–12 weeks to fade. Your surgeon will probably advise you to avoid any activities (such as ball sports) that could cause a bump to your face for at least two weeks. If you swim, stick to indoor pools to avoid sun and wind, and keep your face out of chlorinated water for at least four weeks. It will be at least three to four weeks before you can drink alcohol without experiencing a flush of redness. Above all, it's important to protect your skin from the sun until the pigment has completely returned to your skin – as long as 6–12 months. When the new skin appears, it generally has a smoother and refreshed appearance.

MICRO-DERMABRASION This is a milder form of dermabrasion. A small micro-dermabrasion machine bombards the skin with thousands of sterilized aluminium oxide crystals, then a vacuum suction pump removes the particles along with dirt and dislodged skin. The force at which the crystals are propelled determines the depth of the treatment.

There is a small risk of hyper-pigmentation and bleeding, but it is safe if done by a trained doctor. It should be done once a month maximum and is comparable to a light chemical peel. Several treatments are required and although it will probably improve your skin's circulation and unblock your pores, don't expect miracles – it is unlikely to do anything for your wrinkles. The treatment is not painful. Initially, you may feel a mild scratching sensation as the crystals make contact and redness may occur for 30 minutes to one day.

Lasers

Lasers have pretty much taken over from chemical peels because they are so much more effective. However, it is worth bearing in mind that they have not been used for long enough to determine the effects of repetitively reheating collagen so there is some concern that, over time, the use of lasers, particularly non-ablative lasers, could actually increase the ageing of the skin. Many women don't realize that the side effects of serious laser treatment are often worse and last longer than those of a peel or dermabrasion. Laser resurfacing doesn't cause charring, bleeding or whitening, as a strong peel can, but the skin scabs over and looks very inflamed (like a bad case of sunburn) for about three to four months afterwards. In the right hands, they can give great results with little or no scarring, but everyone's skin responds differently. And because they require great precision, it is essential that you find an expert practitioner who uses the latest equipment. One way of doing this is to find a surgeon who performs laser resurfacing at an accredited hospital. This at least ensures that the doctor has been reviewed by the institution's experts.

Lasers work by aiming a beam of amplified light at the skin. The colour and energy of the light is adjusted according to the blemish being removed. The heat from the laser doesn't actually burn the skin, because there's very little heat transfer involved. Instead, it vaporizes the skin surface by making the water inside the skin boil. During the process, the treated skin changes in a way that allows the doctor to wipe off the top layers with a wet gauze pad revealing new fresh skin underneath. On deeper blemishes, the laser will be passed several times over the same wrinkle, gradually smoothing it out. Selecting the right wavelength and pulse allows the laser to deliver energy faster than the surrounding tissues can conduct the heat, so they remain undamaged. But the small amount of heat that creeps into the underlying skin appears to slightly shrink the collagen, promoting the production of more collagen, giving the skin a tighter, smoother look. For superficial or medium resurfacing, the laser can be limited to the epidermis and papillary dermis, but several treatments may be required. For deeper resurfacing, the upper levels of the reticular dermis can also be removed. Laser treatments are usually performed with topical anaesthetic, though full face resurfacing is done under a general anaesthetic.

Lasers are generally safe if used correctly but they can cause burns, scarring and obvious lightening or darkening of the treated skin. Laser treatments can cause pigmentation changes to olive, brown or black skin. They are not advisable for women who have taken Accutane in the past 12–18 months; those prone to keloid scarring; women with active skin infection and women who have had herpes (unless they take a low dose of Acyclovir before and after treatment). And remember, new skin is not immune to the effects of ageing. In the months and years following laser treatment, natural facial movements will eventually cause any 'expression' lines to

I wish young women would realize how pointless all that anti-ageing stuff is. Don't they know that at some point they will have to give up because you can't fight it and then they will wonder why they threw so much money down the drain. They have pills and creams and injections for everything if you have enough money but when you get to my age you don't care what your skin looks like you care that your bones and your brain are intact. A very clever and beautiful lady I know is so badly crippled with arthritis. Three weeks ago she said I wish ... I said I know what you wish and it is up to the Almighty. She is coming out of rehabilitation but she has to have everyone looking after her. She can't eat or pick up a pencil by herself. A few weeks ago when I said my prayers I asked for the best for her. It is heart breaking when someone has a good brain but their body breaks down and beauty doesn't matter a damn then. You are really better off having senile dementia because the people who have it don't know what they are doing, unlike my friend.
Catherine, 78, UK

recur. You will need to wear sunscreen every day to protect your skin from sun damage and, if resurfacing was performed around the eyes, it's best to wear sunglasses with UVA and UVB 100% filters.

CARBON DIOXIDE LASERS (CO2) Sometimes called a 'laser peel', the CO_2 laser is most commonly used for full face resurfacing to minimize the appearance of fine lines around the mouth and the eyes, to remove scars or uneven pigmentation, and it can also be used to treat warts, shallow tumours and certain pre-cancerous conditions. Erbium(Er):YAG Laser, FeatherTouch and SilkTouch are attachments for CO_2 lasers, which have been designed specifically for skin resurfacing and to treat fine lines and wrinkles.

Total skin resurfacing can be done with local anaesthetic for sections of the face, or a general anaesthetic if you are having your whole face done. Treatment of the whole face takes around an hour and a half. When the imperfections are especially deep, your surgeon may recommend the resurfacing be performed in two or more stages. When the procedure is over, the resurfaced skin is treated with applications of protective creams and ointments until healing is complete. Some surgeons will apply a bandage to protect the healing skin for the first five to ten days.

You will be able to go home about four hours after the operation but your face will be red and swollen and you will need to take antihistamine tablets to calm down the irritation. Over the next eight to ten days, you will begin to look even worse with red, raw, weeping, peeling skin and a fat puffy face. During this phase of healing, it is very important that you don't pick the crusts off the treated area or scarring may result. After about two weeks you can begin to wear a bit of make-up, though your skin may be very sensitive. By the third week, residual swelling makes you temporarily completely wrinkle free. In the fourth week, your wrinkles will reappear, but your skin should continue to improve over the next few months.

NON-ABLATIVE LASERS Non-ablative or sub-surfacing lasers require little to no healing time. Instead of heating and removing the top skin tissue, these lasers bypass the surface of the skin and work beneath the surface layers to improve skin tone, minimize fine lines and encourage the growth of new collagen. Recovery times are much quicker and side effects are less serious. However, multiple sessions are required, and it can take several weeks for results to be seen. Anticipate a 20–30% improvement in the appearance of wrinkles and acne scars.

N-LITE (aka Cool Touch, Smooth Beam, Auira and Lyra Laser) In all these treatments, a hand-held laser gun shoots pulses of concentrated red light into the dermis, deep under the skin surface. The cells are briefly heated to 80°C, which causes them to start manufacturing new collagen. Just before the laser fires, the gun shoots a jet of freezing spray on the skin, which stops it burning and protects the sensitive nerve endings. Four to six treatments are given about six weeks apart. For best results, a top up treatment session should be repeated every 6–12 months after that. These treatments are good for removing fine lines from around the eyes and mouth and also act as a preventative measure to slow ageing effects. However, they will not banish laughter or frown lines, which are caused by muscle movement rather than collagen loss. The treatments work best for people in their 30s and 40s who have not yet lost too much collagen. The treatment helps combat the effects of sun, smoking, stress and neglect, and helps reduce acne, scars and stretch marks.

YELLOW LIGHT LASERS Pulsed yellow light is more precisely absorbed by haemoglobin than other colours, so these lasers are more effective in the treatment of blood vessel disorders, such as port wine stains, red birthmarks, enlarged blood vessels, rosacea, hemangiomas and red-nose syndrome. Certain yellow light lasers may also be used to treat stretch marks. They are a safe and effective option, which can be used on infants and children without anaesthetic.

GREEN LIGHT LASERS Green light lasers are used for the treatment of benign brown pigmented lesions, such as liver spots. Green light lasers are also used for the treatment of small blood vessels on the face and legs.

RUBY LASERS The red light spectrum is emitted in extremely short, high-energy pulses in a technique known as Q-switching. The Q-switched ruby laser system was initially used to remove tattoos, but is now commonly used to treat many brown pigmented lesions, such as freckles and liverspots.

TATTOO REMOVAL LASERS These lasers shatter the tattoo ink pigments without destroying the surrounding skin. The type of laser used generally depends upon the pigment colours. Professionally applied tattoos penetrate deeper layers of the skin at uniform levels. This allows dermatologists to remove broader areas of inked skin at the same depth. However some of the newer inks and pastels and homemade tattoos which are often applied with an uneven hand are more difficult to remove. In many cases, multiple treatments may be required.

IPL FACIAL (aka Fotofacial, Photorejuvenation Photofacial, EpiFacial) This uses a multitude of wavelengths at low energy. It is not very powerful but it is good for hyper-pigmentation, freckles, ruddiness, broken blood vessels, early sunspots, large pores, fine lines and lax skin. Treatment is once a month for four months.

If you are planning to get a tattoo, you should check with council authorities to see if the tattoo parlour and the tattooist are registered. The person who is tattooing has to hold a license from the local authorities. On a technical level you need to see examples of their skill. Some show photos but you cannot be sure that it is really their work so word of mouth is often best. Walk-in clientèle need to make sure that the artist can actually draw and that they have a sterilizing unit. You can usually tell if someone is any good. Awards don't mean much because they are rigged so you should go by instinct. If you are worried about whether you might want to lose your tattoo, you should get something small done to start and stick to lighter colours, which are easier to laser off. You should also think about positioning. The hands and neck are not usually a good idea. I know a guy who decided to really push the boat out. He tattooed himself solid black from top to bottom and then tattooed himself white again.
Leslie, 36, Chinese

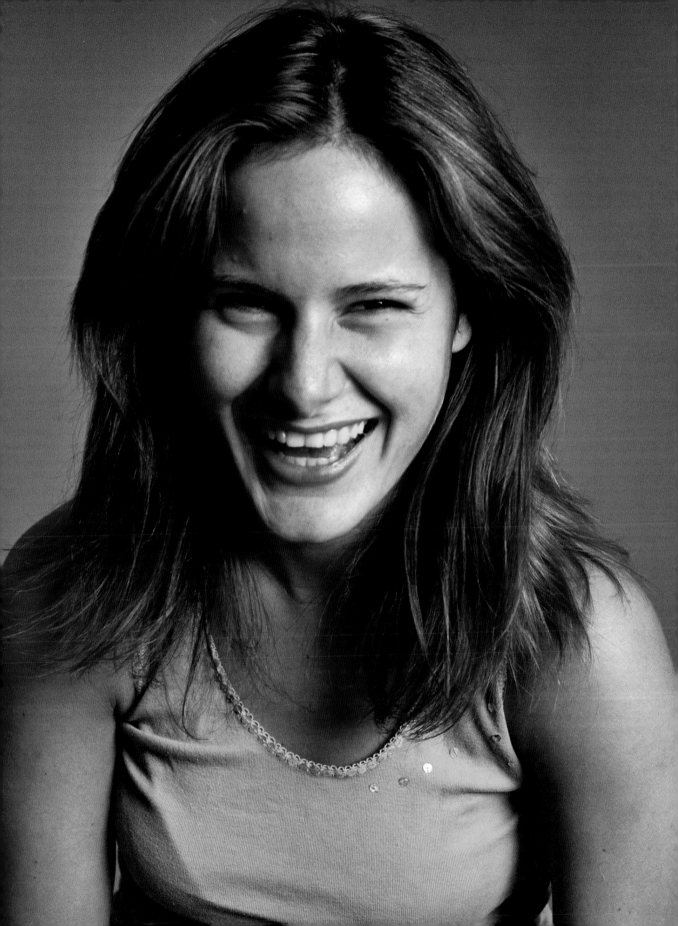

THE Cosmetic

SURGERY CHAPTER

From necessity to invention

Throughout history, the more reputable members of the medical profession have struggled with the moral contradictions of cosmetic as opposed to reconstructive surgery because the procedures appear to directly contravene the Hippocratic oath. Elective surgery on physically healthy patients who suffer from a disease that can only be called 'perceived ugliness' does not sit well with an oath that promises doctors will not put their patients' lives at risk unnecessarily. However since the early 1900s, for every principled surgeon preaching caution there has been a scalpel-wielding quack only too happy to promise the moon and charge the earth.

At the turn of the last century, youth and good looks had long established their social value, and the financial potential for anyone who could promise to extend or enhance either was enormous. Women willingly volunteered for painful cosmetic procedures, but the techniques were terribly primitive and completely untested and the results were often disastrous. Early practices such as the injection of paraffin into the breasts or nose lead to the development of hideous cancers and post mortems on women who had died following facial peels revealed large quantities of phenol having leached into their brains. However there was little sympathy for the early victims of botched cosmetic surgery. The medical profession – and society in general – took the view that any woman dumb enough to risk her health in the pursuit of physical perfection deserved what she got.

Surgical techniques improved dramatically during the First World War when reconstructive surgery saved the faces of thousands of young men who had sustained head injuries as tanks rolled over the trenches. The commitment and skill that went into restoring their appearance was a huge boost to the morale of disfigured soldiers who might otherwise have been prevented from getting jobs and fully re-entering society on their return from the front. The understanding that facial reconstruction was economically important to these men gave plastic surgery some new found credibility, though enhancing female appearance still had no medical or economic justification.

However, by the 1920s and 30s, the relatively recent science of psychology finally provided women who wanted it with the perfect excuse to have plastic surgery. Alfred Adler's 'inferiority complex' theory proposed that women and men who were severely lacking in confidence as a result of some perceived physical inadequacy (e.g. an enormous nose or a weak chin) were unable to live normal lives, because their low self-esteem made it difficult for them to socialize, find a partner, get married or get jobs. Because job or marriage prospects were adversely affected, doctors were then able to argue that the perceived physical imperfection or deformity was having a negative psychological and economic impact on the patient.

This suitably pseudo-scientific theory created the perfect hook on which to hang the practice of cosmetic surgery. By linking physical imperfection to psychological trauma, principled plastic surgeons were no longer restricted to pure reconstruction. They were absolved of their responsibility to the Hippocratic oath because cosmetic surgery had reinvented itself as 'psychiatry with a scalpel'.

As society became increasingly competitive, attitudes to cosmetic surgery continued to soften. Early 20th century advertising sold everything from vacuum cleaners to spot treatments by reinforcing the importance of making a good 'first impression' and 'getting on in life' became increasingly synonymous with physical self-improvement. If reconstructive surgery offered hope of normality and acceptability, cosmetic surgery promised all the advantages enjoyed by the 'beautiful people'. Beauty has always opened doors, particularly for women. Attractive females are more likely to find a husband, and according to a study by economists at the National Bureau of Economic Research in Massachusetts, they earn close to 6% more than average-looking individuals. At the opposite end of the spectrum, unattractive women (and men) get paid 9-25% less.

Not surprisingly, the socio-economic benefits of being beautiful create an undercurrent of dissatisfaction amongst more average-looking women who feel incapable of competing on a playing field that simply isn't level. And many have concluded that since they can't change the way the world works, they can only change themselves. Naturally, the cosmetic surgery industry is only too happy to help, and the industry has grown exponentially. However, there is now a glut of cosmetic surgeons and consultants and since they are all competing for the same business, prices have had to drop to allow the market to expand and accomodate them. 50 years ago most procedures were so prohibitively expensive that they were naturally restricted to the few who could afford them. Today, any woman who can afford to go on holiday can afford a facelift. In fact a recent UK study has shown that among working women, plastic surgery is the third most common reason for asking for a bank loan – behind buying a car or paying for a holiday.

As mass media continues to heighten female insecurity, TV programmes such as *Extreme Makeover, The Swan* and *Nip Tuck* continue to normalize surgical intervention. Their existence reflects the growing desire for, and acceptance of, cosmetic surgery, but the danger is that the more powerful the surgical promise becomes, the more faith women put in it. This chapter provides a thorough and realistic appraisal of the pain, the gain and the totally insane because although there is no doubt that cosmetic surgery has positive benefits for many women, for others it is simply a form of masochism rooted in insecurity.

It's easy to criticize women who have cosmetic surgery but for me it was the life changing experience I had hoped for. It was very painful and took much longer to recover from than I expected but the long-term rewards have been huge for me in terms of self-confidence. My face lift was a gift to myself.
Rose, 60, UK

I think cosmetic surgery sucks. Anyone who has unnecessary intrusive surgery must be raving mad. I had to have an operation because of a burst eardrum two years ago and it was a horrible experience. Don't people realize that anaesthetic itself is really bad for you, let alone surgery, recovery, the risk of infection, the risk of anything going wrong? With all the real illness in the world, I think it's an appalling waste of time, money and medical talent. If someone has suffered first-degree burns or something, fine. But surgery for the sake of surgery is stupid.
Caroline, 40, UK

In programmes like *Extreme Makeover* they make it look like all the procedures happen in a single day. In fact they take weeks, sometimes months.
Ellen, 37, UK

Things are not always what they seem

All I want is to get better, to feel good about myself and my life, but I just see ugliness staring back at me in the mirror, in my reflection in shop windows, in my sleep even. I hate meeting people. I try to remember that their first impressions of me are what count, but I'm constantly paranoid that when they look at me they see a monster. I hate myself. I can't even enjoy the odd moment of feeling better because I panic about when I'm gonna feel bad again. My arms and hands ache so much because I've been trying to pull the muscles on my face in an attempt to alter its shape. It's so pathetic, and I feel totally stupid saying it, but it's what I do. My parents are always asking me why my face has bruises on it, well like I'm gonna tell them the truth! They'll think I've totally flipped. This afternoon I was looking at my face and I've realized my jaw sticks out more on one side than the other; I'd always thought my face looked strange, but could never pin down exactly what was wrong with it; well now I know. My life's totally ruined. I just wanna sleep and sleep and sleep ...
Anon, 17, US

BODY DYSMORPHIC DISORDER (BDD) Many women seeking cosmetic surgery are actually suffering from a psychological illness which distorts their perception of what they look like. When most people think about body image they think about aspects of physical appearance. But body image also concerns the mental picture a woman has of herself. Negative body image alters perception, influences behaviour, impacts self-esteem and often causes difficulties in other areas, including sexuality, careers and relationships. For some women, negative body image is so severe that they develop 'cognitive distortions' and become abnormally preoccupied with a real or imagined defect in their physical appearance. Women with BDD may worry endlessly that their legs are too fat, their skin is too pale, their hair is too curly, their nose is too long, or their eyes are too small. And when others tell them they look fine, they don't believe it.

BDD affects approximately one in 50 people. It often starts in adolescence, possibly as a result of difficulty adjusting to physical change, but it is also very frequently found in children who have been bullied or who have high-achieving parents who have high expectations for their child. Like many people with eating disorders, BDD sufferers are often perfectionists, but although the vast majority of people with eating disorders are female, BDD appears to affect males and females equally. It can follow or be triggered by psychiatric problems and may be associated with a chemical imbalance in the brain, however it may also have a genetic basis because it occurs more frequently in families with a history of depression, anxiety or obsessive-compulsive disorders. Warning signs are: constant comparison of a perceived defect; camouflaging it with clothing, make-up, hats, or strange postures; seeking reassurance about it or attempting to convince others of its ugliness; avoiding mirrors; frequently touching it; picking the skin; measuring it; reading about it; avoiding social situations in which it might be exposed; feeling anxious and self-conscious around other people because of it; seeking cosmetic, amputative, dermatological or other medical treatment against doctors' advice.

BDD is often mis-diagnosed because doctors don't know much about it, but awareness is growing, particularly in the cosmetic surgery industry. In 2003 a woman in New York filed a malpractice suit against surgeons who failed to recognize that her mental state made her unfit to consent to more than 100 cosmetic operations. However studies show that cosmetic surgeons still don't discourage patients from seeking unnecessary surgery as much as they should and as a result, thousands of women undergo surgery that will not have the desired effect because they are taking a surgical approach to a psychological problem. The only treatment for BDD which has demonstrated any evidence of effectiveness is cognitive behavioural therapy carried out in conjuction with anti-depressant medication.

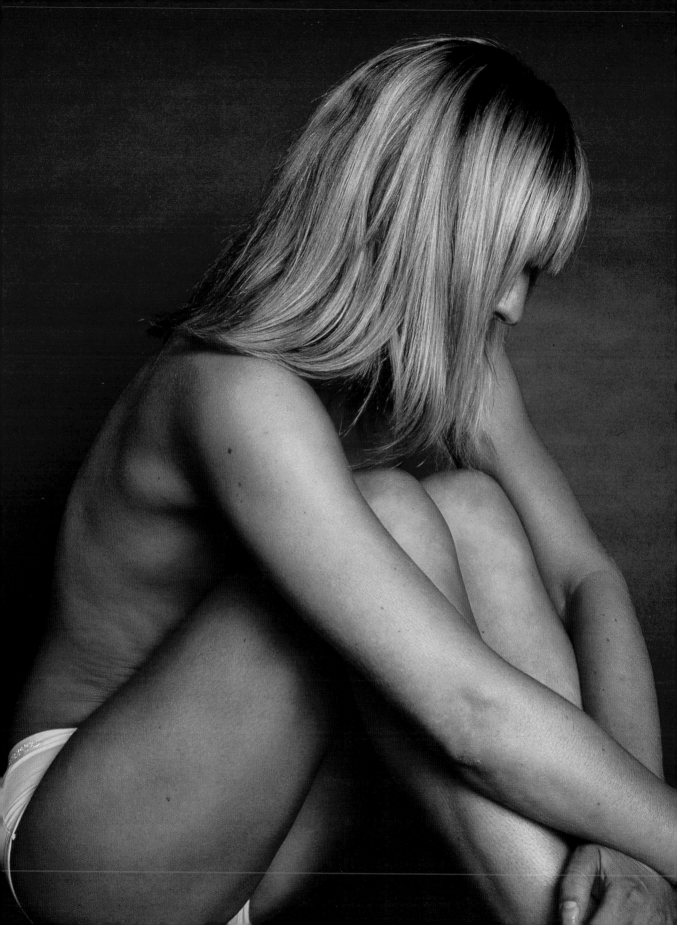

Choosing a surgeon

IT'S A LOTTERY As things stand, the cosmetic surgery industry is a lottery. What you get depends almost entirely on the advice you receive and the expertise of the person you choose to treat you, so it is absolutely essential that you check whether your surgeon is properly qualified and has significant experience in the procedure he or she plans to carry out on you.

Athough one would presume that standards of cosmetic surgery are closely monitored, this is not the case. At the moment, any doctor with a medical degree can call himself a 'cosmetic surgeon', advertise those services, and perform them, regardless of whether he, or she, has any training. And there is no law preventing an ear, nose and throat surgeon carrying out breast augmentation, even if he has never performed the operation before in his life. Many surgeons are not even doctors at all. They call themselves consultants and set up in private practice, and as long as they don't pretend they are a doctor, and they get you to sign a consent form allowing them to operate on you, they can.

EXPERIENCE AT YOUR EXPENSE There is still no specific medical qualification in cosmetic surgery. Many doctors learn their skills by crash courses and watching videos, and begin their surgical careers operating on human guinea pigs using technology that they don't fully understand. Lasers, which are the new big thing in surgery, are a very specialist product; however, laser manufacturers are so keen to sell their wares that they offer two-day courses to obstetricians, gynaecologists, family doctors and even dentists in the hope that they will buy a machine and offer laser surgery.

It's difficult for doctors to resist the temptation to add another string to their bow. The combination of a lucrative market and inadequate regulation make it an irresistible money spinner but avarice and medical ethics make lousy bed-fellows. Horror stories of botch jobs abound, but very few bogus surgeons get their come-uppance and they can usually carry on practising while they are being investigated. In the UK, David Herbert, 62 (nicknamed the 'flying doctor' because of the speed with which he carried out his procedures), is the first doctor ever to be suspended by the General Medical Council (GMC) during investigation, though the Department of Health had to give special permission to impose the interim ban because the GMC still don't have enough power to do this. Herbert, who worked privately at the Cromwell Clinic in Huntingdon, was said to carry out facelifts, which colleagues said would normally take four hours, in about 40 minutes. One of his patients allegedly nearly died after a bowel infection following a tummy tuck. He performed a facelift without using enough anaesthetic and numerous women had to have corrective surgery.

REGULATION It's clear that regulation will have to be improved but this will take time. Until that happens, women in the UK should get their GP to recommend a registered cosmetic surgeon and ensure that the surgeon they choose is certified by the British Association of Plastic Surgeons (BAPS), which carries out National Health Service (NHS) reconstructive surgery, or the British Association of Aesthetic Plastic Surgeons (BAAPS), which carries out private cosmetic surgery. Both these bodies are approved by the GMC, recognized by the Royal College of Surgeons and are part of the International Society of Aesthetic Plastic Surgery. Members of these two bodies have to have had six years of specialist training in plastic and reconstructive surgery. However, it is still important to check that your surgeon has experience in the particular operation you are undergoing. Using NHS reconstructive surgeons sounds reassuring but, in reality, a lot of them don't get a huge amount of cosmetic practice so they may not actually be as good as a surgeon who specializes in your particular procedure.

Some UK private clinics advertise that their surgeons are Fellows of the Royal College of Surgeons (FRSC), but this only guarantees that the surgeon has a basic surgical training. The letters FRSC plas means the surgeon has done up to six years training in plastic surgery. Other surgeons are members of the British Association of Cosmetic Surgeons (BACS). Although they have to prove they have cosmetic surgery experience, they may not have completed any specialist training in the UK.

QUALIFICATIONS In the US, the scale of the industry makes it even more confusing. To be safe, anyone seeking cosmetic surgery needs to ensure that their surgeon has the appropriate credentials and is certified by the American Board of Plastic Surgery (ABPS), the only certifying board for plastic surgery recognized by the American Board of Medical Specialties (ABMS). The ABPS has only certified 6499 plastic surgeons. However, there are more than 50,000 cosmetic surgeons practising in the US, many of whom declare themselves board certified. Letters after a doctor's name can lull patients into a false sense of security, but with more than 100 other so-called 'certifying boards' that are not recognized by the ABMS nor approved by the Council of Medical Education of the American Medical Association, clients are well advised to stick to ABPS surgeons.

EXPERIENCE It is worth remembering that, as with anything in life, long-term experience and a good track record in a particular procedure can count for more than qualifications. A recommendation from a friend who has had a positive experience is a good bet. You should also, ensure that your surgeon is accredited to use equipment in major hospitals, particularly if you are thinking of having liposuction, laser treatment or abdominoplasty.

Liposuction on my thighs was brilliant – painful but worth it to take away the saddle-bags. Ten years on it hasn't come back!
Di, 48, UK

Cosmetic surgery is dangerously tempting if there is a part of the body you are not happy with, but I am not at all convinced that the procedures are safe. I would never consider it for something like bigger boobs or anti-ageing, but a reduction on the stomach could tempt me if I was convinced it was safe and painless!
Alice, 35, UK

I am terrified by it. I don't think it's always successful. I think I would only undergo it if it were vital or after a disfiguring accident.
Rosalyn, 56, UK

I can understand why men and women want cosmetic surgery. Friends of mine have had their boobs done, but I don't want it. I just deal with my imperfections because, God knows, everyone has them!
Charley, 38, Aus

I wouldn't do it myself but if people want to do it then go ahead. It's a free country.
Judith, 26, US

Your pain, their gain

GENERAL SURGICAL COMPLICATIONS Any surgery that involves anaesthesia carries considerable risk, particularly for patients who are obese or have heart or lung problems. Most complications occur with general anaesthesia, which can sometimes irritate air passages, causing the vocal cords to spasm and airways to block. The anaesthesiologist may need to insert a tube down the throat or cut into the windpipe if this happens. Aspiration occurs if a patient vomits during surgery and the vomit is forced into the lungs. It can also lead to chronic cough, lung obstruction, pneumonia or infections.

A sudden drop in blood pressure due to blood loss can lead to an irregular heart beat and possibly heart attack. Brain damage can occur if blood circulation is depressed to dangerous levels. Excessive bleeding after surgery can lead to blood accumulating under the skin and this can require additional surgery. Loose sutures can lead to internal bleeding or a hernia, which can require additional surgery. Malignant hyperthermia is a rare (possibly inherited) complication where body temperature, blood pressure and heart rate all rise to hyperactive levels. If not recognized and treated quickly, it can lead to death.

Extensive surgery, greater blood loss, smoking, taking steroids or certain vascular conditions increase the likelihood of post-operative infection, though antibiotics reduce the risk. Extensive surgery and longer operating times also increases the risk of a deep vein thrombosis (DVT) blood clot. Liposuction in the legs also increases the risk of DVT, though compression garments help to reduce it. Temporary paral-ysis can occur if muscle relaxants have not fully worn off after surgery.

COMPLICATIONS WITH COSMETIC SURGERY Each cosmetic surgery procedure has its own set of specific dangers. These are dealt with in more detail later on in the chapter but in brief, liposuction can lead to pain, numbness, bruising, discoloration, and de-pigmentation, face lifts can damage nerves, leaving a woman's face permanently numb or even partially paralysed, while breast augmentation can cause hardening as fibrous tissue grows around the implant, loss of nipple sensation or nipple death, not to mention leaking silicone.

SAFETY The majority of cosmetic surgery procedures are carried out in the surgeon's private office. Although surgeons believe that the risk of infection is smaller than it would be in a hospital setting, if anything should go wrong, there is not as much life-saving equipment available as there would be in a hospital. These issues are not usually explained to potential patients who are often assured that they are undergoing 'a simple office procedure'. Medical experts are also very concerned about the growing tendency to offer discounts on multiple procedures, e.g. combining a face lift and eyebrow lift with liposuction, because this practice keeps patients under anaesthetic on the surgical table for too long, which increases the risk of complications.

DEATH RATES Though the given death rate for cosmetic surgery is 1% this is probably an underestimation and the 'correction rate' for all cosmetic surgery may be as high as one procedure in ten. Anyone considering cosmetic surgery should bear in mind that the generally accepted death rate for any kind of elective surgery, the type not needed to save someone's life, is meant to be one in 100,000, but according to a study in *Plastic and Reconstructive Surgery* magazine (2000), one in 5224 patients who underwent liposuction between 1994 and 1998 died and over the last three years at least 21 people have died during or immediately after undergoing cosmetic surgery in the state of Florida.

SURGICAL SPIN Your surgeon has a duty to make you aware of any potential complications. Yet independent research in both the UK and the US shows that the serious nature of cosmetic procedures is often glossed over by consultancies, literature and advertising. For example, cosmetic surgery brochures often portray serious procedures, such as chemical peels (p.179), as little more than a salon facial. In reality the treatment involves burning the outer layer of skin off the face which leaves the face raw, bruised, swollen, crusty, oozy and scabbed for up to ten days or more and when the wounds heal the skin on the face can be several shades lighter than the skin on the neck, leaving a tide mark around the jaw. Any woman who is planning to undergo cosmetic surgery should be given both best and worst case scenarios beforehand, but it is estimated that up to 90% of patients are ill prepared for the pain, swelling, discomfort, the potential complications and the lengthy healing and recovery times.

OPPORTUNISM AT YOUR EXPENSE Before you fall for a reassuring bedside manner, remember that cosmetic surgeons are in the business of making money, not saving lives, and unfortunately, far too many are willing to perform a nose job on anyone that has a nose. Although surgeons generally advise women that starting surgery earlier means that less invasive techniques will be required and fewer people will notice a dramatic change, the truth is, the sooner women start having surgery, the more often the procedures have to be carried out. Ageing doesn't stop, implants can't stay in forever and lifts eventually droop. In general, results only last between five and ten years and, according to the president of the American Society for Aesthetic Plastic Surgery, the cosmetic surgery industry thrives on repeat business, ie. once a woman has one surgical procedure, she is unlikely to stop there.

In the States they have a TV programme called Extreme Makeover that takes people and gives them a complete surgical overhaul. They get these women who are overweight and not very attractive and they do the works on them – lipo, face lifts, tummy tucks, Botox, everything. It is really pretty gross but then they do the before and after and although I don't agree with it and think it is way too much and totally voyeuristic, there is no doubt that the women look a hell of a lot better afterwards and they say that they feel more confident and that people treat them better too. I would like to see what the people look like a year later without the diets and hair and make-up though. I imagine them with chips in their veneered teeth!
Penny, 38, Cayman

I imagine that once you have done it once it becomes less terrifying and it is easier to consider doing it again. It's a case of pushing your boundaries a little. For me, believing I will wake up after the anaesthetic, that is the bit that freaks me out the most. But like child-birth I guess once you have a good result you forget the pain.
Erin, 32, US

Scalpel safaris

A CULTURE OF SECRECY Though the market grows annually by about 10%, there is still a culture of secrecy surrounding cosmetic surgery. Some women are happy to flaunt their face lifts, but a greater percentage are less than keen to advertise the fact that they have had anything done. Arguably, undergoing a face lift and hoping no one will notice the change is an ironic illustration of how unnecessary many procedures are in the first place. But since the industry began, women have been prepared to travel abroad to undergo their operations and recovery anonymously. Over the past ten years, this tradition has been picked up on by canny tour operators and surgical package deals are now widely advertised in the back of health, beauty and fashion magazines.

SUN, SEA, SAND AND SURGERY Operators tend to concentrate on less developed regions such as Eastern Europe, Cuba, Turkey, Asia and South Africa, where favourable exchange rates cut the cost of surgery. Last year hundreds of British women were operated on in South Africa, where a face lift costs only £3000 compared to an average price of £5000–£10,000 in London. Holiday packages which include flights, 12 days at a five star hotel in Cape Town, face lift, eyelid surgery, laser treatments and a tour of the Cape's famous wine region cost about £6,500. The hotels are set up to accommodate recuperating patients and clients can slip in and out of their hotel without passing through a central lobby. Theoretically, by the time the bruises have healed, it is time to return home and no one is any the wiser.

CHEAP SURGERY COSTS MORE Though they are unlikely to bump into the neighbours in Budapest, women who are tempted by surgical package holidays are taking a risk, particularly if they do so in countries where English is not the spoken language. Having serious surgery – and cosmetic surgery really is serious – in a country where it is virtually impossible to check out the credentials of your doctor (whom you generally only meet once before the operation), is very naive, because if anything goes wrong it can be very difficult to pursue a case through the courts. To take a case against a foreign company or surgeon you need to find, and pay, a lawyer from that country. You may also need a translator and you will have to find a local expert to call as a witness.

Doctors in the UK who have had to repair botch jobs carried out abroad have no records to work from and warn that 'cheap plastic surgery' is the most expensive kind because correcting mistakes is much more difficult, more likely to lead to permanent disfigurement and obviously generates huge medical bills. Before choosing to have surgery abroad it's worth remembering how hard it is to find a legitimately qualified plastic surgeon in the UK or the US.

If things go wrong ...

LOOK BEFORE YOU LEAP After your initial consultation your surgeon must secure your informed consent. You will be asked to sign a piece of paper agreeing that you fully comprehend the procedure and any risks involved. If, for example, you had a breast reduction and your nipple died and your surgeon had not pointed out that this was a possibility, you could sue him because you were not given enough information. However, if you were told that nipple death was a possible complication, you would not be able to sue. Before you sign anything you should ensure that your surgeon is fully insured and find out what will happen if there is a problem and who will pay to correct it. It's important to check your surgeon's insurance because some doctors have had so many legal actions made against them for medical negligence that companies refuse to insure them.

CORRECTIVE SURGERY If you have surgery and you are not happy with the results, your first step is to go back and see the surgeon who carried out the operation. A reasonable surgeon will normally correct the fault for free, though you may still have to pay for hospital care, anaesthetics, etc. If things have gone wrong, you may not want to have the same surgeon to carry out the operation. Some have gentlemen's arrangements with other surgeons, but you need to clarify who will pay for consultations and corrective work. Corrective operations generally can't be carried out until scars have softened. This can take at least a year and secondary procedures are likely to cause even more scarring.

LEGAL ACTION If the complications are very severe, you may have no choice other than to take legal action. You can only sue a surgeon on grounds of either 'negligence' or 'assault and battery'. A surgeon is negligent if their work falls below an expected standard of advice, operative performance or aftercare. Assault and battery is used if a surgeon carries out a procedure that you haven't agreed to. If you decide to take legal action, Action for Victims of Medical Accidents in the UK will help you to find a solicitor who specializes in the appropriate area. In the US, the Federation of State Medical Boards may be able to help, but patient complaints are usually directed to the State Medical Licensing Board where the physician in question practises. Taking legal action is always a gamble and, if you are not entitled to legal aid, the cost can be prohibitive. Claims have to be filed within three years and your solicitor will go through your medical notes with an expert to establish your case. If you have a strong case, it will probably be settled out of court but, if you lose your claim, you will be left to carry the costs. In 1998, the cosmetic surgery industry in the US turned over $5 billion dollars in revenue. In the same year, there were also over 5000 lawsuits issued against cosmetic and plastic surgeons. Of the 35,000 US doctors who have been responsible for two or more negligence settlements since 1990, fewer than 8% have been disciplined.

When I wanted to get my breasts enlarged I was put off by the fact that most surgeons charge about £50 for an initial consultation. I found a surgeon who gave a free consultation providing I went ahead with surgery and since I was dead set on it I spoke to him on Friday and had the operation on the following Tuesday. I wish now that I had taken some time to think about what I was doing and had talked to other doctors. It would have been a small price to pay. My surgeon was qualified and he covered himself by getting me to sign consent forms but I am very unhappy with the result of the operation. My left breast is higher and smaller than my right breast and unless I pay for further surgery I will have to stay like this. It seems like a small thing to other people but not when you have to live with it, particularly since there was nothing really wrong with my breasts before. I now feel that I was impulsive and so determined to have the operation that I didn't want to listen to anything negative. I have learned the value of patience and making informed choices the hard way.
Louisa, 32, UK

Liposuction

Introduced in the US in the early 1980s, liposuction is now the most popular cosmetic surgery procedure and 89% of clients are female. Though it is considered to be fairly safe, some studies show risk of death to be between 20 and 100 deaths per 100,000 (US deaths from car accidents stand at 16 per 100,000). Though it leaves fairly small scars, women generally underestimate the seriousness of this procedure. Liposuction is a major internal assault and it can lead to serious complications and even death. Surgeons need to have specific liposuction training and privileges to work at an accredited hospital. Procedures that involve the removal of more than 5 litres (8¾ pints) of fat require a doctor with advanced surgical skills.

THE PROCEDURE Liposuction on smaller areas (up to 1.5 litres (2½ pints)) can be carried out using local anaesthetic as a day case. Larger areas require a general and an overnight stay in hospital. During the procedure your body loses a lot of fluid so you need to be carefully monitored and given intravenous fluids to prevent the body going into shock. Liposuction takes anywhere between an hour and four hours depending on the technique and the amount of fat being removed. The surgeon will try to take out as much fat as possible but some has to be left so that the skin does not stick to the muscle. Once he has done one side, he measures the amount of fat removed and takes the same amount out of the other side.

TECHNIQUES *Traditional liposuction* involves inserting a 3mm tube known as a cannula through several tiny incisions, then pushing and pulling it through the fat layer to break up the fat cells. Once the cells have been separated, they are sucked out through the tube using either a vacuum pump or a syringe. The fat that is removed should be white, not red with blood. The *wet or tumescent technique* involves injecting the area to be treated with a mix of saline fluid, local anaesthetic (lidocaine), adrenaline to stop bleeding and a drug called Hyalase, which allows the fluid to penetrate the body's fat cells. As the liquid enters the fat, it causes the compartments of fat to become swollen and firm or 'tumesced'. The expanded fat compartments allow the liposuction cannula to travel more smoothly beneath the skin as the fat is removed, but it takes significantly longer than traditional liposuction. If the solution's lidocaine content is too high, it can cause lidocaine toxicity. If too much fluid is administered, it can lead to the collection of fluid in the lungs. *Ultrasound assisted lipoplasty (UAL)* uses a special cannula that produces ultrasonic energy, which heats the fat and makes it liquid. The fat is then removed with the traditional liposuction technique. UAL has been shown to improve the ease and effectiveness of liposuction in fibrous areas of the body, such as the upper back. However, there is concern that the heat from the ultrasound device may cause burns to the skin or deeper tissues and the long-term effects of ultrasound energy on the body are not yet known.

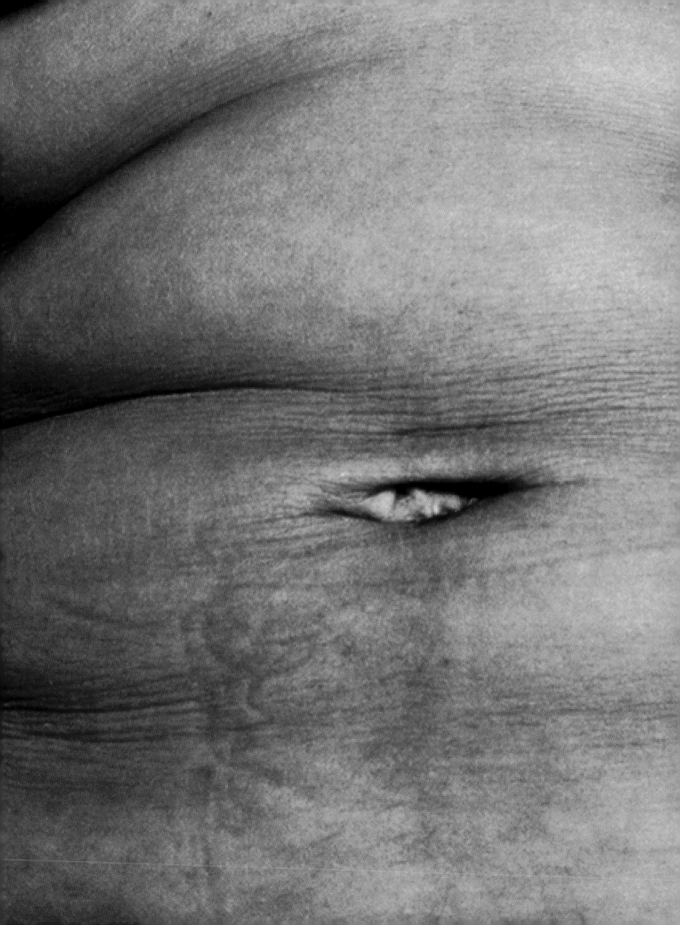

AFTER SURGERY You will probably require drains to prevent fluid retention and you are likely to experience some pain, burning, swelling, bleeding and temporary numbness. To control swelling and to help your skin spring into shape you will be fitted with a snug elastic garment to wear over the treated area for a few weeks. Your doctor may also prescribe antibiotics to prevent infection and you will be advised to start walking around as soon as possible to reduce swelling and help prevent blood clots from forming in your legs, however strenuous activity should be avoided for about a month as your body continues to heal. Stitches are removed or dissolve on their own within the first week to ten days. Post-operative swelling can mean that treated areas are even larger than they were before the procedure and this can take six months to settle down completely, so you won't really be able to judge the results until then. If you have any unusually heavy bleeding or a sudden increase in pain, call your doctor immediately.

ELIGIBILITY As techniques have improved, the age at which women can have liposuction has risen to 50 or 55, but it is best performed on women who are normal weight with firm, elastic skin who have pockets of excess fat that don't respond to dieting and exercise. These bulges are most commonly found in the thighs, hips, abdomen, buttocks, knees, ankles, calves, upper arms and facial areas such as the chin, cheeks, jowls and neck. Patients should be healthy, psychologically stable and realistic in their expectations. Women who want to have liposuction are advised to diet before surgery and it is very important that this weight is kept off after surgery. Post-op weight fluctuations can leave the surface of the skin lumpy as the sucked out fat cells won't grow back but the cells around them will expand and this can leave you looking pretty weird, e.g. a woman who has had liposuction on her upper arms may get fat lower arms if she gains weight. As such, liposuction is considered unsuitable for teenagers whose weight has not stabilized.

RISK Liposuction won't tighten loose skin or eliminate cellulite because it sucks fat out from a deeper level under the skin and imperfect end results are not uncommon. The skin surface may be irregular or even baggy, especially in very overweight patients or those with older, less elastic, skin. In some cases, patients have to have excess folds of empty skin surgically removed, which means more operations and scarring. The scars from liposuction are small but skin pigmentation and temporary or long-term numbness can sometimes occur. Complications include delayed healing; the formation of fat clots; blood clots, which can migrate to the lungs and cause death; excessive fluid loss, which can lead to shock; fluid accumulation that must be drained; friction burns; damage to the skin or nerves; perforation injury to vital organs such as the abdominal wall or bowel; and unfavourable drug reactions, particularly to lidocaine.

Breast augmentation

Breast augmentation or enhancement is the second most popular cosmetic surgery procedure. The number of women and teenage girls in the US who underwent augmentation surgery more than doubled between 1997 and 2002 (101,176 in 1997 vs 249,641 in 2002). However, these procedures don't necessarily represent new implants. Many are actually repeat operations to replace old implants that have broken or caused problems. Though implants have been around since the 1960s, the US FDA did not have the authority to regulate them until 1976. Despite the fact that there had never been any studies on safety, by 1990, almost one million American women already had breast implants.

Breast implants consist of a soft silicone shell filled with either silicone gel or a salt-water solution called saline. Silicone implants have the same consistency as body fat so they are by far the most popular option, however there has been a great deal of controversy about their safety. Claims have been made that leaking silicone causes breast cancer, birth defects and a range of connective tissue and autoimmune disorders such as ME, lymph node swelling, fatigue, fibromyalgia, scleroderma, rheumatoid arthritis and memory loss. By 1992, reports of complications and illnesses concerned the FDA enough to limit availability in the US to clinical trials, women who wanted to replace existing silicone implants, women who had had mastectomies or those who suffered from breast deformities. Silicone implants for cosmetic purposes are still not allowed in the US.

In the UK, the Department of Health set up the Independent Review Group to review the safety of silicone implants. Though they found no scientific link to illness or immune reactions and silicone implants are still available, the report did point out that, 'there is some risk associated with the use of any implant'. So, although research has not proven that autoimmune disease is caused by *silicone* implants, several European studies have indicated that any form of breast surgery (whether for breast implants or to reduce the size of breasts) may be associated with an increased risk of neurological or autoimmune disease. If this is the case, then there would be a risk associated with all breast implants, regardless of what they are made of. Since autoimmune diseases take many years to develop, in this context, many people believe the studies on implants have been too short term to establish that there is no risk.

Women, quite rightly, question why, despite 25 years of usage, there is still so much confusion about the long-term risks that implants might pose to female health. That such inconclusive evidence of safety is tolerated suggests that vanities like 'breast implants' don't appear to merit the usual rigorous testing to establish whether these procedures are safe or not.

I had no idea how much I missed out on by being flat as a board. I never had a man return a shopping cart for me when I was an A-cup. Then suddenly the men were falling over themselves to help me with things, when I didn't want or need their help. Because of some boobs. Crazy!
Nic, 35, US

Breast implants are so common now but they don't look anything like real breasts, they look like small footballs, and are nothing like the soft tissue of a natural breast.
Barbara, 43, UK

All through my teens I was teased because I was so flat chested. I was very self-conscious. If I had had the money, I would have had a boob job at 16 but luckily I was skint. I now love my skinny shape and wouldn't want boobs if you paid me to have them.
Carla, 24, UK

I personally have saline implants, which were inserted through my armpits, the shells put in first and then filled with saline through a valve, then the valve closed so my scars are pretty small and I know they are safe.
Lorraine, 44, UK

Breast implants

I had my breasts done as a fortieth birthday present. My partner was against it but I really wanted to do it. The operation was fine because I had a general anaesthetic but it was more painful afterwards than I had anticipated. I was due to go on holiday shortly after-wards and I had hoped that would provide the perfect opportunity for recuperation but I was sore and bandaged and, quite frankly, pretty uncomfortable for the whole trip. I was eventu-ally quite happy with the results but I do think that although my chest looks good, now I feel as if I should get my face done to match. I have these big, bouncy, youthful boobs and then I look at my lined face and think it looks a bit incongruous.
Karen, 41, UK

I have implanted breasts and although they do not feel 'natural' per se, men seem to find them very erotic and exciting. I think subconsciously they process my desire to have big breasts as a desire to appeal to them. Implanted breasts suggest a woman who is willing to capitalise on her sexuality and I believe men find this to be a turn on. I have no problem with this interpretation.
Monica, 44, US

THE PROCEDURE In your initial consultation, your surgeon should evaluate your health and explain which technique is most appropriate for you. If your breasts are sagging, your doctor may also recommend a breast lift (p.221). Breast augmentation can be performed with a local anaesthetic and a sedative to make you sleepy, but in the UK it is usually carried out under general anaesthetic. The method of inserting and positioning your implant will depend on your anatomy and your surgeon's recommendation. The incision can be made either in the crease where the breast meets the chest, around the aureola or in the armpit. The implants are then centred behind your nipples. Working through the incision, the surgeon will lift your breast tissue and skin to create a pocket, either directly behind the breast tissue or underneath your chest wall muscle (the pectoral muscle). Some surgeons believe that putting the implants behind your chest muscle rather than behind your breast tissue, reduces the potential for capsular contracture (hardening of the breast), though this has not been proven. This placement may also interfere less with breast examination by mammogram (breast x-ray) though it will not fill out the breast as much and when you flex your muscles the breast sometimes moves in an odd way. Placement behind the muscle may be more painful for a few days after surgery than placement directly under the breast tissue.

New techniques that make an incision under the armpit leave a scar of just 5cm (2in). If saline implants are inflated inside the body, the scar is only 2cm (¾in). The disadvantage with these techniques is that it is difficult for the surgeon to stop internal bleeding. And if the implant has to be removed, the surgeon cuts beneath the breast making a second scar. There is also a risk of blood clots forming between the armpit and elbow and numbness to the inner arm.

The surgery usually takes one to two hours to complete. Stitches are used to close the incisions, which may also be taped. A gauze bandage may be applied over your breasts to help with healing and drainage tubes may be used for a couple of days. You're likely to feel tired and sore for a few days, but you'll be up and around in 24 hours and pain can be controlled by medication. If you have nursed a baby within the last 12 months, you may produce milk for a few days, but drugs can counter this. When the gauze dressings are removed, you will be given a surgical bra to wear around the clock. Your nipples may have a burning sensation for about two weeks, but this will subside as bruising fades. Your stitches will come out in a week to ten days, but the swelling takes three to five weeks to disappear. Your breasts will be sensitive for two to three weeks and your scars will be firm and pink for at least six. They may remain that size or even appear to widen, but after several months, they will begin to fade, although they will never disappear completely. Follow your surgeon's advice on when to begin exercises and normal activities.

Implant complications

RISK About three out of four reconstruction patients and almost half of all first-time augmentation patients experience some difficulties with their implants. The most common complication is a bad result – the implants appear lopsided, one breast is higher than the other or the amount the breasts stick out varies.

Another common complication with breast implants is capsular contraction. All implants are 'foreign bodies' and women's bodies react by forming a capsule of fibrous scar tissue around the implants. Sometimes these become too tight for the implant and this can cause the breast to feel hard and the edges of the implant can become quite pronounced through the skin. It can be treated in several ways. Sometimes the implant has to be replaced or the scar tissue has to be scored away. A late complication of augmentation is that when the breast eventually droops with age, the implant is left high up so the nipple is actually below it. This can only be corrected with a breast lift or the insertion and repositioning of a new implant.

More serious health risks include infection and the accumulation of clotted blood, which has to be surgically removed. In some cases, the implant may need to be removed for several months until the infection clears. Some women lose all or partial sensitivity in their breasts and nipples, and others become overly sensitive. This cannot be corrected, though sometimes the condition improves over time. The bigger the implant, the more likely it is that there will be some kind of nerve damage or loss of sensation.

According to the Institute of Medicine, women with any kind of breast surgery, including breast implant surgery, are at least three times more likely to have an inadequate milk supply for breastfeeding. There is some concern about the safety of breastfeeding because of the risk of bacteria around implants transferring to infants but there is insufficient research at present.

Breast implants can interfere with the detection of breast cancer, because implants can obscure the mammography image of a tumour. Although mammography can be performed in ways that minimize the interference of the implants, approximately 30% of the breast tissue is still obscured and mammograms are less accurate if the woman has capsular contracture. There is no evidence that implants cause breast cancer, but a delay in diagnosis could necessitate more surgery or be fatal.

RUPTURE All breast implants eventually break. Rupture can occur as a result of injury, but normal compression and movement may also cause the implants to leak. It is not known how many years the breast implants that are currently on the market will last. Most implants last 7–12 years, which means some women undergo

Complication rates

A survey of saline implants in 1,264 women after three years by Mentor, US showed:

- *21% had wrinkling*
- *13% needed another operation*
- *10% lost nipple sensation*
- *9% had hardening*
- *8% needed removal*
- *7% asymmetrical*
- *5% felt intense nipple sensation*
- *5% felt breast pain*
- *3% had leakage or deflation*
- *2% could see the implants' outlines*
- *2% had infections*
- *2% had sagging*
- *2% had bad scarring*
- *2% had haematoma.*

Findings on silicone implants by Dr Gregory Hetter found that hardening occurred in 74% of women with silicone implants and 40% of women with saline implants. 41% of all patients reported some loss of nipple sensation, 15% had some numbness and 15% were dissatis-fied with the shape. However, in a disturbing triumph of hope over experience, 91% said they felt better about themselves and 96% said they would do it again.

as many as six or more surgeries as their implants are replaced over the years. However, some implants break during the first few months or years. In a study conducted by researchers at the FDA, most women had at least one broken implant within 15 years. All breaks can require a second operation to replace the leaking implant and additional surgery carries considerable costs. Even if the implant itself is replaced for free, which is sometimes the case, the costs of the doctor, the medical facility and anaesthesiology are not. Cosmetic surgery is not covered by health insurance and problems resulting from cosmetic surgery are also excluded from coverage.

SILICONE BREAKS If the shell of a silicone implant breaks, there may be a change in the shape or firmness of the breast. If the shell breaks, but the scar capsule around the implant does not, a woman may not detect any change. In 21% of women with silicone implants, the scar also breaks or tears, and the silicone filler migrates outside of the breast capsule and leaks into the surrounding tissue. Though women are often unaware that this has happened, the migrating filler may cause a new scar to form around it wherever it collects and it is not always possible to remove all of the gel from the breast tissue. The health risks associated with broken implants are unclear (p.219), but higher rates of lung cancer in women with silicone implants may be related to their proximity to the lungs.

SALINE BREAKS Saline implants don't appear to pose the same health risks because if fluid leaks out it is simply absorbed by the body. However one in ten saline implants ruptures and they have a very high complication rate in the first three years. The most common complication with saline implants is wrinkling and this is the main reason that surgeons prefer to use silicone despite the risks. The bag that contains the fluid creases and the ripples can be seen through the skin. Some women believe saline implants leave breasts looking or feeling unnatural or asymmetrical, and the saline can make a 'sloshing' sound.

IMPLANT REMOVAL Removing an implant can be much more complicated and expensive than putting one in, especially if a gel implant has broken. Most surgeons who specialize in removal recommend that the implant and the natural scar tissue surrounding it and any leaked filler are all removed together in order to try and remove as much of the silicone gel as possible. However this means that women with ruptured silicone implants often lose breast tissue as part of the removal surgery and because the breast tissue is also stretched, the breast is unlikely to be as attractive as it was before the implant surgery. In some cases, this may result in a surgical result that looks similar to a mastectomy (p.281).

Breast lift and breast reduction

BREAST LIFT Sagging breasts can be raised and reshaped by a breast lift or mastopexy. The best results are usually achieved in women with small, droopy breasts and a lift can also reduce the size of the aureola. Breast lifts are usually performed under general anaesthestic. The procedure takes one to four hours. Techniques vary, but the most common procedure involves an anchor-shaped incision that circles the aureola, extends downwards, and follows the natural curve of the crease beneath the breast. Excess skin is removed and the nipple and aureola moved to a higher position. The skin surrounding the aureola is then brought together to reshape the breast. Stitches are usually located around the aureola, extending down from the nipple area and along the lower crease of the breast. Some patients, especially those with relatively small breasts, may be candidates for procedures requiring less extensive incisions such as the 'doughnut mastopexy', where circular incisions are made around the aureola and a doughnut-shaped area of skin is removed. Post-surgical procedures are much the same as those for augmentation. Stitches will be removed after a week or two and you can expect some loss of feeling in your nipples and breast skin. This usually fades as the swelling subsides over the next six weeks or so. However, it may last a year or more, and occasionally it may be permanent. Although you may be up and about in a day or two, you will need to take it easy for three to four weeks. Pregnancy after a breast lift is likely to stretch the breasts again and may also interfere with your ability to breastfeed so this procedure should only be carried out when you have finished having children.

BREAST REDUCTION Most women who have reduction surgery are impeded by very large, sagging breasts that cause physical discomfort and restrict activity. The procedure removes fat, glandular tissue and skin, making them smaller, lighter and firmer and it can also reduce the size of the aureola. The goal is to give a woman breasts that are more in proportion with the rest of her body. Breast reduction is not recommended until the breasts are fully developed and it is not advisable if you intend to breastfeed because the surgery removes many of the milk ducts leading to the nipples. Your surgeon may require you to have a mammogram before surgery and most good surgeons will suggest that their patients diet before the operation and control their weight after surgery.

Breast reduction can be performed under local or general anaesthetic and usually takes two to four hours. An anchor-shaped incision circles the aureola, extends downwards, and follows the natural curve of the crease beneath the breast. The surgeon then removes excess glandular tissue, fat and skin, and moves the nipple and aureola into their new position. Then the skin from both sides of the breast is brought down and around the aureola, shaping the new contour of the breast. In

If you do plan to get plastic surgery, research, research, research! After your research on the procedure itself is done, research the doctors thoroughly. I saw a Dateline show a while back about a woman who died during a plastic surgery procedure by a non-plastic surgeon in Mexico. Women are lured by the great deals they can get. As the saying goes, 'You get what you pay for.' I've seen lots and lots of boob job results. I don't think a $10,000 boob job is necessarily any better than a $5000 boob job – I've personally seen $3500 boob jobs that look far superior to $12,000 ones – but if someone is offering you breast augmentation for less than $2500 (assuming you don't work for that person, aren't related to them, and aren't providing a service in exchange for the procedure that warrants a price break), just say no.
Bettina, 31, US

I had my breasts reduced when I was 20 because they were so heavy. Carrying so much extra weight around killed my back and left me exhausted. I really cannot see why women would pay to have them put in.
Linda, 28, UK

most cases, the nipples remain attached to their blood vessels and nerves. However, if the breasts are very large or pendulous, the nipples and aureolas may have to be completely removed and grafted into a higher position. Stitches are usually located around the aureola, in a vertical line extending downwards and along the lower crease of the breast. In some cases, techniques can be used that eliminate the vertical part of the scar. Liposuction may be also used to remove excess fat from the armpit area.

Post-surgical procedures are the same as those for augmentation and the breasts may be painful for a few days, though this can be helped with medication. The bandages will be removed after a day or two, though you will continue to wear a surgical bra around the clock for several weeks, until the swelling and bruising subside. A small amount of fluid draining from your surgical wound or some crusting is normal. Some patients develop small sores around their nipples; these can be treated with antibiotic creams. Your stitches will be removed in one to three weeks. Your first menstruation following surgery may cause your breasts to swell and hurt. You may also experience shooting pains for a few months. You can expect some loss of feeling in your nipples and breast skin, caused by the swelling. This usually fades over the next six weeks or so, though it may last a year or more, and occasionally, it can be permanent. Your breasts may ache for a couple of weeks and you should avoid lifting, pushing or anything other than gentle contact for three or four weeks. Much of the swelling and bruising disappears in the first few weeks, but it may be six months to a year before your breasts settle into their new shape. Even then, their shape may fluctuate in response to your hormonal shifts, weight changes and pregnancy. If you have any unusual symptoms, such as bleeding or severe pain, call your doctor.

RISK Breast reduction is not a simple operation, but it is normally safe when performed by a qualified surgeon. The specific risks include extensive and perma-nent scarring. Poor healing and wider scars are more common in smokers. Bleeding and infection are uncommon, but can cause scars to widen. The procedure can also leave you with slightly mismatched breasts or unevenly positioned nipples. Some patients experience temporary (or ocasionally permanent) loss of feeling in their nipples or breasts. Occasionally, the nipple and aureola may lose their blood supply and the tissue will die. This requires further surgery to rebuild the nipple and aureola using skin grafts from elsewhere on the body. Breast reduction does not usually require a blood transfusion however, if a large amount of breast tissue will be removed, you may be advised to have a unit of blood drawn ahead of time. A breast reduction or lift won't keep you firm forever and the effects of gravity, pregnancy, ageing and weight fluctuations will eventually take their toll again.

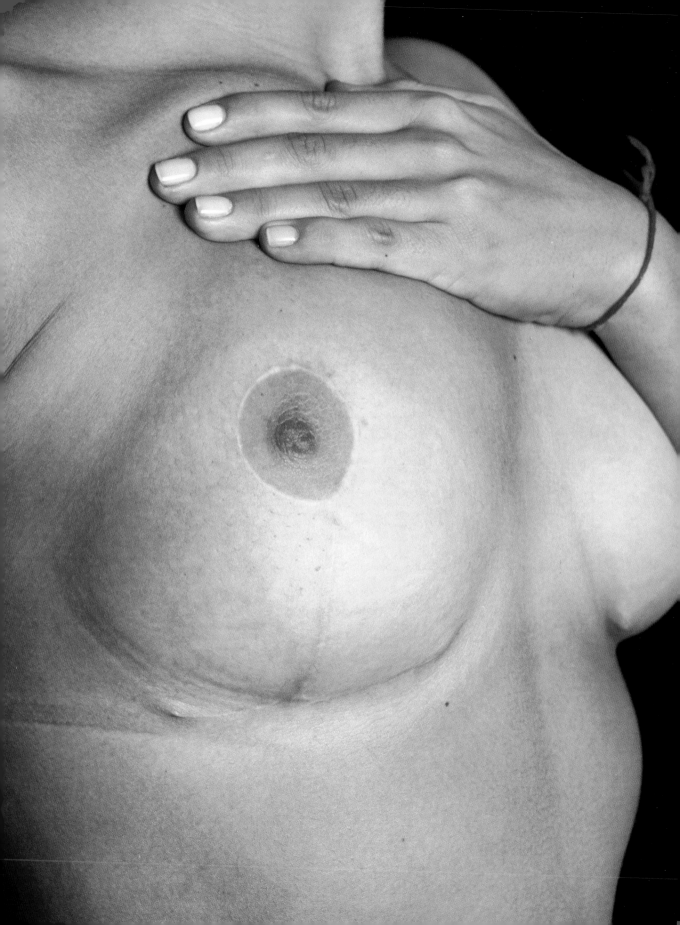

Nose jobs

When my flatmate's grandmother died she left my flatmate some money in her will to have a nose job. She felt she had suffered all her life because of her big nose and she didn't want her granddaughter who had the same nose to have the same experience. My flatmate is a very unhappy person and over the years she had decided that everything in her life would be better if she had a different nose. She didn't look bad to me but it became such a huge issue. In the end she had a nose job and it was awful. She looked like a pig, much worse than she had done before, but she was really happy about it. It hasn't improved her life much though.
Caterina, 29, Italy

One of my friends, who was happily married, decided to have a nose job. Her husband thought she was ill advised to do it, but let her go ahead because she had a fixation. Then, once she'd had it done, she turned up at a party – and none of us even noticed! She had to point out that she'd already had the operation and that she was pleased with the result. It was ridiculous.
Carmine, 52, US

Surgery to reshape the nose can reduce or increase the size, change the shape of the tip or the bridge, narrow the span of the nostrils, get rid of lumps or bumps, change the angle between your nose and your upper lip, correct birth defects, injuries, or help relieve breathing problems. Sometimes a person's profile needs to be balanced with a chin implant after rhinoplasty. Because the nose only really begins to grow at about the age of 13, surgeons prefer to wait until girls are about 15 or 16 before they operate.

The nose is a difficult structure to work with. Surgeons can't simply plane down the nasal bones to make them smaller. They have to break them, either from the inside, or by inserting little chisels through nicks in the skin between the eyes and on the cheeks, and then push both sides together. Most good nose reductions involve adjusting the cartilage in the tip first and then cutting down the bone to suit it, but surgeons can't remove too much cartilage because, without it, the nose would collapse, making it impossible to breathe. Though bone is easy to work, cartilage is a delicate, springy substance, which tends to return to its original position. To add cartilage, surgeons can use grafts taken from the ear, rib or bone or they can also use implants.

CLOSED RHINOPLASTY Closed rhinoplasty is usually performed under general anaesthesia. It takes between one and two hours, and requires an overnight stay in hospital. It is the most straightforward operation because it is carried out on the inside of the nose (when there isn't a problem with the tip or the bone) and it leaves no visible scar. The surgeon makes an incision inside the rim of the nostrils, then the skin of the nose is separated from the supporting framework of bone and cartilage and sculpted to the desired shape. If your nostrils are too wide, the surgeon can remove small wedges of skin from their base, bringing them closer together. The surgeon removes humps using a chisel and brings the nasal bones together to form a narrower bridge. Trimming the septum improves the angle between the nose and upper lip and cartilage is trimmed to reshape the tip of the nose. Internal problems, such as breathing obstructions, can be improved by removing or changing the shape of the obstruction. Finally, the skin is redraped over the new framework.

OPEN RHINOPLASTY This is a bigger operation with a longer recovery time. The operation involves making a small incision across the base of the nose through the strip of tissue that separates the nostrils. This leaves patients with a small scar but it is not usually visible unless you are looking up. When the nose is also narrowed there will be tiny scars hidden in the creases where the nostrils join the cheeks.

TIP SURGERY When full rhinoplasty is not required, tip surgery is carried out to remould the tip of the nose.

AFTER SURGERY The surgery takes around two hours and after the operation you will have a plaster of Paris splint taped to your nose. Your face will feel puffy, your nose may ache and you may have a dull headache. Keeping ice packs over your nose and remaining upright help to reduce bruising and swelling round the eyes. This begins to subside after about three days, though healing takes longer for smokers. A little bleeding is common during the first few days following surgery, and you may continue to feel some stuffiness for several weeks. If you have nasal packing, it will be removed after a few days and you'll feel much more comfortable.

Stitches are taken out after about four days and the plaster is removed in ten days. Most of the swelling and bruising should disappear within two weeks and the rest can be covered with camouflage make-up. Some subtle swelling will remain for several months and you will have to breathe through your mouth for some time. Your surgeon will probably ask you not to blow your nose for a week or so, while the tissues heal. Don't fiddle with your new nose, use cottonbuds to clean it or peek in under the splint. You'll also be advised against activities that make your nose run, such as eating spicy food or taking hot baths and you should avoid any activity that increases your blood pressure for two to three weeks. You will have to be gentle with your nose and avoid hurting it or getting it sunburned for a couple of months and, although you can wear contact lenses, glasses are a no no until the nose has healed completely. The final results may not be apparent for a year.

RISK It is impossible to predict how nose reshaping will turn out because it depends entirely on the thickness of the skin. Some surgeons take photographs and use computer enhancement to show you what you could look like with a different nose, but don't buy this. Although rhinoplasty usually improves nose shape, drastic change is not normally possible and any surgeon who brags that they can 'give' you a particular nose is lying. There is always a possibility of complications, including infection, nosebleed or a reaction to the anaesthetic. After surgery, small burst blood vessels may appear as tiny red spots on the skin's surface; these are usually minor but may be permanent and require treatment (p.201). Because rhinoplasty is complicated, there is a higher incidence of corrective surgery. About one in 10 people who have rhinoplasty need additional surgery though this often cannot be done for a year. Sometimes touch-up surgery can be done under local anaesthetic if it is just a question of shaving off a little more bone. However, it can sometimes be quite complicated, particularly if it involves putting things back rather than taking things away.

At the young age of 15, I begged and pleaded with my parents to let me get my nose done. I was sick of years of agonizing over my profile, adjusting the angle I stood as I spoke to people, and just the overall lack of self-confidence. My pre-op era of life is still evident today when I watch TV or a movie – I still catch myself unconsciously angling my head in a manner that my profile is less obvious. It is over 14 years after my surgery and it was the best thing I could have done. The biggest shock I had was after years of agonizing, no one at school realized I had had it done. I went back to school with some minimal bruising and people asked me if I had had my eyes done or whether I had had a chin implant.
Yalda, 29, Iran

One has to question the ethics of an industry that allows people like Michael Jackson to turn themselves into freaks and then charges them for it. It should be illegal for people to volunteer to get themselves cut up and sewn back together for no reason other than vanity.
Holly, 32, UK

Face lifts

My mother-in-law, a notorious self-publicist on the subject of cosmetic surgery, invited my seven-year-old son to visit her following a full reconstruction job. She said that she had had an appendix out to avoid explaining her vanity to him. She was mummified in bandages from the neck down. Her breasts were strapped into couture cone shapes like a Gaultier frock and these swaddling bands ended at the knees. My son ate chocolate ice cream and was promptly very sick at the sheer horror of this display. This woman in her late 60s enjoyed a month of reclaimed youth. She received me at the United Universities Club in Pall Mall via a back door whereby she answered the door stark naked but for a pout in the full knowledge that I had been shown to her room by a young doorman. The scars that remained of rolls of waist, thigh and bust were reduced to pink marks that could have been the marks left by tight bikini elastic and bra straps. For a time her skin was stretched and taut but she then proceeded to fill that body up all over again and the excercise ended with an even larger woman who was (continued next page)

There are now several different options to choose from when it comes to face lifts though all the procedures require operative incisions and stitching so none of them could be considered minor surgery. The best candidates for face lifts are women who still have a degree of elasticity in their skin. Women with a strong bone structure are also likely to achieve better results. Face lifts are effective at correcting sagging and tightening slack and jowly jaw lines. Some, but not all, procedures can get rid of deep creases between the nose and mouth, but no face lift will remove all folds and eliminate all lines. If you smoke, it's especially important to stop at least a week or two before and after surgery as smoking inhibits blood flow to the skin, and can interfere with the healing of your incision areas. If your hair is very short, you might want to let it grow out before surgery, so that it's long enough to hide the scars while they heal. Most surgeons advise women who want to have the procedure to lose any excess weight first.

Women who opt for face lifts are generally aged between 40 and 60 but, as with all cosmetic surgery, the results don't last forever. Surgeons prefer operating on younger women because the change in appearance is not so dramatic, but face lifts don't last forever and too few women are warned that they will probably be back on the operating table within ten years. For a 40-year-old woman this may mean that she will have three or four operations before she is 70.

THE MINI LIFT This is the simplest skin tightening procedure and can be carried out under local or general anaesthetic. The surgeon cuts a line in the skin from the temples down in front of the ears and then behind the ears and behind them across the base of the scalp. The skin is then lifted up off the face and pulled taut and any excess is trimmed off and the wound is stitched. The obvious advantage is that it doesn't cut into the muscle and is a less invasive form of surgery. However, the effects don't last very long and in some cases, as scars contract, it can lead to the ears being pulled downwards after about six months. The mini lift has no effect on nose to mouth grooves and it can leave bad scars behind the ears and create lumps under the skin. Repeated lifts can leave the face looking 'tight'.

THE SMAS LIFT This is also known as the standard face lift. It involves deeper cuts into the skin and aims to pull up both the skin and the layer of tissue and muscle underneath. The incisions are similar but the muscles in the lower part of the face are tightened and attached to underlying bones if possible. The skin is redraped and pockets of fatty tissue can be removed. Facial implants may also be inserted to increase the volume of the face. This operation can help turkey gobble neck and gives a better, longer lasting effect but it does not have much effect on nose to mouth grooves. It requires a general anaesthetic and you will look like road kill for at least three weeks after the operation. It can result in a taut look, bad scarring and, occasionally, damage to the facial nerve can result in either temporary or permanent paralysis.

THE EXTENDED SMAS LIFT During this procedure the surgeon cuts further in towards the nose to lift the skin, muscle and underlying tissue right off the cheek ligaments. He then pulls it up to improve the look of the middle of the face, perk up sagging cheeks, flatten nose-to-mouth grooves, reduce jowls and tighten the neck. Though it sounds hideous, it produces less swelling than a standard lift and has a shorter recovery time. It is carried out under a general anaesthetic and some women are fully recovered within two weeks. The disadvantages are that there is a greater risk of damaging the facial nerves and incurring paralysis.

THE COMPOSITE LIFT This is a much larger and longer operation (four to six hours) and combines an extended SMAS lift with a brow lift and lower eyelid surgery to treat drooping brow, eye and cheek bags as well as the middle and lower face. It is mainly used on much older patients and it takes a lot longer to recover from. The swelling can take up to six months to go down and there is an increased risk of damage to the facial nerves and paralysis. Patients may also feel an altered sensation in their scalp and it can affect the shape of the eyes too.

THE MASK LIFT This technique involves cutting from inside the mouth to free the cheeks and cutting across the top of the head and then tunnelling under the covering of the bone to remove the deepest layers of fat so that everything can be pulled upwards. The mask lift can have a very dramatic effect and it works well on lines around the eyes and mouth but it can give you an unnatural appearance because it flattens the face and gives the eyes an Oriental slant. It requires a general anaesthetic and it can take three months or longer for swelling to go down. There is an increased risk of infection in the cheek area and hair loss may occur around the incisions. Sensation in the scalp may be altered permanently.

THE KEYHOLE LIFT The use of endoscopes means that the mask lift can now be carried out through five very small cuts in the scalp and via the lower eyelids and mouth. A narrow fibre optic light and camera are inserted through the incisions so that the surgeon can see what he is doing. Through another incision, a long-handled curved chisel dissects beneath the covering of the bone to avoid damaging nerves and other structures. The procedure is relatively new and only certain surgeons are trained to do it and not all hospitals have the equipment. However, although it reduces scarring it is no less invasive than an ordinary mask lift. It requires a general anaesthetic and it will take just as long for the swelling to

even more depressed about her self-image. The saddest thing of all was that she is old, frail and needs the care and comfort that old age deserves. She should be helped across the road, and one would show sympathy for tiredness after lunch and offer her a bed but for the fact that her face is as smooth as a young girl and her expression conveys none of that. She has made herself an alien, one that no-one, least of all herself, can communicate with, who is destined always to be alone and unhappy in her tortured skin.
Georgina, 17, UK

My mother had a face lift about 20 years ago. She was not at all into make-up and looking after her skin but one day just decided to have this done and went ahead without telling any of us. It looked very good, just like she had been on a holiday and relaxed. I still have the receipt I found, after she died – it was approx £340!
Theresa, 54, UK

Anyone who is going to consider meddling with mother nature should check www.awfulplastic-surgery.com. It is the antidote to cosmetic surgery culture.
Juliette, 34, Canada

go down. At the moment, surgeons are still unsure as to how long the effects will last and, because this lift produces a radical change in appearance, it is not generally carried out on older patients.

POST OP Bandages are placed about the head and face for 24 hours and you have to keep your head elevated and as still as possible for two days to keep the swelling down. A small, thin tube may be placed under the skin behind your ear to drain any blood that might collect there. The drainage tube will be removed after one or two days. Bandages are usually removed after one to five days and most stitches will be removed after about five days. Your scalp may take longer to heal, and stitches or metal clips in your hairline may be left in longer.

Your face will look swollen, pale, bruised and puffy and this often gets worse before it gets better. Your features may be distorted from the swelling and your facial movements may be slightly stiff. Bruising may persist for two to three weeks but swelling can last up to six months. Some numbness of the skin is normal; it will disappear in a few weeks or months. The hair around your temples may be thin and your skin may feel dry for several months. You'll have some scars, but they're usually hidden by your hair, or in the natural creases of your face and ears.

RECOVERY Plan on taking it easy for about three weeks after surgery. Be especially gentle with your face and hair. Avoid hair tinting or colouring until your surgeon says it is OK. You can probably have a blow dry on a cool to medium heat after about two weeks, but don't allow anyone to pull on your hair or roughly massage your scalp. Don't wear earrings until sensation has returned to your earlobes and avoid strenuous activity, alcohol, steam baths and saunas for several months. Make-up may be applied over the skin of the face up to the edge of the surgical scars approximately seven to 14 days following surgery. Special camouflage make-up such as Jane Iredale's Mineral Make-up or Amazing Base can be used to disguise bruising and swelling and neutralize colour in reddened or yellowish skin.

RISKS AND COMPLICATIONS Complications can occur with all surgery but the specific risks with face lifts are injury to the nerves that control facial muscles (usually temporary), enduring pain in the cheeks or ears, a lop-sided smile, an asymmetrical appearance and drooping ears. Additional side effects are changes to the colour of the skin, a darkening over sites of bruising, the development of spider veins and a change in hair-growth patterns. Scars are normally hidden by the ears, but they can look red for some time and become itchy and lumpy. In rare cases, necrosis, a form of gangrene that affects skin that has lost its blood supply, occurs behind the ears. Poor healing of the skin is most likely to affect smokers.

Other facial procedures

THE NECK To get rid of turkey gobble on the neck the surgeon makes an incision under the chin to lose the vertical bands of skin that hang down. The surgeon can also reach in to the platysma muscle, which runs across the neck. If cut and tightened this can restore a right angle to the jaw. It may also bring some improvement to horizontal lines around the neck. The skin on the neck is very delicate so bruising is extensive and recovery takes between three and six months. Scars under the jaw take much longer to soften and mature and they feel stiff and lumpy for up to 12 weeks.

THE CHIN Where there is a double chin, surgeons may use liposuction to restore the shape of the jawline. A helmet of elasticated bandage then has to be worn for two to three weeks. Liposuction only works for people with skin that is elastic enough to spring back into shape and it can leave the area feeling numb. There is also an additional risk that it can damage the nerve that works the lips, leaving a lopsided smile. Older people who have liposuction under the chin may be left with worse jowls and turkey gobble than before.

FACIAL IMPLANTS In addition to a facelift or rhinoplasty, some women opt to have an implant in their cheek, jaw or chin to balance their profile, increase definition or fill out their face. Several different materials are used. Gore-tex is FDA approved and has been in use since the 1960s. However, it has been associated with ulceration and infection and there is some concern that it has a tendency to migrate from the site of implant over time. If a facial implant shifts out of alignment, a second operation may be necessary to move it back into its proper position. New versions are Softform and Ultrasoft, which come in strips and are also used to treat depressed scars, lip atrophy, and deep furrows, such as nasolabial folds and marionette lines. They are considered more effective because the materials are porous which allows your collagen to grow into them, preventing migration. Implants are inserted through existing incisions if they are carried out with a face lift or new incisions if they are being done alone. The operation takes up to an hour and is usually carried out with a general anaesthetic. The site of the implant is bandaged for about a week to keep it in place. Stitches are removed in five to seven days. There will be significant bruising and swelling and it can take several months for the swelling to subside.

RISKS Over time, implants can put pressure on the bones beneath them. This can cause the bones to dissolve and recede and sometimes the end result is worse than the pre-operative one. Infection can occur around facial implants and if it does not clear up with antibiotics, the implant may have to be temporarily removed and replaced at a later time, which means additional surgery and scarring.

I have always thought that I might have a face lift at some point but recently I saw a TV programme on a group of women who had had surgery and I was horrified. It was absolutely brutal. I think anyone who wants to have surgery should be forced to watch it because it made me realize that nothing is worth putting yourself through that amount of trauma for. It really is major surgery and even if you get the result you want, which not all of them did, you put your body through such violence and shock and surely that must age you quicker than anything.
Vicky, 52, UK

I think women who have had face lifts don't look younger. They get a kind of taut, stretched look, which might pass unnoticed in a city where not many women have access to cosmetic surgery, but in any major capital, forget it. You can spot a lift a mile away.
Justine, 40, US

Weight loss left my face looking like a rotten apple, all collapsed and sunken. Facial implants have given me back my bone structure. I love them.
Carole, 50, UK

Eyes

The number of women having eyelid surgery has soared in the last ten years. Eyelid surgery can alter the shape and symmetry of the eyes, remove fat, tighten skin and, in the case of Oriental women, widen the eyes to make them appear more Western. It will not remove crow's-feet or wrinkles, but surgeons can tighten the muscles that cause them. Although the operations sound relatively simple, it is essential you choose a highly skilled surgeon. Overtightening, inaccurate incisions and scarring can leave patients unable to close their eyes or suffering from muscle damage and drooping. Sometimes, fluid accumulates under the mucus membrane covering the front of the eye, making the eyes water for up to six weeks. If it is serious, the surgeon may have to nip the membrane to release the fluid.

UPPER EYELID SURGERY The operation takes about an hour and is usually done with a general anaesthetic, though it can be carried out with local anaesthesia as a day case. The doctor makes an incision along the line of the eyelid crease. Excess skin and fat is removed, then the skin is sewn together with very thin plastic sutures, left in for three days. The scars will leave a thin line along the upper eyelid creases, which rarely causes problems though it can cause the formation of lumps or cysts. It takes about two weeks to recover and some patients feel their eyelids are numb for up to six weeks but the final result won't be seen for two months. Because excess skin tends to regenerate, the operation is generally performed with slight overcorrection. However, the skin contracts when it scars, so if the surgeon over°corrects too much, the patient may have difficulty shutting their eyes.

EYEBAG SURGERY Eyebags run in families and sometimes develop in much younger women, so lower eyelid surgery for young people removes only fat, whereas older women need both skin and fat removed. If fat alone is removed, the operation can be done from inside the lid, which means there will be no scars. If skin has to be removed, too, then the incision has to be made on the outside just below the eyelash line out into the laugh line by the side of the eye. Excess fat is taken away, then the skin is straightened and the overlapping skin is removed. If the surgeon removes too much fat, it can lead to a gaunt, staring look, so the latest techniques leave some fat in the eyebag and then redrape the skin. It takes longer to recover from but looks more natural. If the surgeon takes too much skin away, the lid comes away from the eye and the eye dries out or the whites of the eye show too much. The eyes may also change shape. Eyebag removal is permanent, but any wrinkles that are ironed out are likely to recur. Stitches are removed after five days. Swelling and bruising takes up to two weeks to subside but it can take four to six months to see the real result. Eyes will water and feel gritty and itchy and there will be a loss of sensation in the lids until the nerves grow back, which takes around six weeks. Scars must be protected from the sun for several months.

Japanese women are very admiring of Western culture. Most Japanese women would prefer to have big wide eyes and a high nose and many actresses and hostesses have their eyes surgically widened. In the West, women make their eyes dark but in Japan they make them lighter, wider. Blue eyes are popular and tinted contact lenses are worn by girls who don't need glasses. Japanese men like whiter women with blonde hair and lots of girls use peroxide or get hair extensions because if you look right, you get a boyfriend. At high school, the fashion is to have very dark skin. Japanese girls use tanning shops and they wear a lot of white eyeshadow. To be skinny is a big deal. I am bigger than my mother because the culture and the diet has changed. Teenage girls try not to eat fatty food and fashion magazines are all about diet. In this country I look OK but when I go back to Japan I have to reduce my weight because I feel fat. Everyone stares and I feel uncomfortable because people are so tiny and I feel out of place.
Kana, 27, Japan
(Pictured right)

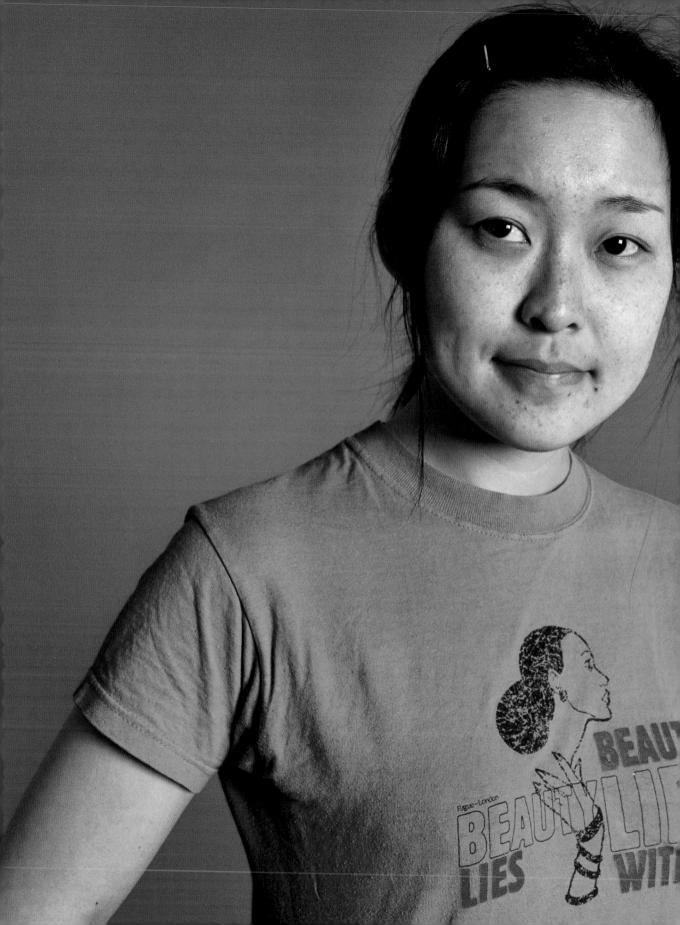

Tummy tucks, staples and bands

TUMMY TUCK A tummy tuck, or abdominoplasty, is a major surgical procedure to remove excess skin and fat from the middle and lower abdomen and to tighten the muscles of the abdominal wall. The best candidates for a tummy tuck are women who are in relatively good shape but are bothered by a large fat deposit or loose abdominal skin that won't respond to diet or exercise. The surgery is particularly helpful to women who, through multiple pregnancies, have stretched their abdominal muscles and skin beyond the point where they can return to normal. Women who plan future pregnancies should wait before they have a tummy tuck as vertical muscles in the abdomen that are tightened during surgery can separate again during pregnancy. Older women who have less elastic skin as a result of slight obesity can also see an improvement, though patients who are very overweight will be told to lose weight before they can have surgery. It produces a permanent scar, which can extend from hip to hip, so if you have scarring from previous abdominal surgery, your doctor may recommend against the procedure.

THE PROCEDURE Complete abdominoplasty takes between two to five hours. The surgeon cuts an incision from hipbone to hipbone, just above the pubic area. A second incision then frees the navel from surrounding tissue. Next, the surgeon separates the skin from the abdominal wall all the way up to your ribs and lifts a large skin flap to reveal the vertical muscles in your abdomen. These muscles are tightened by pulling them close together and stitching them into their new position. This provides a firmer abdominal wall and narrows the waistline. The skin flap is then stretched down and the extra skin is removed. A new hole is cut for your navel, which is then stitched in place. If your fat deposits are limited to the area below the navel, you may require a less complex procedure known as a mini tummy tuck. The incision is much shorter and the navel may not be moved, although it may be pulled into an unnatural shape as the skin is tightened and stitched. Finally, the incisions will be stitched, dressings will be applied, and a temporary tube may be inserted to drain excess fluid from the surgical site.

RECOVERY For the first few days, your abdomen will be swollen and painful. Though you may not be able to stand straight at first, you should start walking as soon as possible. Surface stitches will be removed in five to seven days, and deeper sutures, with ends that protrude through the skin, will come out in two to three weeks. The dressing on your incision may be replaced by a support garment. It may take you weeks or months to feel like your old self again. Some people return to work after two weeks, while others take three or four weeks to rest and recuperate. Exercise will help you heal better. Even people who have never exercised before should begin an exercise program to reduce swelling, lower the chance of blood clots and tone muscles. Vigorous exercise, however, should be avoided until you can do it comfortably. Your scars may actually appear to worsen during the first three to six months as they heal, but this is normal. Expect it to take nine months to a year before your scars flatten out and lighten in colour. While they'll never disappear completely, abdominal scars will not show under most clothing, even under bathing suits. Poor healing and conspicuous scars may necessitate a second operation.

STOMACH STAPLING AND GASTRIC BANDS These procedures are only intended for severely obese people, those who are at least 45kg (100lb) overweight, those who are at least twice their ideal body weight or those who have failed to reduce their weight by other methods. Severely obese people usually have serious health problems such as hypertension, gall bladder disease, and diabetes so the medical profession does not view these procedures as cosmetic and they are often available on the NHS.

STOMACH STAPLING Stomach stapling involves cutting through to the stomach and sealing off a small portion of the stomach with staples. The doctor then re-attaches the intestine to the new, smaller, stomach and the thinking was that if the stomach was smaller, patients would eat less.

GASTRIC BANDING Stapling has now largely been replaced with gastric banding because it is less invasive. An inflatable band is placed around the upper stomach to create a small gastric pouch. This limits food consumption and creates an earlier feeling of fullness. The band is implanted by laparoscopic 'keyhole' surgery and is then adjusted over time – either tightened or loosened – to meet the patient's needs. Once the band is in place, it is inflated with saline. Subsequent adjustments are made through a portal under the skin. The band is intended to remain in place permanently but, if necessary, it can be surgically removed. A three-year study in the US of 299 patients aged 18–55 who were given gastric banding showed they steadily lost weight. However, they were all on a severely restricted diet and exercised at least 30 minutes a day. By 36 months they had lost on average 36% of their excess weight but 5% stayed the same and 2% put on weight. Some 89% of patients experienced at least one side effect. These included nausea and vomiting (51%), heartburn (34%), abdominal pain (27%) and band slippage or pouch enlargement (24%). A further 9% of patients needed to have another operation to correct a problem with the device and 25% had their band removed, mostly because of adverse side effects. In about one-third of those patients, insufficient weight loss was also reported as a contributing factor to the decision to have their band removed. People who have a gastric band need to diet and exercise in order to maintain their weight loss.

I had been seriously overweight since my teens and my quality of life was just awful. My home life and my diet were partly to blame and my Mom was very heavy right up until she died in '94. When she passed away I inherited a small amount of money and did two years of psychotherapy in the hope that I could address my issues with food but I only managed to reduce my weight by a few kilos. Then I read a magazine article about a woman who had lost a large amount of weight through gastric banding and I decided to spend the money on having the operation. I would not say it has been perfect. I have some ongoing problems and it is difficult for me to eat in company owing to the risk of vomiting. I can only eat in restaurants if I limit myself to a small first course usually. My life has changed I suppose but it has taken time, more time than I anticipated. Nevertheless, I am pleased that I had the operation because my weight has dropped from 149 to 108 kilos and I have improved my eating habits and now exercise regularly.
Cynthia, 40, US

Thigh and arm lift

THIGH LIFTS A thigh lift is most often carried out on people who were once very obese but have since lost a lot of weight. It is also sometimes performed on people who have had a large amount of liposuction on their inner thighs. The skin on the thighs is thin and has little, if any, tone. If it has been stretched over a vast expanse of fat for a number of years, when the fat is removed it leaves empty sacks of skin, which were once filled by fat. A thigh lift is a serious procedure that requires a general anaesthetic and a three to four day stay in hospital. It takes three to six months to recover and the scars are permanent.

There are three different types of thigh lift. In the first procedure the surgeon cuts into the thigh and removes as much fat as possible and then sews up the cut, which runs from the front of the thigh between the legs and round into the crease behind the buttocks where they meet the thigh. The second type of operation is carried out on more extreme cases where people have skin running all the way down to the knee. The surgeon makes the same cut in the groin and a second cut running vertically down the inside of the thigh to the knee, which will leave a noticeable scar. The third type is for people who have been left with empty buttocks after weight loss. This is also known as a bottom lift and involves making a cut in the crease below the buttocks which runs all the way round and up to the hip bone.

Catheterization of the bladder is often required and you may become constipated after the operation. You will have to wear a pressure garment for some time to prevent DVT. Scars may become infected and the risks of fat dying off and the development of seroma – clear fluid collecting – are higher than for other operations. Nerves are sometimes cut, leaving areas of numbness, and there may be significant swelling of the thighs and lower legs. Scarring is the main problem. Initially they may be concealed by folds of flesh but over time, as skin becomes looser, the scars will start to show. Sometimes patients complain that the scar on the inner thigh pulls on the vaginal lips.

ARM LIFT This removes extra skin and fat from the upper inner arm and the upper chest near the armpit. The procedure takes about two hours and is usually under a general anaesthetic. The incision is placed on the inner and under surface of the arm and often curves or zigzags. Drains may be required for two days. A padded bandage is left on for two weeks. Bruising can be quite marked and can make tracks down the arm. Swelling is usually controlled by the bandage. Recovery takes up to four weeks and the real result won't be seen for a year. Often some fat may be liposuctioned out at the same time. The main specific problem for this operation is the long and sometimes heavy scar, though there can also be transient numbness in the arms. The scar may not heal kindly and may need revision.

Vein removal

VARICOSE VEINS One in three people get varicose veins in their lifetime and unfortunately, the 'one' nearly always wears a skirt. They occur when there is damage to the one-way valves that pump blood around the body. When a valve fails, gravity pulls blood flows down instead of up and this puts pressure on the valve below. Blood starts to pool in the veins and varicose veins begin to build up. It takes years for them to become severe but they can cause major damage if they are left untreated in either the groin or the lower leg. New technologies are making surgery less invasive but the problem can return. Very occasionally the operation causes damage to the superficial nerves leaving areas of numbness in the foot or upper thigh.

Surgical removal involves an incision in the groin which allows the major vein (long saphenous vein) to be removed completely. If the damage is situated in the lower leg, tiny cuts are dotted around the leg and the affected veins are disconnected and pulled out through the incisions. After surgery your leg will be bandaged for the first day and you will need to keep it elevated as much as possible. You will then be advised to wear heavy elastic stockings and encouraged to walk as much as possible to get your circulation moving.

Transilluminated powered phlebectomy (TIPP) is a relatively new method of vein removal that minimizes the number of incisions. Fibre optic technology illuminates the varicose vein through the skin, then suction draws the tip of the vein into a rotating blade, which effectively removes the vein. Large clusters of varicose veins can be accurately removed and recovery time is quicker.

SPIDER VEIN REMOVAL Spider veins are clusters of small, thin red, blue or purple veins that start showing up on the cheeks, nose and legs as we get older. They are much more common in women but they can be removed quite easily though treatments don't prevent new veins from surfacing in the future.

Pulse dye lasers (p.201) are the best treatment for any red blotch or blood vessel in the skin, though they may not be appropriate for blue veins and varicose veins. Each vein is treated within a couple of seconds. The site will probably come up as bruised, swollen and numb for a few days, but will be completely normal within about ten days. *Sclerotherapy* is when a chemical solution is injected into each spider vein to create a small clot, which stops blood flow and makes the vein disappear. Anywhere from five to 40 injections are required per treatment and you need two or more sessions one month apart to achieve optimal results. Residual brownish pigmentation may take up to a year to completely fade. *Electrolysis* from beauticians does not guarantee good results. It can leave tiny pitted scars and can provoke a new crop of thread veins.

I don't think that varicose vein removal can be considered to be cosmetic surgery because the veins are a medical condition that can actually be dangerous. There is obviously a cosmetic aspect because they are very unsightly and it stops women wearing skirts but I would recommend any woman who has them should have them removed.
Dierdre, 36, Wales

Laser treatment for thread veins is hyped as being quick and painless but I can assure you that it is neither. I had laser treatment for broken veins on my cheek and although they put cream on to numb my skin, the sensation of the gun was like millions of needles pinging my skin and burning me. The treatment did work but I have noticed that the skin that was treated appears to have lost all its pigment, which I was not warned about and it will not tan in the sun, so I now have white areas that look a bit like a skin disease. As such I think I have swapped one problem for another at great expense.
Sandra, 39, UK

The bits below the waist

As elective surgery goes, having a buttock implant or a designer vagina has got to be high on the list of unnecessary, ridiculous and dangerous options.
Alison, 43, UK

My labia are extremely sore and I get a burning feeling off and on and I am bruised by the incision and cannot wear pants. I am 16 days post-op and the bruising started three days ago. I have been more mobile in the last three days.
Janet, 39, US

Jesus H, I've been feeling perpetually miserable and ugly for 25 years. I hate my genitals, and I am terrified if a man starts going down on me in case he discovers my hideous deformity (labial turkey gobble). I'm 38 and single, for God's sake. When past boyfriends haven't recoiled and said, 'Oh my God, what's that?' I believe — no, I know — they're keeping stumm so as not to hurt me. My labia are ugly as hell! I've got therapy coming out of my ears, but this never goes away. But surgery might render me totally insensitive.
L, 38, UK

BUTTOCK IMPLANTS These are soft, silicone implants placed into each buttock through a single incision overlying the tailbone. Since this is an area of the body that is required for so many movements, patients can experience greater pain during the recovery period than with other cosmetic surgery procedures and the recovery time is usually longer. Pain medications are prescribed to help with the discomfort, but after approximately five to seven days the patient shoul be up and about; moving, walking, and sitting a little more comfortably. There is generally very little swelling and bruising after buttock augmentation so the results may be seen very soon after surgery. Full physical activities are usually permitted within a month after surgery. Surgical risks are few, but may include infection, bleeding, nerve and/or muscle damage, slippage and asymmetry.

LABIAPLASTY / LASER VAGINAL REJUVENATION
Women with big or flappy labias can suffer from friction during sex and discomfort when wearing tight clothes. Others just feel unattractive or think they will enhance their sexual experiences by removing some of the skin that covers the clitoris. *Labiaplasty* reduces or reshapes the labia minora — the skin that covers the female clitoris and vaginal opening. The surgery takes one to two hours and the inner lips are cut and trimmed back to a more usual size. *Laser vaginal rejuvenation (LVR)* is widely hyped as being able to enhance vaginal muscle tone, strength and control and decrease the internal and external vaginal diameters. In fact, the only difference between LVR and labiaplasty is the use of a laser scalpel instead of a knife. Using a laser scalpel during surgery is a common method of cauterizing and insuring smooth incisions, resulting in less tissue trauma (shock) and controlling bleeding. However, the procedure has the same end result and the same side effects.

After surgery, patients experience pain and swelling for two to three weeks and must abstain from sex for six weeks. In some cases there are still likely to be irregularities in the inner lips and there is risk of injury to the bladder and rectum. Overcorrection can result in painful sex and, in some cases, women who have previously been able to orgasm easily find it difficult to achieve post-operatively.

HYMEN REINSTATEMENT There is growing demand for hymen reinstatement from women wanting to reclaim their virginity. It is a relatively low-tech procedure but it requires a general anaesthetic and is very expensive. The surgeon stitches the remnants of the old hymen back together again with six dissolvable stitches leaving a small hole for menstruation. Alternatively, if the hymen is totally shredded, the surgeon tightens up the back rim of the vagina to create a narrower orifice. Whichever method is used, when penetrative sex next takes place the tissue will be torn and blood will be spilt. And then you have to get it done all over again.

Teeth

Most dental decay occurs before the age of 25 but greater emphasis on brushing means more people reach adulthood with fewer fillings so the entire profession of dentistry appears to have focussed on cosmetic whitening and treatments to straighten, mend or contour imperfect teeth.

RECEDING GUMS Receding gums are often a sign of gum disease caused by a build-up of plaque. Regular brushing helps, though overbrushing can actually make receding gums worse so it is best to consult a dentist. If the top of the tooth is very exposed, your dentist may put a white match filling over the top to protect the nerves and make the tooth look more complete. Gum surgery is still in its infancy though dentists have experimented with transferring gum tissue from one area to another or cutting away gums that are too big.

STRAIGHTENING Though wearing braces is synonymous with adolescence, teeth straightening amongst adults has had a bit of a renaissance since stars like Tom Cruise started wearing train tracks. It is a major commitment. If your jaw is overcrowded, you will have to have teeth taken out and the brace that repositions the teeth can be uncomfortable. Cleaning becomes a huge issue and it can take up to two years, after which a retainer has to be worn at night for a further year or more. Orthodontists cannot give any guarantee about the results but most people who wear train tracks are eventually pleased with the result. Costs approximately £1500–5000, though severe cases may be eligible for NHS treatment.

CROWNS OR CAPS Crowns or caps are used to disguise heavily filled or broken teeth. They are essentially false covers which are fitted over the damaged tooth, which is usually drilled into a cone shape. The strongest ones are made of gold with a porcelain veneer. Hand made to a mould of your tooth, the crown is cemented into place over the stump of the cone and they can last for years. The cost is approximately £500.

IMPLANTS These are essentially single false teeth that are anchored to the bone and work just like a normal tooth. The surgery requires a general anaesthetic while a titanium stud is inserted into the jaw bone. The wound is then stitched up and takes about a week to heal. The bone then fuses around the stud, which strengthens the jaw over a period of about six months for the top jaw and three months for the lower jaw. When the jaw is healed, a titanium post is screwed into the stud and, finally, a false tooth is attached to it. One implant will support ten to 12 teeth. It is a long-term process and requires great commitment, but the procedure has a 90% success rate. It is a very expensive procedure – up to £2000 per tooth – particularly if you are replacing more than one tooth.

I have no use for the whiteners on the market but I do on occasion pour some peroxide on my toothbrush to get rid of tea and coffee stains.
Allison, 37, Canada

Five years ago doing anything to whiten your teeth was considered quite an indulgence. I notice that attitude has changed substantially and teeth whitening is now considered to be a routine as opposed to a cosmetic process. My teeth have yellowed as I have gotten older so I think that I might investigate some of the cosmetic whitening procedures.
Carolyn, 54, UK

When I looked into having veneers I was really shocked by how much they cost – £250 per tooth. Actually the dentist wouldn't do it for me because he said my teeth were healthy and that they don't last more than five years anyway so I opted for teeth bleaching instead. I have had it done twice and my teeth are a lot whiter than they used to be. I would now like to try laser whitening which I believe is even more successful.
Rebecca, 32, UK

VENEERS Custom veneers are modelled in thin sheets of porcelain or plastic from a mould of your own teeth. The perfect veneers are then bonded over your imperfect teeth to change their colour or shape. They are ideal for teeth that are oddly shaped, chipped, gappy, crooked, too small, too big or have uneven surfaces though celebrities often get their entire mouth veneered to ensure a permanently perfect smile. If teeth are very uneven, the dentist may have to file the teeth back so that the veneers form a straight line. Teeth are prepared for veneers by lightly buffing to allow for the small added thickness of the veneer. Your dentist places the veneers with water or glycerin on the teeth to verify their perfect fit and the shade or colour. The colour cannot be changed after the veneers are adhered to your teeth. The tooth is then cleansed with chemicals to achieve a durable bond. Once the glue is between the veneer and your tooth, a light beam is used to harden the glue/cement. Veneers don't stain, are strong and very durable, last from ten to 15 years, and come in a range of colours. They are occasionally available on the NHS but most of this work is carried out privately and is incredibly expensive. Porcelain veneers cost about £450 per tooth and require two or more visits, one to two weeks apart. Plastic veneers cost significantly less, around £100 per tooth, but only last from five to seven years typically.

LASER BLEACHING The latest whitening treatments involve using a laser with a whitening gel as an in-office bleaching system. A translucent bleaching gel is applied to the teeth and a laser light is used to activate the crystals to absorb the energy from the light and penetrate the teeth enamel to increase the lightening effect on the teeth. The length of time in the cosmetic dentist's chair depends on the degree of discoloration you have, but it usually takes about an hour and a half in total. One visit is usually all it takes to substantially brighten your smile, but the procedure is more expensive than other whitening options (approximately £350).

TEETH BLEACHING Teeth bleaching involves the use of hydrogen peroxide gel to lighten the colour of the tooth enamel. The procedure can be carried out in the cosmetic dentist's office in about three hour-long treatments or it can be performed at home over a two-week period. Before whitening can begin, the dentist creates a custom mouth tray for the patient, which ensures that the correct amount of whitening solution is used and that the patient's teeth are properly exposed to the hydrogen peroxide. There are no real side effects though some people report that their teeth become increasingly sensitive. The long-term effects of having hydrogen peroxide in your mouth are not known and teeth whitening is not a permanent procedure. Results can last for one or more years, depending upon your personal habits. In most cases, the whitening procedure is very effective and the patient is pleased with the results.

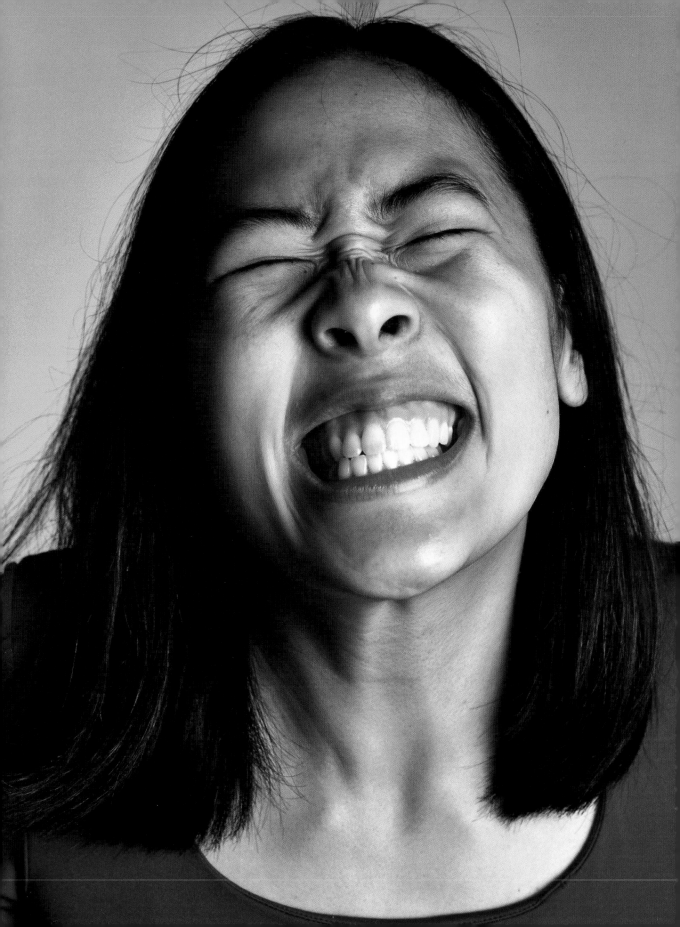

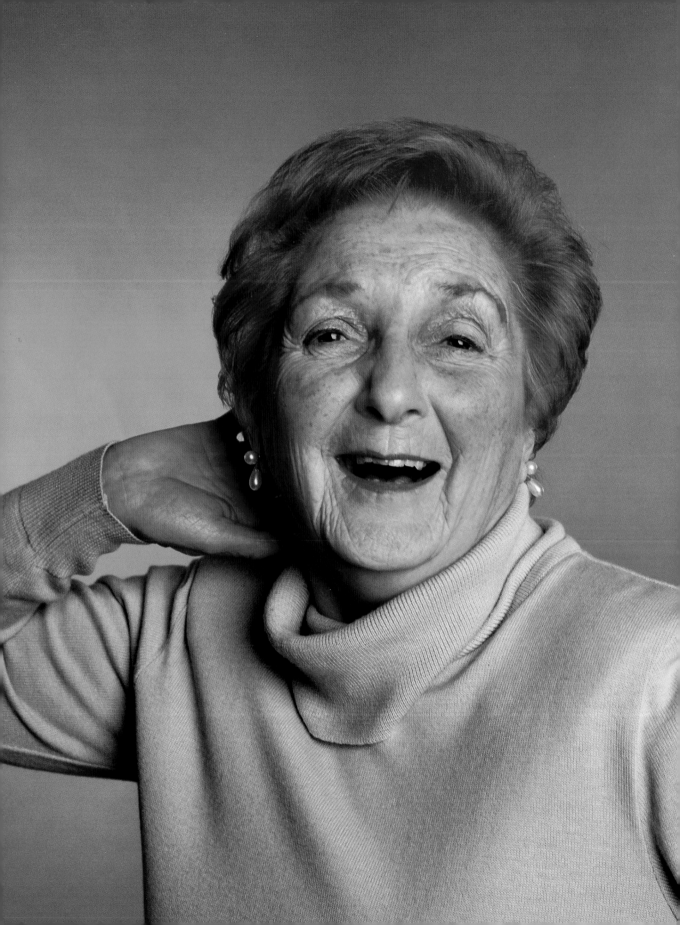

THE
Health
CHAPTER

From life span to health span ...

When I was younger I was always on the move and had buckets of energy. I managed the kids and my elderly father and and I used to fit in running around picking up antiques for my business in between. 16 years ago my hubby had a triple bypass so I had to watch his diet and as a result I eat very healthily. I can walk for two hours without any problem and I keep myself very busy. I want to go on for as long as I can but the way we live now, they have so many drugs to keep you going that you have to make a choice. I don't want to get to the point where I sit in a chair all day just waiting to be fed. That's not living. I have a living will because if I don't have any quality of life I want to be allowed to go. The problem is knowing when the cut off point is. My cousin is a very clever lady but her body is crippled with arthritis. She can't eat or pick up a pencil . It is heart breaking when someone has a good brain but their body gives up on them. Senile dementia is probably better because the people who have it don't know what they are doing, unlike my cousin . It is much harder for her because she is so astute.
Blanche, 76, UK
(Pictured previous page)

The average life expectancy for a woman living in a developed country is now between 76 and 80 years and within 60 years that figure is expected to have risen to 100 years. But extending lifespan isn't proving to be all it was cracked up to be because studies show that, for women, greater life expectancy carries no real advantage in terms of healthy additional years. Although the things that used to kill women sooner – having children, infectious diseases and acute illness – don't any more, they have been replaced by chronic diseases and degenerative illness such as cancer, heart disease and osteoarthritis, which kill later, but make old age a misery.

One of the biggest challenges for the medical profession now is how best to prevent and postpone disease and disability in order to maintain the health, independence and mobility of an ageing population. And one of the biggest challenges facing governments is how to pay for it. By 2030 the worldwide population aged 65+ will have reached 973 million, yet relatively wealthy countries already acknowledge that they have insufficient provision to meet the healthcare needs of their existing populations. This situation will inevitably get worse as greater numbers of elderly people consume increasing quantities of medical and social services. Long-term illness costs money. Immobility necessitates constant care. And as the family unit falls apart, responsibility for public welfare falls to the state. Where you are in the world and how much money you have plays a significant part in how well you will be looked after. Globally, poverty and discrimination continue to deprive many millions of women of basic healthcare. And even in developing and industrialized countries, women who are poor are less likely to be healthy. Lack of education, a diet of cheap fatty foods and a sedentary lifestyle all predict an old age plagued by obesity and ill health.

Since two-thirds of the population over 75 is female, degenerative illness is a much bigger issue for women than it is for men, and medical research, healthcare policies and social service facilities are of even greater significance to them. More research into causes and cures for degenerative diseases is vital, but gender bias appears to be rampant in medical research. Studies show that men have better access to curative care during their lives, whereas women are primarily exposed to preventative care during their reproductive years. Though high quality family planning and obstetric services are of paramount importance, women could be forgiven for concluding that medical research is only really concerned about their capacity to reproduce. Statistically, if an affliction affects both genders, there is a better chance of a cure being found for it, but studies show that women's health issues are not researched either as much, or as effectively, as health issues that affect men. This is particularly apparent when you look at areas that are fundamental to a woman's quality of life but not considered life threatening. Although the anatomical intricacies of the penis have been known for centuries, the full extent of the clitoris was only discovered in 1997. By a woman. Viagra already has competition in the form of Cialis and Levitra, but there is as yet no comparative drug for women who suffer from sexual dysfunction. And as for the male pill? It's still at least five years away.

Everyone hopes that one day there will be a magic bullet to eliminate age-related illnesses such as arthritis, osteoporosis, cancer and Alzheimer's, but the reality is, that like any machine, after a certain amount of time the body starts to malfunction, slow down, clog up and eventually conk out completely. How long your machine lasts depends on how well you have serviced it in the past. But decades of under-utilization and filling up on cheap fuel have led to a situation where, globally, cases of diabetes are predicted to reach 300 million by 2025, obesity is already an epidemic and approximately 59% of people over 65 in the US are disabled by chronic arthritis. Unless lifestyle factors are addressed right now, painful, debilitating and incurable illnesses will rise in virtually all industrialized countries. Although women cannot predict or control the socio-economic or hereditary factors that add to their risk of ill health, women can exert a positive influence over negative risk. There is no doubt that quality of life after the age of 75 is directly related to the quantity of effort invested in good health, diet and fitness before that age. Many of the degenerative conditions that place such a burden on both the affected individuals and the healthcare system that has to support them, are largely avoidable. For example, everyone knows that smoking causes lung cancer but people, particularly women, continue to smoke.

Although it's true that society has a responsibility for us, we also have a responsibility to society. Any woman who wants to have a reasonable quality of life when she is older must adopt pro-active strategies for health, nutrition, wellbeing, strength and stamina while she is still young enough to believe they don't matter. Unfortunately, we're not very good at preventative measures, (if we were, the birth rate would go right down and none of us would ever need to go on a diet, or pay a parking fine) but if the number of old, unhealthy and immobile women continues to grow, the pot of money with which to treat them will shrink proportionately, and media reports are already drawing attention to the fact that within the next 20 years cancer drugs will be too expensive to be given out free on the NHS. Given the chance again most elderly women say they would pay more attention to nutrition, fitness and good health, but hindsight is always 20 20. It is too late to regret the impact of smoking, obesity and inactivity when you are already suffering from the debilitating condition that will undermine the last 20 years of your life. As anyone suffering from a long-term illness will tell you, it's not 'life span' that counts, but 'health span'.

Reproductive and sexual health

When a girl hits puberty she spends the next three years or so engaged in an ongoing battle with her hips, her hormones and her heartstrings. From child to woman is an explosive transition and how well a girl adapts to the change can make or break her self-esteem. It can be difficult for parents too. Learning to communicate through a slammed door is no mean feat but girls who are given a sound understanding of what is happening to them, when and why, fare better physically and emotionally. For a young girl, knowing that what she is feeling and experiencing is natural and normal helps her to feel more comfortable in her new skin.

WHAT HAPPENS WHEN Puberty is triggered when the ovaries and the adrenal glands begin to increase the production of the female sex hormones, oestrogen and progesterone. The first sign of change is the swelling of the aureola (the dark brown area around the nipple). The nipple then enlarges and the breast bud grows, though the breasts are often unequal in size and shape at first. The rate at which they grow and their eventual size is partially genetic, but hormone levels also play a major role. If a girl starts taking birth control pills, her breasts may become bigger because the pill contains oestrogen.

One of the first signs of puberty is a sudden growth spurt, usually around the age of ten. Fat is laid down beneath the skin, especially on the breasts, upper arms, stomach, hips, buttocks and thighs. Affectionately referred to as puppy fat, it is regarded with anything but affection by young girls. Because this increase in body fat usually happens before there is any noticeable skeletal growth or height difference to offset the imbalance, it is often misinterpreted as actual weight gain but it should disappear naturally as soon as a girl gets taller. She should not cut out any food groups, particularly dairy (p.111), though she may want to choose low fat versions. Pubic hair usually begins to appear 6 to 12 months after the growth spurt. Hair starts to grow on the pubis, legs and arms, in the armpits, around the nipples and sometimes above the upper lip. It is longer, darker and coarser than other body hair and not necessarily the same colour as the hair on your head. It starts to grow on the vulva before spreading out in an inverted triangle to the pubic mound. As the sweat glands become more active, it can sometimes lead to body odour, and hormonal changes make hair more greasy.

SPOTS Spots almost always break out during puberty when male hormones called androgens become more active in the body. These hormones stimulate the sebaceous glands to produce sebum, the gunk that clogs up pores and causes spots. Blocked pores occur when abnormal cells at the entrance to the pore trap sebum, which then creates blackheads or whiteheads. The whole condition should really be regarded as a hypersensitivity to testosterone and treatment has to concentrate on getting rid of the blockage to the pores rather than just cleaning the surface of the face. Chronic acne (p.148) sufferers are hyper-sensitive to the bacteria, which gets trapped in hair follicles causing surrounding tissue to become inflamed and develop red and pussy spots and deep nodules and cysts. Contrary to popular opinion, eating fatty foods and chocolate doesn't contribute to spots, though greasy creams, perspiration, headbands and other things that can plug up pores can make acne worse. When washing, use a mild soap, avoid scrubbing and avoid squeezing, which can spread the problem and may lead to scarring.

PERIODS A girl's first period begins, on average, two to two and a half years after she begins to show the first physical signs of puberty. Periods are erratic to begin with and it can take as long as two years, and in some cases up to seven years, for periods to become regular, hormones to settle down and the reproductive system to mature fully. As the menstrual cycle becomes regular, a vaginal discharge, which helps to keep the vagina healthy, starts to appear. At least 20% of women have irregular cycles which makes constant contraception an imperative. Illness or eating disorders can make periods temporarily disappear, though it is still possible to get pregnant so always use protection.

Menstruation generally follows a 28-day cycle but everyone is different. Getting to know your own cycle helps you avoid pregnancy while you are young or increase your chances of getting pregnant when you are a bit older. The first day of your period is day one of your cycle (periods usually last about four or five days). During the first 14 days of your cycle, oestrogen hormones promote the growth of an egg within the ovary and the uterine lining thickens in preparation for 'potential' pregnancy. Ovulation occurs on approximately day 14 of a 28-day cycle. During ovulation, hormonal reactions make the egg burst out of its sac and travel from the ovaries, down the fallopian tube and into the uterus where it waits to be fertilized.

WHEN YOU CAN GET PREGNANT Sperm can live in the vagina for up to three days so if you have unprotected sex between day 11 and day 16 of your period, you are likely to get pregnant. Though this is the critical period there are cases of women getting pregnant at all times of the month so to be safe your partner should always wear a condom. If you don't have sex and the egg is not fertilized, approximately eight days after ovulation the lining of the uterus breaks down and is shed with blood as a period. Periods can last between two and seven days and will typically discharge about half a cup of blood and tissue. A dip in hormone levels at this point can adversely affect your mood. Your breasts may feel tender and swollen and spots may break out on your face. The decrease in hormone levels triggers increased hormone production and the cycle begins again.

As a child I always felt tall and awkward for my age and I developed a bit of a hunch because I wouldn't stand up straight. I never felt fat exactly but was never satisfied with the shape of my body or skin discoloration. My ears stuck out. I hated my feet. My boobs were always droopy, even at a young age.
Louise, 36, UK

I had my first period at the age of eight, which was so young. It was 1950 and people were very reluctant to take something like that on board. My mother was a nurse but we didn't really talk about body changes. She took me to a doctor who told me I had precocious menstruation and my mother warned me that I could get pregnant, which was pretty terrifying for an eight-year-old who knew nothing about sex. She gave me some books to read and I managed to figure out what was happening to me, but looking back I can see that it had a big effect on my confidence. I was the only child in my class dealing with a period and I just felt very different to the other girls.
Angela, 53, US

If you like your eggs unfertilized ...

My mother put me on the pill when I was 15 which was a very progressive thing for her to do given that Ireland in the 1970s was so vehemently opposed to the notion that anyone had sex unless they specifically wanted to create another mouth to feed. Thankfully she was broadminded and insightful enough to realize that my relationship with an older local boy was unlikely to remain as innocent as the church would have wanted. And how right she was.
Maeve, 45, UK

I hit a low about two days before my periods come and I just want to burst into tears at the slightest provocation. When I told my doctor he suggested that I go on the progesterone pill and it has actually alleviated the problem. I also used to suffer from painful swollen breasts and the pill has improved this too.
Kat, 28, UK

I was a bit drunk and this guy said that I shouldn't worry that we had no protection because we could get the morning after pill in the morning. That sobered me up pretty quickly. It stinks that women are expected to be responsible for everything.
Nadia, 19, UK

All methods of birth control have advantages and disadvantages. While they all offer protection against pregnancy, the condom and femidom are currently the only options that offer protection against sexually transmitted infections (STIs). A doctor, family planning clinic or health centre will help you decide what is most appropriate for you, but anyone who changes partner should use both condoms and additional contraception. If the contraceptive that you are using doesn't suit you or causes side effects, tell your doctor. Some women believe that using the pill or the coil will make them gain weight, but this hasn't been proven. In the UK, contraceptives and contraceptive advice are free from doctors and family planning clinics – private clinics may charge a fee. British law says that people under 16 can access medical treatment confidentially and can consent to it without informing their parents as long as the doctor believes they fully understand what they are doing. Most contraception is very effective if used correctly. If something is 99% effective, it means that one woman in 100 will get pregnant in a year, even if they follow the instructions. A contraceptive device inserted by a doctor should conform to the maximum success rate. Anything that allows human error – pills and condoms – generally won't.

EMERGENCY CONTRACEPTION WITHIN 72 HOURS

Previously called morning-after pills, two tablets are taken within 12 hours of each other and within 72 hours of unprotected sex. Estimated to be 75% effective, if taken sooner rather than later. Possible side effects include nausea and vomiting. If you are over 16 in the UK, you can buy them without prescription. If the pill fails, there is an increased chance of ectopic pregnancy.

EMERGENCY CONTRACEPTION WITHIN FIVE DAYS

If you are worried about pregnancy your doctor can insert a small plastic and copper device called an IUCD into your womb up to five days after sex as a form of emergency contraception. It is uncomfortable to have fitted but it is almost 100% effective. If used as emergency contraception it can be removed following your next period. Alternatively, it can be left in or inserted specifically to provide long-term contraception. Not recommended for teens. Risks of infection, pain and bleeding.

MALE CONDOM
Condoms are 98% effective for people who follow the instructions. 86% for the rest. Made of very thin latex or polyurethane, the condom is put over the erect penis before foreplay to stop sperm from entering the vagina. Condoms are widely available and are one of the only forms of contraception that also protect both partners from STIs. However, condoms need to be put on before any genital contact occurs and a new condom should be used each time. In the UK, use a condom with a BSI kitemark (BS EN 600) and CE mark on the packet. Check the expiry date. Oil-based lubricants erode latex condoms.

FEMALE CONDOM (FEMIDOM) Effective for 95% of people who follow instructions. 79% for the rest. The female condom is a soft polyurethane sheath that is inserted into the vagina and hangs down over the labia to stop sperm from entering the vagina. It offers better protection from STIs because it covers the vulva, but you need to follow the instructions carefully. In the UK, female condoms have a CE mark. They are more expensive and many women complain that they are very noisy – comparable to having sex with a crisp packet inside you.

DIAPHRAGM/CAP WITH SPERMICIDE 80+% effective. A flexible rubber/silicone device used with spermicide is put in the vagina to cover the cervix. Your doctor will fit you for the correct size. Fitting should be checked every 12 months and also if you gain or lose 3kg (7lb), have a baby, a miscarriage or an abortion. It can be put in any time before sex (if more than three hours, add extra spermicide) and must stay in for at least six hours but no more than 30 hours after sex. May protect against some STIs and cancer of the cervix. Can cause cystitis.

CONTRACEPTIVE INJECTION Effective for 99% of people and you don't have to remember to take a pill. The injection lasts eight weeks (Noristerat) or 12 weeks (Depo-Provera), offers some protection from pelvic inflammatory disease and may protect against womb cancer. Periods often become irregular or stop. It may take up to seven months for regular periods and fertility to return after stopping injections. Possible side-effects include weight gain, headaches, acne, tender breasts, depression, mood swings and water retention/bloating. Before having the injection, go on a course of the progestogen-only mini pill to check side effects. The injection cannot be removed, so side effects continue as long as it lasts.

CONTRACEPTIVE IMPLANT 99% effective. A small, flexible tube is placed under the skin of the upper arm under local anaesthetic. No stitches required. It works for three years and, when the implant is taken out, normal levels of fertility should be re-established immediately. Some women gain weight. Temporary side effects include headaches, mood changes and breast tenderness. Most women can feel it in the skin, but it can't be seen. Removal is simple and leaves no scar.

EVRA CONTRACEPTIVE PATCH No error statistics available but not idiot-proof. Recent concerns about safety have not been proven. A 7.5cm (3in) waterproof patch is worn on the buttocks, upper-outer arm, lower abdomen or upper torso, but not the breast. Women replace the patch weekly on the same day for three consecutive weeks, then go patch-free for a week. Efficacy may be reduced in women who weigh more than 90kg (14st 2lb).

If you are older and a smoker, your options for contraception become increasingly limited. My doctor is quite unsympathetic because he simply tells me to give up smoking so that I can go on the combined pill. The progesterone pill doesn't seem to agree with me. It is all very well saying that but if I could quit, believe me I would have done it by now.
Fi, 42, US

I had a contraceptive implant put in before I left because I knew I was going to be travelling for at least two years. Well I haven't had as much sex as I would have liked but it seems to have done the trick. The only thing I don't like about it is the fact that I can feel it like a hard square under my skin on my arm.
Ellen, 23, Aus

I think any contraception that has to be thought about doesn't work. I had a cap but I kept forgetting to put it in and then, if you try and insert it quickly, you get butterfingers and it is a disaster. I also felt wierd carrying it around in my handbag just in case I found someone to have sex with. Way too calculated and unromantic.
Rowan, 27, UK

NUVARING A flexible ring impregnated with progestin and oestrogen is inserted into the vagina for three weeks, then removed for one. It has to be taken out on the same day and at the same time as it was put in. Position is unimportant. 99% effective despite the fact that it delivers substantially lower doses of hormone.

PROGESTOGEN-ONLY PILL (MINI PILL) Generally about 95% effective. Progestogen thickens cervical mucus making it difficult for sperm to enter the womb or for the womb to accept a fertilized egg. In some women it prevents ovulation. Suitable for older women who smoke, have migraines or high blood pressure or women who are breastfeeding. May be less effective in women who weigh over 70kg (11st). It is important to take this pill at exactly the same time every day because it is not effective if taken more than three hours late. Vomiting or severe diarrhoea can also make it ineffective. Some drugs stop the pill working.

THE COMBINED PILL Generally about 95% effective. Contains oestrogen and progestogen, which stop ovulation, thicken cervical mucus and alter the lining of the womb. Often reduces bleeding, period pains and PMS, and gives some protection against ovarian and uterine cancer and some pelvic infections. Suitable for most healthy non-smokers up to the menopause. It is not suitable for all women, depending on their medical history. Rare but serious side effects include blood clots (thromboses), breast cancer and cervical cancer. Can cause acne, weight changes, tender breasts, nausea and headaches. Not suitable for smokers over 35 years. Not effective if taken over 12 hours late. Some drugs stop the pill working.

SEASONALE A new pill that limits the number of periods you have to four a year. Researchers estimate that women now have three times as many periods (450 over a lifetime) as our ancestors and many doctors believe cutting back on the number of periods we have would be a good thing. Currently US FDA approved, and a UK licence has been applied for. May reduce the risk of ovarian cancer but the risks for breast cancer and blood clots are the same as the pill.

INTRAUTERINE SYSTEM (IUS) – THE MERENA COIL 99% effective. A small, plastic, T-shaped frame with a tiny reservoir containing 52mg of a progesterone hormone delivers about 20 micrograms a day to the lining of the uterus. It works as soon as it is put in, lasts for five years and can be taken out at any time. Periods are much lighter and shorter so it can be useful for women with very heavy periods. Some women don't get any periods at all. The disadvantages are irregular bleeding, which is common for the first three months or so. There may be temporary side effects, such as breast tenderness and acne. In the early months of use there is a small chance that the IUS may dislodge and come out.

Promises, promises ...

THE MALE PILL We've waited years for a male pill, but now it looks like two might come along at once. The most promising one could be available within five years but how many men are going to queue up for an implant of the female hormone progestogen which has to be supported by three monthly testosterone injections to counter the 'feminising effects' of man breasts, a squeaky voice and a penchant for Manolos? The implant lasts for a year and reduces sperm production from 20m-200m sperm per millilitre to less than 1m/ml. This renders men temporarily infertile though normal sperm production is resumed within three to six months after the implant is removed. It won't offer any protection against STIs.

The second drug (NB-DNJ) was originally tested on mice but is already licensed for use in treating a rare human genetic disorder called Gaucher's disease. In studies, after three weeks of treatment the mice became completely infertile which makes it, at the very least, a revolutionary new rodent control, at the very best, a fully reversible male contraceptive pill. Since it has already been tested for side effects on humans fast-track development is more likely. Once off the treatment fertility is regained within about 40 days. It won't provide protection against STIs (and would have to be taken daily by a gender that struggles to remember events that only occur once a year ie. birthdays, anniversaries etc.).

MICROBICIDE GELS Currently being developed in the UK, the US and France, microbicides are gels, creams, foaming tablets and films that aim to provide protection against both pregnancy and sexually transmitted infections. There are three different types at present. Carreguard, a seaweed gel that lines the cells of the vagina, is the most advanced. It works by putting a sticky coating around viruses and bacteria as they enter the vagina. It is put in two hours before sex, lasts for about eight hours and with the addition of a strong spermicide becomes a contraceptive too. The second type of gel works by increasing acidity levels in the vagina to neutralize sperm, which are alkaline. However, too much acid can burn the skin and cause lesions, which obviously makes infection more, rather than less likely. The third option puts anti-retrovirals – HIV drugs – in a topical gel to deliver the drugs directly to the virus. It's at an early stage but would either prevent the replication of the virus once it has entered the host cell, or render it non-infectious beforehand. Assuming microbicide products can be further developed, they would be greatly welcomed by women in the West, but their real impact would be felt in less developed countries where they could help to halt the spread of HIV. However, the first generation of these products are only 50% effective against STIs and HIV so there is a long way to go. With sufficient investment these products have the potential to save millions of lives, but they also offer the first chance of a contraceptive alternative to condoms which will protect against STIs and HIV.

It's typical that there is no male pill. There would be no market for it because men would simply refuse to take it. Men see contraception as an entirely female responsibility and they are not likely to change that view.
Claude, 31, UK

I went on the pill for six months but I put on loads of weight and I just felt slightly wierd. I know they say it does not make you fat but it does. I was switched to a lower dose pill but I don't feel that my doctor really listened to what I was saying because it seemd to have the same effect on me. When I split with my boyfriend I came off the pill immediately but I now don't feel safe. If I meet someone, what do I do? Condoms are just awful and, to be honest I don't trust them. Until I have children my doctor refuses to give me a coil and a friend of mine who used a diaphragm ended up pregnant. What are women supposed to do?
Sarah, 26, UK

I have tried pretty much everything when it comes to contraception and reckon that there is still no perfect form of protection. Right now I use a diaphragm but I think it is fiddly.
Bryony, 34, US

Beginner's gynaecology

The importance of Smear Testing

Smear tests prevent between 1100 and 3900 cases of cervical cancer each year, so all women over 20 should be tested every three years. Results are more accurate if the test is done in the middle of your menstrual cycle and the result will either be normal (negative) test, or abnormal (positive). Unfortunately, the test itself is not perfect and in up to one in four positive tests there is actually no disease present ('false positives'). Similarly, in up to one in five negative tests there are cancerous cells present ('false negatives'). Innacurate results have led to a huge loss of faith in the smear test in the last ten years and doctors are as concerned about false positive tests that lead women to undergo unnecessary intensive treatment, as they are about false negatives where women who have cancerous cells that could be nipped in the bud are told that there is nothing wrong with them. Smear tests are clearly beneficial but it seems a bit bizarre that scientiists can clone sheep and grow human ears on mice, yet they can't make an accurate screening system for cervical cancer.

PREMENSTRUAL SYNDROME (PMS) The sudden falls in the levels of progesterone and oestrogen just before a period can alter emotional and behavioural patterns and cause PMS. Symptoms include crying, depression, fatigue, irritability, sensitivity, forgetfulness, apathy, feeling bloated, spots, breast tenderness, headache, food cravings, fluid retention and swelling and a deep dissatisfaction at having been born female. In bad cases doctors may prescribe the combined pill, mild diuretics, hormone therapy or anti-depressant drugs. Report all serious pain or abnormal or heavy bleeding to a doctor as it may indicate gynaecological problems.

URINARY TRACT INFECTIONS (CYSTITIS) If you experience pain, irritation or need to urinate more often, you may have a urinary tract infection (UTI). UTIs can cause kidney damage or other serious health problems if left untreated for more than 48 hours, so it may save time to go directly to a Genito Urinary (GU) clinic, where diagnosis and treatment (with antibiotics) will be swift. Recurrent UTIs, such as cystitis, are more common in women. Attacks often coincide with new, more frequent or more vigorous sexual activity, hence the term 'honeymoon cystitis', but they can also be triggered by thrush, dehydration or even by wearing tight underwear in a hot environment. The decrease in lubrication and thinning of the vaginal walls at menopause may also trigger recurrent cystitis.

To avoid UTIs wear clothes that allow air to circulate, avoid synthetic underwear and drink lots of water. Use extra lubrication, and urinate before and after sex to clear your urethra. At the first hint of an attack, drink as much water as you can (even if it is in the middle of the night). Cranberry juice contains a mystery ingredient that prevents the bugs that cause cystitis from latching on to the bladder wall and eases the symptoms. If it really hurts to urinate, sit in a bath of lukewarm water and pee, or pour warm water over yourself while you pee.

THRUSH (CANDIDA ALBICANS) A common yeast infection that infects the vagina and can also infect the mouth, creating a very itchy area and creamy patches of a curdy, non-smelly discharge. Thrush is simple to treat with antifungal creams, pessaries or a single over-the-counter pill. The problem may be triggered by antibiotics, which is why cystitis and thrush often follow one another.

BACTERIAL VAGINOSIS (BV) This develops when naturally occurring bowel bacteria multiply in the vagina. The most noticeable sign is a strong fishy smell. This may be accompanied by a thin, watery, white-grey discharge, soreness and occasionally itching or swelling around the vagina. It may be contracted as a result of having sex without a condom or hand-to-vagina contact. Many women develop BV as a result of over-cleaning. Vaginal deodorants, bath products or clothes conditioners can destroy protective bacteria and alter the acid–alkali balance in the vagina, allowing germs to multiply. Diagnosis involves testing the vaginal lining and swabbing discharge. Treatment is by antibiotics, creams or pessaries.

HAEMORRHOIDS (PILES) These are varicose veins in the anus that can bleed and be painful. The extra weight of pregnancy and pushing during labour makes women who have had children particularly prone to them. Treatment is by cream or pessaries, from your doctor or a pharmacy. Generally, they shrink in two to three days, and then it helps to gently push them back up inside the rectum. Taking exercise and increasing the amount of fibre and water in your diet may help. Persistent, painful piles can be injected to shrink them, or surgically removed.

SKIN IRRITATIONS ON THE VULVA Skin conditions, such as eczema, scabies and lichen sclerosis (which can manifest as scarred white or pigmented skin or as open wounds) are relatively common and need medical treatment. But women often mistakenly believe that their condition is due to lack of hygiene and use DIY methods to clean (household antiseptic) or cure (inserting garlic cloves) their problem. In fact, these remedies can severely aggravate the skin.

POLYCYSTIC OVARY SYNDROME (PCOS) A common condition caused by a hormone imbalance that often starts during the teenage years. Symptoms include irregular periods, hair growth on the face and other parts of the body, weight gain, patches of dark skin and acne. The most common treatment is the combined contraceptive pill, which can help to balance hormone levels, lower the risk of endometrial cancer and lessen hair growth and acne. Your doctor should monitor your condition as it can affect fertility.

PELVIC INFLAMMATORY DISEASE (PID) Inflammation of the uterus and fallopian tubes is usually caused by an infection (such as chlamydia or gonorrhoea) that has not been treated properly. It can also develop when the cervix dilates during an IUD fitting, miscarriage, childbirth or an abortion. It is often symptomless, but acute PID can cause severe abdominal pain, a high temperature, heavy periods, nausea, a change in vaginal discharge, a fast pulse and pain or discomfort during sex. The diagnosis is made by an internal pelvic examination or by ultrasound. In severe cases, a gynaecologist may need to carry out a laparoscopy under a general anaesthetic. A small cut is made to allow the doctor to see the internal organs through a tiny fibre-optic device incorporating a camera. Treatment is with antibiotics, bed rest and painkillers. In severe cases, a stay in hospital is necessary so that antibiotics can be given intravenously. Sexual partners need to be treated too.

I knew something was wrong because I was having to go to the bathroom every 15 minutes from four to eight times in a row. When I went to the doctor I got the usual spiel about cystitis, cotton knickers and cranberry juice, but I knew I needed treatment. I eventually went to see a new general practitioner who did a dipstick test and told me I had a UTI. He gave me Bactrim and told me to take it for three days. Well, I took it for four and the infection seemed to be gone. Then three days later, it was back. I went back to the doctor and he gave me Cipro, a seven-day course. I was on the antibiotics but about two to three days after I finished the course it was back again. Then I was given some other kind of antibiotic and some Pyridium (my first experience with orange wee wee). Nothing seemed to work. One night I had to pee every five minutes for over an hour. Eventually I was put on a month's worth of Amoxycillin and that seems to have worked, but who'd have thought a lousy infection could be so hard to treat?
Nicky, 34, US

ENDOMETRIOSIS   10-15% of women of childbearing age have endometriosis, a condition where the cells that normally line the uterine cavity grow outside the uterus creating tissue growths such as fibroids and polyps on the ovaries, fallopian tubes, uterine surface and the lining of the abdominal cavity. This causes pain and abnormal menstrual bleeding, and fertility can be negatively affected. Diagnosis requires a laparoscopy examination under a general anaesthetic. Surgery or hysterectomy may be required to remove the tissue.

CERVICAL CANCER   Abnormal bleeding patterns may also be a sign of cervical cancer. It is thought to be more common in women who have had genital warts, those who smoke and those who start having sex at an early age. It affects about 4000 women in the UK every year, the vast majority of whom have never had a smear test. It can be successfully treated if it is caught in the early stages, but women who don't have smear tests don't usually find out they have the cancer until it is too late. Cervical cancer takes several years, even for severely abnormal cells to progress to cancer, but studies show that if women with early signs of cancer are not treated, 36% will develop an invasive tumour within 20 years.

ENDOMETRIAL CANCER   Abnormal vaginal bleeding, especially after the menopause, can be a sign of endometrial cancer. It is rare in women under 50 and less common in women who have taken the pill. Women who are over 50, childless, obese or are late starting the menopause have more risk. Early diagnosis has a high success rate. Treatment involves hysterectomy and possibly radiation.

OVARIAN CANCER   This affects about 5000 women a year in the UK and 4000 of them die because it is difficult to detect and doesn't cause specific symptoms until it is quite advanced. It can be picked up by vaginal examinations or ultrasound scans but there is still no reliable screening procedure so women who have a family history of ovarian cancer should inform their doctor so that they can be monitored. It generally doesn't cause abnormal bleeding but it can cause abdominal pain, bloating, nausea, vomiting, eratic bleeding, diarrhoea or constipation. The treatment involves surgery to remove growths, further surgery to remove the womb, ovaries and tubes, and chemotherapy to kill the cancer.

HYSTERECTOMY   In the UK, one in five women, mainly aged between 40 and 50, has to have a hysterectomy: the removal of the uterus, fallopian tubes, cervix and sometimes the ovaries. It is a serious procedure and most woman take about six weeks to recover. Following a total hysterectomy, a woman will automatically go through the menopause. Women who are left with one or both of their ovaries intact have a 50% chance of entering menopause within five years of this operation.

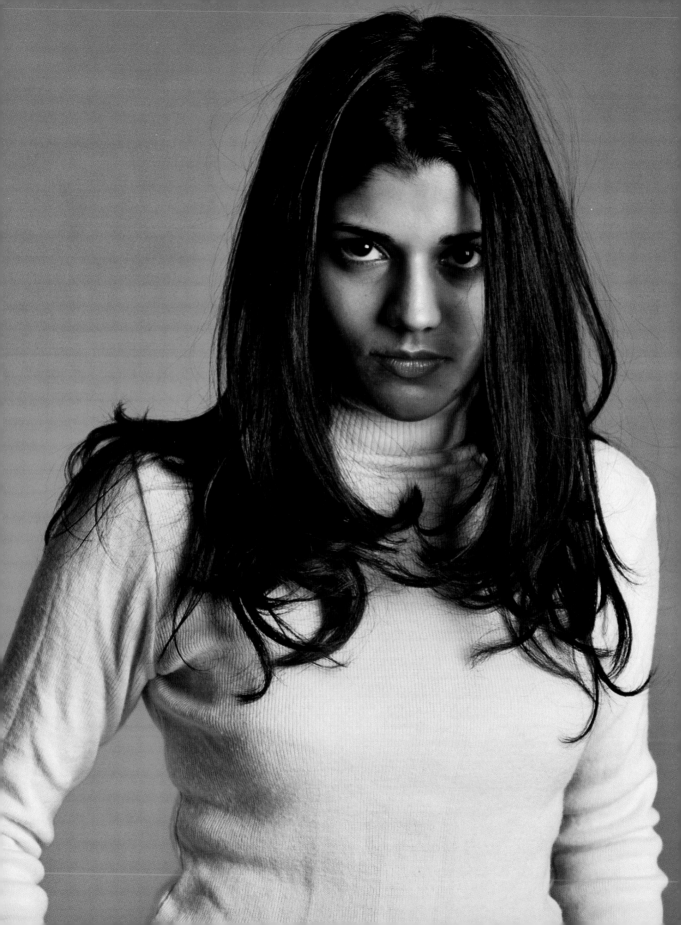

Sexually transmitted infections

STIs DON'T DISCRIMINATE Though sex education campaigns often target young people, recent research has shown that as older generations become increasingly sexually active (a result of divorce, better health and increased longevity), the rate of STI infection in later years is rising. Though women are routinely screened for infection, men are not, yet they are statistically more likely to carry infections like chlamydia and less likely to consult health professionals. So, any female who is sexually active needs to simultaneously protect herself from pregnancy and infection.

VISIBLE SIGNS Though exposure to an STI doesn't automatically mean that you will contract one, some infections don't have any visible symptoms so you should get yourself tested if you have had unsafe sex with a new or risky partner. Symptoms of an STI may include: a change in the consistency, smell or appearance of discharge; pain or burning when peeing; needing to pee more often; sore, swollen genitals; itching, rashes or lumps or blisters on the genitals or the anus; and a persistent dull ache or sudden, acute pain in the lower abdomen. It is vital both to avoid sexual contact while waiting for test results and during treatment. And you must contact all your recent sexual partners and encourage them to be tested as well.

TELLING YOUR PARTNER Most people accept that their partners have a sexual history when entering into a relationship, but disclosure can be very difficult because it raises so many questions. Was your partner infected before your relationship started, or is this STI an indication of recent infidelity? Did you have the STI without knowing it and have you passed it on to your partner? Whatever the answers are, it is important that you both see a doctor without delay to prevent re-infection and that you tell anyone that you have recently had sex with, as they will need to be tested and treated before they spread the infection further. Because telling partners is awkward, GU clinics have come up with a clever system to limit embarrassment. You are given a contact slip with a code written on it. You can either pass this on to partners you might have infected or you can get the GU clinic to post them the slip anonymously. The slip can then be presented at any GU clinic, and the code will let the doctors know exactly which STI they are looking for.

CHLAMYDIA This is the most common but treatable STI but if left untreated it can lead to pelvic inflammatory disease (PID) and eventually infertility. It also increases the chances of having an ectopic pregnancy. It is contracted during sex and can pass from mother-to-child during birth. It affects the cervix, urethra, rectum and eyes. In women, signs and symptoms include increased vaginal discharge; frequent or uncomfortable peeing; pain in the abdomen; irregular periods; and pain or bleeding during deep penetrative sex. However, often there are no symptoms at all which is why regular sexual health screening is important. To test for chlamydia a doctor will take urine samples and take swabs from the sites of infection. You may need to have an internal examination too. Results usually take about a week and treatment is with antibiotics. Doctors advise against penetrative sex until you have been given the all-clear and your partner should also be tested.

GENITAL WARTS Genital warts are caused by the human papilloma virus (HPV). They are transmitted via skin-to-skin contact or vaginal or anal intercourse and appear in the genital region one to three months after infection, either as small pinkish-white lumps or larger cauliflower-shaped lumps. They may itch, but are usually painless. A doctor or nurse will be able to tell just by looking, but a vaginal or anal examination may also be required. A brown liquid (podophylotoxin) is prescribed and applied to the warts at home. It may take from four to six weeks of repeated applications to be effective. The warts can also be removed by freezing them or by laser treatment. Avoid sex and keep the infected area covered.

GONORRHOEA (THE CLAP) A bacterial infection transmitted via penetrative sex, rimming or touching the infected area and then touching your own vagina, mouth or anus without washing your hands in between. It infects the cervix, urethra, rectum, anus and throat. It can be symptomless. however women may have a yellow discharge. Peeing may be painful, too, and the anus can become irritated or produce a slight discharge. The test involves a genital examination, an internal swab and a urine sample. Treatment is by antibiotics and you must abstain from sex until the course has been completed.

HERPES This is a virus (herpes simplex) that hides away in the body, undetected and symptomless, after the initial outbreak. Some people never have another episode; others do, especially when they are feeling run down, stressed or depressed. There are two types: HSV1, which infects the mouth or nose as cold sores; and HSV2, which infects the genital and anal area. The infection can be transmitted through skin-to-skin contact but the strains cross over, so a woman with a cold sore can give her partner genital herpes if she performs oral sex and vice versa. Oral herpes can be easily cleared up with creams like Zovirex. Genital herpes is more complicated. The virus stays with you for life and the blisters and sores are highly infectious during an outbreak, so any direct contact will spread the virus. Medical treatment is required to clear up first-time bouts of genital herpes but people who suffer severe recurrent bouts may need continual treatment. Between outbreaks the chances of infection are reduced, so sufferers can resume their sex lives as long as they use condoms. Genital herpes can cause flu-like symptoms, backache, headache, swollen glands and fever. Small, fluid-filled blisters develop,

Information about sexually transmitted infections and even pregnancy goes out the window when you fall for a bloke. The heat of the moment is so much more persuasive and powerful and emotional than some lukewarm government sponsored advertising campaign. I have had mornings where I have woken up and looked at the guy beside me and thought shit!!!!! but generally I have never had a problem so far and I think the statistics don't really relate to me and my peer group. We don't do drugs and share needles and no one is bi. My guess is that people who are very promiscuous and doing drugs are far more likely to screw up and catch something. I might be wrong of course.
Esme, 26, UK

An old boyfriend of mine had really bad herpes but we managed to work around it. He wore condoms and was careful whenever he had an outbreak and we were fine the rest of the time. Eventually I just got fed up of it and I felt depressed about the thought of catching it and I thought, 'I'm not putting up with your disease' so we split up.
Rachel, 32, UK

causing itching or tingling in the genital region. They then burst and turn into sores which can be very painful, especially when urine passes over them. They eventually dry out, scab over and heal in two to four weeks. Testing involves an internal examination and swabbing of the genitals. Results take about two weeks.

HEPATITIS A (HAV) A viral infection that causes damage to the liver. Hepatitis A is one of three of the more common types of hepatitis. The virus is transmitted through oral and anal contact and faeces and causes damage to the liver. Signs and symptoms are fever, nausea, jaundice, fatigue, weight loss and a distaste for fatty foods, alcohol and cigarettes. The virus is detected by a blood test. A vaccination is available but it is not commonly given to women. There is no treatment for HAV, though avoiding alcohol and plenty of rest are advised. 99.9% of people recover completely and are then immune to subsequent infection.

HEPATITIS B (HBV) A viral infection that can cause ongoing damage to the liver. HBV is transmitted through infected blood or bodily fluids in the same way as HIV, though HBV is more infectious than HIV. About a third of people infected have no symptoms at all, but when they are present they include nausea, fever, vomiting, aching, jaundice, yellow eyes, dark urine and pale stools. In the majority of cases, flu-like symptoms pass after a few weeks, often without lasting liver damage. The virus is detected by a blood test. Post-diagnosis patients need lots of rest, no medication, no alcohol and a low fat diet. Chronic carriers may have injections of interferon, either daily or three times a week, or combination therapy.

HEPATITIS C (HCV) HCV is transmitted in blood and possibly semen. Signs and symptoms are the same as for HVB. The virus is detected by a blood test and affects the liver. The treatment is injections of interferon, three times a week for 6–12 months. Combination drugs (ribavarin and interferon) are becoming available. Vaccination is not possible. About 80% of people with HCV become chronic carriers.

HIV AND AIDS HIV can be transmitted via blood (including menstrual blood), seminal fluid, vaginal fluid and breast milk. The virus generally passes from one person to another through the internal lining of the sex organs and rectum during penetrative sex without a condom. It can also be transmitted by sharing needles and from a mother to her child during birth or breastfeeding. A simple blood test can pick it up, but it may not be detectable for up to three months after exposure, so if you have unprotected sex during that time, the result might give you a false negative. Testing is usually done at a GU clinic and some clinics can give results on the same day. Since 1996, highly active anti-retroviral therapy (HART), a life-preserving cocktail of drugs, has lowered the AIDS-related death rate by 75 per cent. However, levels of drug-resistant HIV have increased five-fold in the last four years as the virus mutates rapidly. The disease can lie dormant for ten years, so it's quite possible that anyone (including you) could be infected and not know about it. Never assume that a new partner is free of HIV. HIV can be given, but only to someone who puts themself in a position to receive it.

PUBIC LICE (CRABS) Crabs are tiny parasitic insects that live in pubic hair, but occasionally they are found in underarm, leg, abdomen and chest hair, eyelashes and beards. Symptoms are itching in the infected area; black specks in your underwear (from lice droppings); brown eggs in your pubic hair; flaky skin, like dandruff; and, of course, the little crawling beasts themselves. The lice can be seen, so diagnosis is usually immediate. You must warn everyone you slept with in the two weeks before noticing symptoms and avoid sexual contact for a week after treatment finishes. Pubic lice are treated easily with a medicated lotion available from pharmacists without prescription. Clothing and bedding should be washed. Treatment should be repeated a week after the initial one.

SYPHILIS This bacterial infection has been fairly rare in the UK until recently. However, the incidence in gay men is now described as an epidemic. Transmission occurs via sex or skin contact or mother-to-foetus. It infects the anus, vagina, and mouth, or any skin abrasion. Symptoms may take up to three months to show. There are three phases, and the condition is highly contagious during the first two. In the primary phase, a painless sore appears at the site of infection. The secondary phase starts about four to ten weeks after the sore appears. Symptoms include a non-itchy rash covering the body, flat warty growths on the vulva or anus, flu-like symptoms, swollen glands, loss of appetite, general tiredness, white patches on the tongue and the roof of the mouth and patchy hair loss. But many other symptoms are possible, because syphilis is notorious for its ability to mimic other diseases. Treatment is usually a two to three week course of penicillin injections. Without treatment, syphilis stays latent in the body and can develop into tertiary syphilis, anything from years to decades later affecting the heart, the nervous system and internal organs. The test involves analysing blood or pus.

TRICHOMONAS VAGINALIS (TV) TV is a tiny, single-celled organism that causes an infection in the vagina. It is usually transmitted via penetrative sex and, very rarely, sharing moist towels, washcloths, jacuzzis or baths may spread it. There may be no symptoms or you may notice a change in the look and smell of any vaginal discharge (frothy and greenish); soreness around the vagina; and pain while peeing or during sex. The test involves a urine sample and an internal examination. TV is treated with antibiotics. Avoid sex until you get the all-clear.

I went down on my boyfriend and I was giving it my best when I suddenly saw something moving in his pubic hair. I knew what it was and I knew he hadn't caught it from me. We had been together for two years and although he tried to fob me off with a bullshit line about getting it at the gym I am not that dumb. I don't think I had it but I was so repulsed by the idea of having insects in my pubic hair that I shaved it all off anyway. Truly the most gross experience ever and not one that a condom would protect you from either.
Martha, 32, US

I have been married for five years but I recently had a one night stand with a work college while away at a conference. I knew he played around but I never considered the fact that he might have had an infection. We didn't use protection and two weeks later I got an email from him telling me he had gonorrhoea and I had to get tested. That was the worst week of my life. I felt like such an idiot and the thought of telling my husband made me feel sick. I was lucky I was clear but I will never do it again.
Valerie, 28, UK

Body beautiful

I work in a profession where appearance is taken very seriously, but being pregnant means relinquishing any control you may have had over your body. I found that quite liberating. You can't hold your tummy in anymore because your body has a different function. I wanted to continue smoking but I couldn't because it made me feel sick. I didn't drink for several months but I come from a French family so I had the odd glass of wine but it gave me heartburn. I ate well and went organic. I think if you can afford to, you should eat food that hasn't had antibiotics pumped into it. I gained a lot of weight very quickly – four cup sizes in six weeks. The rest caught up later. I was very active during my pregnancy. I swam every day and cycled up to eight months. Because I am over 40 I was advised to have amnio and that was hard because we knew there was a 50% chance of abortion. I think if I had listened to my body, I would have known that everything was fine but doctors overwhelm you with information. They don't make moral judgements but in the end it boils down to whether you could cope with a baby who is disabled.
Liz, 42, U.K., actress

HOW TO GET PREGNANT First you find a guy, and then you have sex. Simple? Not really. It takes an average of six months for any couple to get pregnant but you can increase the odds dramatically by making sure you are healthy, relaxed, the right weight (p.16), and relatively fit (chapter 3). Though pregnancy becomes more difficult once a woman is over 35, for most it's simply a matter of continued persistence. If nothing happens within 12 months, you and your partner should visit your GP to arrange fertility testing (p.263).

BEFORE YOU GO OFF THE PILL BEAR IN MIND If ever there was a test of female body image, pregnancy would be it. Although many women love every minute of being pregnant, others find it very difficult to cope with their changing body. Pregnant women are supposed to 'glow with good health' but many just feel fat, particularly in the period between three to six months when the bump is not really defined. When pregnancy starts to show, uninvited touching makes many women feel as if their bodies are public property, while an abundance of unsolicited advice can be either intensely irritating or downright alarming. Many women object to being treated like an invalid (others love this) by doctors who relate to pregnant women as 'patients' that need monitoring, rather than normal women having babies.

Women report feeling socially invisible as they increase in size and those that already suffer from disordered eating can find it difficult to resolve the internal conflict that occurs when their own eating patterns are at odds with their responsibility to the baby they are carrying. On the other hand, for women who were overweight and self-conscious about their size before they became pregnant, pregnancy can be the one time that they, and others, view their body positively. This can be a big boost to self-esteem and many women find themselves paying more attention to their diet because they feel a responsibility to their baby that they don't necessarily feel towards themselves. If proper eating patterns are developed during pregnancy and maintained after the baby is born, it can be a real turning point for the very many women who struggle with healthy eating.

WEIGHT GAIN Recommendations about weight gain during pregnancy have changed substantially over the last 200 years. In the 19th century, pregnant women were encouraged to eat as little as possible to limit foetal size because mortality during childbirth was so high and Caesarean deliveries were a desperate alternative. By 1989 recommended allowances for energy intake during pregnancy were set at 200–300 extra calories per day and babies were much bigger. But new research now suggests that inactivity and a slower metabolic rate means pregnant women don't need any extra calories at all in the first six months of pregnancy

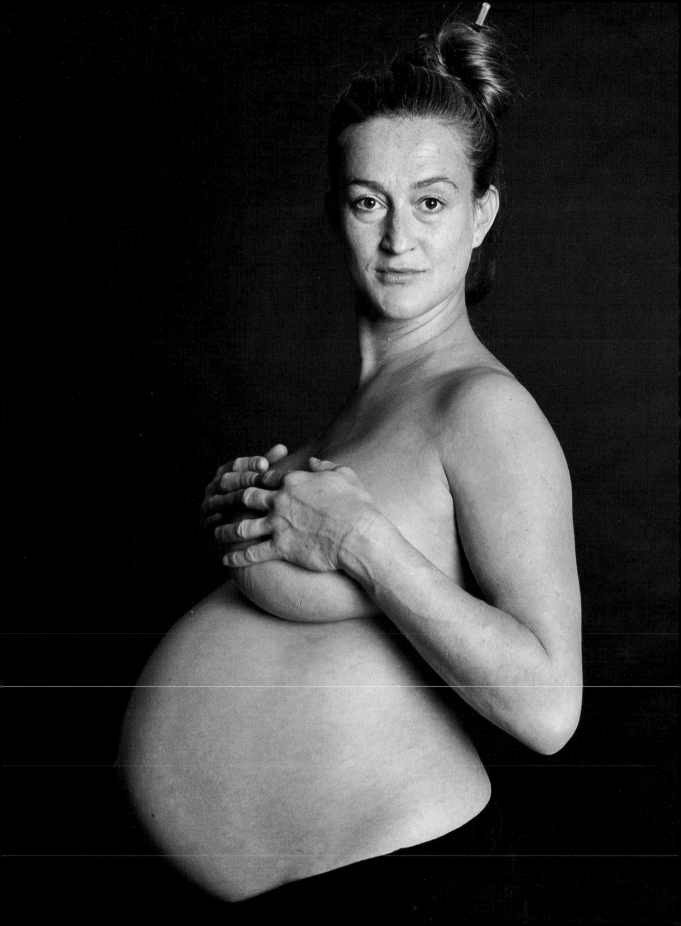

unless they were underweight to begin with. Guidelines suggest women should only increase their food intake by between 50 (half an apple) and 200 calories (a small baked potato) a day in the last trimester. Despite the fact that childbirth is now so much safer, putting on a lot of weight is a bad idea. Besides the fact that it's a night-mare to shift afterwards, it increases the likelihood that you will have to have a Caesarean and is associated with a range of medical conditions such as high blood pressure, gestational diabetes and pre-eclampsia. The American Association for Cancer Research reports that women who gain more than 17kg (38lb) during pregnancy experience a 40% increased risk of breast cancer after menopause, compared to expectant mothers who gain 15–16kg (25–35lb).

EATING FOR ONE Medical experts now say that eating for two is well and truly off the menu, however many women find it hard to let go of such a well established convention because pregnancy has long been viewed as an opportunity to take a short-term break from long-term dietary denial. Pregnant women are expected to eat more. So they generally do. And the sense that their body is controlling their appetite makes it that much harder to say no. Even the excep-tionally disciplined find their iron will no match for nine months of chaotic hormones and social pressure to have 'one for you and one for the baby'. But although women like Catherine Zeta Jones shrink back into shape in seconds thanks to personal trainers and dieticians, it takes most women at least a year to lose the weight they gained in pregnancy and it often becomes a very sensitive issue. In his book *Things that it took me 50 years to learn*, Dave Barry wisely advises his fellow men to 'never say anything to a woman that even remotely suggests that you think she's pregnant unless you can see an actual baby emerging from her at that moment'.

MONITORING WEIGHT GAIN The best way to figure out your optimal weight gain during pregnancy is to determine how close you are to your ideal body weight before you conceive. One way to do that is to calculate your body mass index (BMI) (p.17). If your BMI is less than 19.8, you are considered underweight, so your recommended weight gain during pregnancy would be 12–17kg (27–38lb). If your BMI is between 19.9 and 26, you are considered normal weight, and your recommended weight gain will be 11–16kg (24-34lb). If your BMI is 26 to 29, you fall into the overweight category, and the recommended weight gain will be 6.5–11kg (14–24lb). Women with a BMI greater than 29 need only gain 6kg (13lb) or less. An average woman should expect to gain about 11.5kg (25lb) during pregnancy – about 1.3kg (3lb) in the first three months, 5kg (11lb) in the second, and 5kg (11lb) in the third. If a 27-year-old woman who is 5'5" tall and weighs 65.5kg (145lb) puts on roughly 13.5kg (30lb) during her whole pregnancy, she should gain about 1.8kg (4lb) every four weeks over the last six months. Her total weight gain can be divided out as follows: Her uterus will gain 1kg (2.4lb), her breasts 450g (1lb), the weight of her blood will increase by 1.4kg (3.09lb), water will weigh 1.89 kg (4.15lb), and extra fat will count for about 3.7kg (8.27lb). Her total personal gain excluding the foetus will be 8.6kg (18.9lb). At birth the baby should weigh 3.4kg (7.5lb), the placenta 730g (1.61lb) and amniotic fluid will count for 900g (1.98lb) – a total 5kg (11.1lb).

FOOD FOR THOUGHT Avoid soft ripened cheeses like brie and camembert, raw or lightly done eggs or foods like mayonnaise or tiramisu. Stay away from foods that contain liver, avoid raw or rare meat and shark, swordfish, tuna or mackerel, which can contain mercury. Unwashed fruit, veg or salad, herbal supplements, herbal and Chinese medicines should also be avoided. Cut out the caffeine or get it down to a couple of cups of coffee a day. Guidelines suggest pregnant women should quit alcohol completely, though a glass or two of red wine a week is probably OK. And give up smoking. Morning sickness doesn't affect all women and usually confines itself to the first trimester, but not always. Though it often occurs in the morning it can happen any time, and anywhere. It is thought to be caused by low blood sugar so if you feel sick when you wake up try keeping ginger biscuits or a banana by the bed. Ginger or peppermint tea can help and eating small healthy snacks through the day will minimize nausea. A good diet will ensure the baby gets everything it needs but your doctor will probably prescribe folate supplements and possibly calcium and iron.

EXERCISE Though it's the last thing you will probably feel like, taking some regular and gentle exercise during your pregnancy will boost your blood flow and oxygen levels which will benefit you and your baby enormously (chapter 4). After your baby is born, regular excercise often goes out the window because you are so exhausted, particularly if you don't have help with child care. However, exercise is the best thing for helping to keep your energy levels up. It also boosts the amount of serotonin in your brain, which improves your mood. Doing a home work out (while your baby naps) will speed up weight loss and improve muscle tone (p.115). Try going for a power walk with your baby in either a sling or a buggy and if you want to push yourself a bit harder, attach weights to your arms and ankles (p.130) or get a jogging buggy.

SKIN CARE During pregnancy, some women find that the skin on their stomach, buttocks, thighs and breasts develops stretch marks as it enlarges (they can also occur during adolescence or periods of weight gain). The problem occurs when the tissue under your skin tears from rapid growth or stretching. Massaging

It pisses me off when celebrities like Liz Hurley and Catherine Zeta Jones get acres of publicity for giving birth and turning up at premieres ten minutes later looking like stick insects. The fact that they have had elective Caesareans probably with a tummy tuck and lipo doesn't make it into the papers. The reality for most women is so different and flagging up some fantasy idea of what pregnancy and birth should be puts an unfair pressure on normal women. It used to be OK to be fat when you were pregnant. Now we are meant to wear lycra all during pregnancy and get back on the tread-mill in between breast feeds. Don't journalists ever have children?
Justine, 38, UK

I already have terrible stretch marks on my body because I was overweight when I was younger. I dread the idea of pregnancy because I presume the ones I have will just get worse and since I have tried every treatment under the sun to get rid of them I know that nothing works.
Beth, 30, US

creams, oils or lotions into the skin can help it feel more supple but don't appear to help prevent stretch marks from occurring altogether. At first, stretch marks may show up as reddish or purplish lines, but they will often turn lighter (whitish or flesh-coloured) and almost disappear over time.

Although there are tons of products on the market that claim to eliminate stretch marks, the truth is you can't make them go away without plastic surgery. If you are concerned about your stretch marks, talk to a dermatologist. Stretch marks are more likely to occur in women who uses creams containing steroids (such as hydrocortisone) or ointments on their skin for more than a few weeks.

BREASTFEEDING Exclusive breastfeeding for the first 13 weeks of your baby's life boosts natural immunity and helps protect against illness and allergies. It will help you get back into shape too. Sucking encourages the uterus to contract and manufacturing milk helps burn up body fat. Contrary to popular opinion, however, breastfeeding is not a form of contraception so make sure you use protection when you begin having sex again (p.246).

Many new mums end up with chapped nipples when they start to breastfeed. If you plan to breastfeed, prepare your nipples before the birth by rubbing them with witch hazel. If your nipples do get sore, expose them to the air as much as you can and rub them with a little of your own breast milk or camomile ointment to soothe them. In the early weeks after birth, massage can help prevent mastitis (inflammation of milk ducts). Massage gently, stroking down from the collar-bone towards (never away from) the nipples or in from under the armpits towards the nipples.

Because taking care of a new baby is so demanding and eating well requires forward planning, many women who manage to get through pregnancy within a target weight find that they lose the plot completely when they are breastfeeding. Because it increases appetite considerably, a busy mum who doesn't have time to shop or cook can find herself resorting to cakes and sweets for a quick and easy energy boost and the pounds pile on, rather than off. Breastfeeding mothers do need to increase their nutrient intake (by about 500 calories a day) until their baby is weaned but it is important to stick to nutritious foods. To get the protein, minerals and vitamins that you need, include Bran Flakes, lamb's liver, chicken livers, fresh tuna, eggs, grilled skinless chicken, steamed wild or organic salmon, almonds, tuna, sardines, sweetcorn, plain peanuts, poppy seeds, mixed nuts, raisins, banana chips and sunflower seeds and don't forget to drink loads of water (p.80). Keep the fruit bowl full and ensure your fridge is packed with nutritious foods to make it easier to opt for a healthy snack.

Sod's law

As a young girl you worry about getting pregnant. Then you grow up and start worrying about not getting pregnant. An increasing number of women are finding that as soon as snot-nosed kids start to look like bundles of joy, mother nature seems to bugger off. And no matter how much sex they have, or when, pregnancy remains an enigma. Obviously women who want to have kids should start sooner rather than later, but most aren't in a position to do this. Qualifications and careers come first. Then there's the needle in a haystack task – finding a guy you think will stick around long enough to pass the gas and air. Add the cost of homes and child-care and it's a wonder anyone ever gets around to it at all. A young, fertile couple only has a one in four chance of getting pregnant per cycle and the older they get, the more difficult it becomes, though you can increase your chances considerably by getting to know your cycle (p.245) and making sure you are both fit and healthy. Until now, it has always been thought that female fertility starts to drop significantly in the early 30s, with a big plunge after 35. But a recent study indicates that female fertility begins to slide at 27 – the average age at which women now decide to have their first baby – and male fertility begins to dwindle after the age of 35. By the time a man hits 40, he is 40% less likely to get his partner pregnant in a month than he was at the age of 35. The rising tide of sexually transmitted infections is also a contributing factor. Infections such as chlamydia which can cause infertility, often get left untreated because there are no symptoms.

FACING THE FACTS Though women are more inclined to feel responsible when pregnancy doesn't happen, approximately 40% of infertility is due to the female and 30% is due to the male. In the balance of cases, infertility results from problems in both partners, or the cause of the infertility cannot be explained. Many couples have a hard time admitting that they may have an infertility problem, but if you are over 30, have a history of pelvic inflammatory disease, painful periods, miscarriage, irregular cycles or if your partner has a known low sperm count, you should seek help as soon as you suspect something might be wrong. Your doctor will refer you to a specialist for blood, urine and cervical mucus tests to check for adequate hormone levels; any signs of infection; blocked tubes; scar tissue; endometriosis; fibroids and abnormal shape or position of the womb, ovaries or fallopian tubes (these can be corrected with surgery). Ultrasound scans check if a follicle, which should contain an egg, is being produced. Your partner's hormone levels, sperm count and motility will be tested as will your mucus–sperm compatibility. Scans will also look for blockages and check the blood supply to the testes. Once you are diagnosed you may just need straightforward fertility drug treatment or surgery to help you conceive. If the tests aren't conclusive, assisted conception may still be successful but the techniques are not perfect and women under 35 will always stand a much better chance of a successful pregnancy than women over 40.

I got married when I was 24 and I had irregular periods, so my doctor put me on Clomid to regulate me but it didn't work and later I found that it contributed to my problems. I was diagnosed with PCOS (polycystic ovary syndrome) and I had cysts removed but medication didn't help and finally IVF didn't work so we signed up for adoption. I was miserable and I was overweight. In an effort to make myself feel better I joined Weight Watchers weighing 269lb [122kg]. Over the course of the next year I lost over 100lb [45kg] and as a result of my weight loss, I started to get a period three to four times a year. After I lost another 50lb [23kg], I noticed my periods became more and more regular, and eventually I was down to a pattern of 30-day cycles. I went to my specialist and he checked my hormone levels, which had been way too high. They were 'normal' and an ultrasound identified that I was actually ovulating. I am now 34 weeks pregnant with our first child and so happy! It was losing the weight that did it and I would say to any woman to try that if she thinks she is infertile.
Erika, 38, UK

HORMONE TREATMENTS Fertility drugs stimulate ovulation and aid conception. Success rates are high in properly diagnosed cases but dosage and treatment need to be carefully adhered to in order to avoid multiple pregnancies. In larger doses these drugs can actually prevent conception. A recent study of 2,500 Israeli women showed no increased risk for breast or ovarian cancer among women who have used fertility drugs, but the same study has found a link between fertility drugs and endometrial cancer. The two most popular fertility drugs for women are clomifene citrate (brand names include Clomid and Serophene) and human menopausal gonadotrophin or HMG (brand names include Pergonal and Metrodin), which is used with human chorionic gonadotrophin or HCG. Both drugs prompt the pituitary gland to make more luteinizing hormone and follicle-stimulating hormone to stimulate the ovaries into producing and maturing one or more eggs. Treatment can last three to six months and your doctor can check whether it is is working by testing your hormone levels with a blood test or checking your ovaries with an ultrasound scan in mid-cycle to see if any follicles are developing. Approximately 75% of women who have been diagnosed and put on fertility drugs will begin to ovulate, though the birth rate varies between 20 and 60%.

IN-VITRO FERTILIZATION (IVF) This technique was first used successfully in 1978. Before treatment you will be advised to take a course of fertility drugs to boost ovulation and an ultrasound scan will confirm when your eggs are ready to be harvested. Your doctor will give you a local anaesthetic, and then remove the eggs using a fine, hollow needle. Your partner's sperm is then combined with your eggs and two days later the embryos (fertilized eggs) are transferred into your uterus through your cervix with a thin catheter. No more than three embryos can legally be transferred to avoid the risk of a multiple pregnancy. Extra embryos, if there are any, may be frozen for future use. One cycle of IVF takes four to six weeks to complete and on average it takes three treatments before a woman gets pregnant. Cost is a major factor. Waiting lists and selection criteria mean that 80% of in-vitro fertilization is carried out privately, and each treatment costs £2500+. Outcomes vary greatly depending on your particular fertility problem and on your age, though younger women usually have healthier eggs and higher success rates. The live birth rate per embryo transfer cycle is 31%.

GAMETE INTRAFALLOPIAN TRANSFER (GIFT) GIFT is similar to IVF but the main difference is that it is the gametes (eggs and sperm) that are transferred to the woman's fallopian tubes, so that fertilization occurs inside, not outside, the woman's body. The embryo can begin its earliest development in natural surroundings rather than in an artificial environment. The live birth rate per treatment cycle is 24.5%.

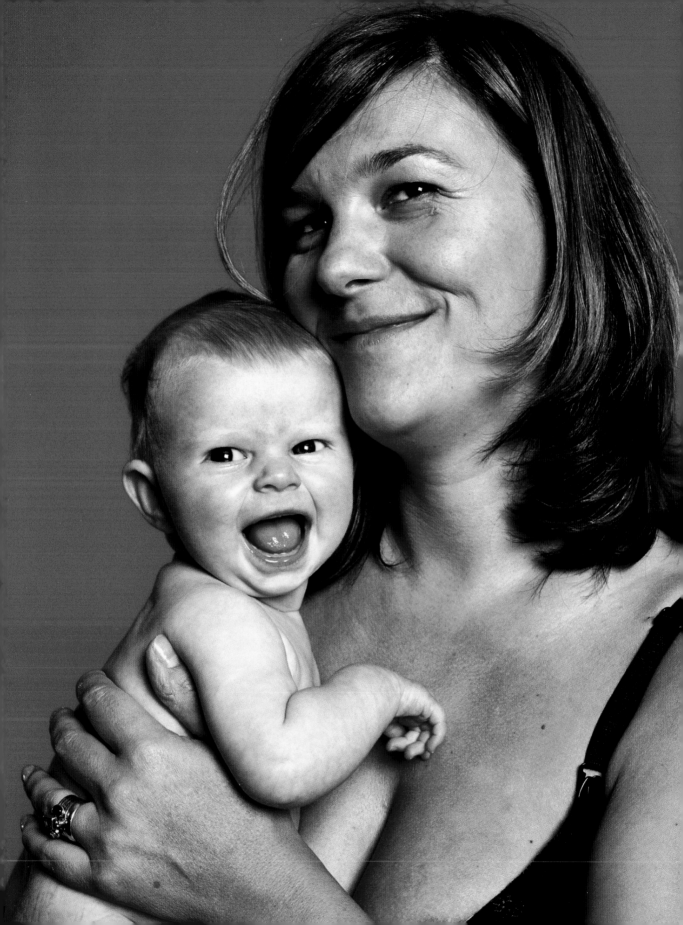

ZIFT (ZYGOTE INTRAFALLOPIAN TRANSFER) This is a similar procedure to GIFT except that it is the newly fertilized egg (zygote) that is returned to the woman's fallopian tubes rather than the mixture of eggs and sperm. This procedure shares the advantage of GIFT in that any resulting embryo will immediately be able to develop in the natural surroundings of your body. The live birth rate per treatment cycle is 29.2%.

DONOR INSEMINATION (DI) If there are problems on both sides, a couple can use donated sperm, eggs or gametes (both eggs and sperm). All egg and sperm donations in the UK are anonymous and regulated by the Human Fertilisation and Embryology Authority. Clinics screen sperm and egg donors carefully and donors are matched as closely as possible to the recipient couple for characteristics such as hair colour, eye colour, occupation and interests. Any identifying information may not currently be given to any child born as a result of the donation. Approximately 5000 couples a year in the UK have DI. Around 50% of couples will achieve a pregnancy following insemination with donor sperm. The live birth rate is around 10%.

INTRACYTOPLASMIC SPERM INJECTION (ICSI) Only one sperm is needed, and this is injected directly into the egg, so this relatively new technique has been embraced as a breakthrough in offering real hope to couples where the man has a very low sperm count or the couples would prefer not to use donor sperm. The success rate per treatment cycle is 28.6%.

ARTIFICIAL INSEMINATION (AI) A much less 'high-tech' process which helps get the sperm nearer to the egg by placing semen directly into the uterus at ovulation. It is most successful for problems with cervical mucus as opposed to sperm quality. The success rate per treatment cycle is 5–10%.

SURROGACY A surrogate mother can be artificially inseminated with your partner's sperm or an embryo that is the biological child of both you and your partner. Surrogacy is legal in the UK, with the main proviso that no fee can be paid to the surrogate; the only money that can be paid is to cover 'reasonable expenses' and it is illegal to advertise for a surrogate or for a surrogate to advertise. Once the baby is born, you will need to legally adopt the baby as it will be registered as the child of the birth mother – the surrogate – whether or not she is genetically related to the child. It's difficult to estimate how successful the process is as so many things can go wrong but the organization Childlessness overcome through surrogacy (COTS), set up by surrogate mother Kim Cotton in 1988, estimates that 97% of the the 200 births they have arranged have had happy and successful conclusions.

Mental health

DEPRESSION Clinical depression is much more than temporarily feeling sad or blue. It negatively affects mood, concentration, sleep, activity, appetite and social behaviour. Some forms of depression are heriditary and 25% of first-degree relatives (mother, father, siblings) of people with depression also suffer from it. Although it can affect anyone at any time, it seems to affect twice as many women as men. Clinical depression is more common in women with low self-esteem, pessimistic views and tendencies towards stress. It can also be triggered by work, family responsibilities, discrimination, lack of social support, traumatic life experiences, and poverty. In one major study, 100% of women who had experienced severe childhood sexual abuse developed depression later in life.

Estimates suggest that one out of every seven women will suffer from depression at some point in their lifetime. Experts are not sure whether this indicates a biological susceptibility or simply reflects the fact that women are more willing to admit how they feel to a doctor. The explanation may be a combination of biological, genetic, psychological, and social factors however the gender gap in depression is most evident during the reproductive years. Some women experience premenstrual mood changes and as many as 80% of women experience the 'baby blues', a brief period of depression after giving birth. 10–15% of women experience serious clinical depression during, or after pregnancy. There seems to be an increase in depression before menopause, but this does not appear to be the case afterwards. Depression is highly treatable with psychotherapy, cognitive/behavioural therapy and antidepressants, but it is often a life-long condition in which periods of wellness alternate with recurrences of illness. Some doctors suggest raising doses of antidepressant drugs premenstrually, as the menstrual cycle may alter drug-absorption rates.

ALZHEIMER'S Two-thirds of all Alzheimer's sufferers are female. It is primarily an age-related illness and there are more older women than men, but hormones may also have an influence. Oestrogen receptors, present in many brain cells, help to improve blood flow and stimulate the growth of nerve-to-nerve connections, so it is thought that the decline in oestrogen production at menopause might be a contributing factor to the higher rates of Alzheimers in women. US research on changes in memory and mental abilities has been unable to establish this link as yet, but current thinking does suggest that excercising the brain strengthens it in the same way as physical excercise benefits other muscles. Studies of older people who stay mentally active by working, studying, reading, pursuing hobbies, etc. show that they are less likely to develop Alzheimer's disease than those who are more mentally passive. Several studies also show that higher education appears to offer protection, although it is not known whether this is because educated people may remain mentally active for longer.

When it started, I found it impossible to get out of bed. I wanted to hide under the covers and not talk to anyone. I didn't feel like eating and I lost a lot of weight. Nothing seemed fun anymore and I just thought being alive was a waste of time. I was tired all the time, yet I wasn't sleeping well at night. But I've got kids and a job so I just had to try and keep going. I started missing days from work, and a friend noticed that something wasn't right. She talked me into seeing a doctor who gave me the name of a psychiatrist. Now I'm seeing the psychiatrist once a month and taking antidepressants. I am not better yet and whereas I used to have highs and lows, now everything is grey and flat, but it is better for my children.
Helen, 43, UK

I struggle every day with trying to like myself, trying to see myself as intelligent, attractive and kind. But I see the opposite – stupid, ugly and selfish. The energy that I spend trying to feel 'normal' is huge, but it is what I want more than anything in the world – to be mentally healthy and emotionally stable.
Ellen, 24, UK

Addictions

I have two cigarettes and a black coffee every morning for breakfast. It wakes me up and gets my bowels moving. In fact, I can't go to the toilet unless I smoke. I would like to give up but everyone I know who has given up smoking has put on weight. I'll quit at 40.
Paula, 34, UK

The last few years have been really stressful - divorce, trying to earn enough to stay in my home and keep the kids in the neighbour- hood they loved. At the end of each day I craved a cigarette and a glass of wine. It was the only way I could relax. A few months ago I met a really great guy. He doesn't smoke and I vowed to quit. We spent New Year together in LA and no one smokes there so I gradually phased them out. Now I don't even think about it but for so long I couldn't live without my Marlboro lights.
Ally, 39, US

To me, alcohol doesn't taste nice but I am also aware that Asian women don't have an enzyme that allows them to process alcohol and I worry that if I did drink I would be sick, or, even worse, act really stupid.
Kim, 22, US

SMOKING For the first time in history, the smoking rate for girls now surpasses that for boys, and women continue to make up the highest proportion of new smokers. Most (38%) women smokers are aged between 20 and 24 and took up the habit when they were 16 years old, and their compelling motivation was not nicotine addiction but weight control. In a survey of 140 adolescent smokers, 15% said they believe that cigarettes help control weight and 40–50% of adult women smoke because they see it as a primary means to control their weight. Some 25% of women smokers will die of a disease caused by smoking and lung cancer now kills more women than breast cancer. Cigarette smoking greatly increases your chances of developing cardiovascular diseases, particularly for women on the pill, and although the risks for this and other smoking-related illnesses are the same for men as for women, women smokers have the added risks of an early menopause, a heart attack or stroke if they are on the pill and an increased risk of osteoporosis.

Nicotine increases the heart rate by 10–20 beats a minute, raises blood pressure, and decreases the amount of oxygen in your blood, causing tar and chemical irritants known to cause cancer to collect in your lungs, leading to smoker's cough. Smoking also causes a build up of fatty deposits in the arteries which eventually leads to heart disease. It depresses the immune system and makes people more susceptible to infection. And since smoking affects the blood vessels in the skin, it gives you a dull complexion and causes your skin to wrinkle and lose its plump natural texture. Women who smoke over a prolonged period will acquire deeply etched lines running between the nose to the lips. That's the bad news.

The good news is that the benefits of giving up kick in immediately. Within 20 minutes of stopping smoking, blood pressure and pulse return to normal. After eight hours, nicotine and carbon monoxide levels in the blood are halved, and oxygen levels in the blood return to normal. After 24 hours, carbon monoxide is eliminated from the body and lungs start to clear out the accumulated tar. After 48 hours, there is no nicotine left in the body and taste and smell are greatly improved. After 72 hours, breathing becomes easier, bronchial tubes begin to relax and energy levels increase. After two to 12 weeks, circulation improves, making walking and running a lot easier. And after three to 9 months, coughs, wheezing and breathing problems improve as lung function is increased.

ALCOHOL There has been a massive increase in female drinking in the last 20 years. A combination of greater freedom and more financial independence has afforded women the luxury of liberating themselves from their inhibitions and, as a result, 1600 women a year in the UK now die from cirrhosis of the liver, a 33%

increase in the last seven years. Until recently, the recommended safe drinking limit for women was 14 units a week but the limit has now increased to a maximum of 21 units for women who are not pregnant (p.261). Women are advised to space the units out through the week so that they can leave two or three completely alcohol-free days. It all sounds reasonable, but unfortunately women (who only graduated from smelling salts and Babycham very recently) don't seem to be following the guidelines. The problem with women is that they tend to binge drink, which does more damage. At the end of the week they may have only had 21 units – but they've managed to cram them all into a Friday night. Binge drinking is defined as seven or more standard units of alcohol for women (ten for men) in one evening. Now, that doesn't sound like a lot but basically if you do this regularly, say three times a week, you put your health at risk.

Arguably, the behavioural changes associated with alcohol pose a bigger threat to female health than the substance itself. Drinking boosts confidence, which makes it attractive to the self-conscious and insecure. But the downside is that lack of inhibition diminishes responsibility. The results can be as unimportant as an inability to say no to a kebab on the way home, or as serious as a bad case of beer goggles which results in unprotected sex with an ugly guy, or pregnancy, or a sexually transmitted infection, or even all three. About 90% of adults drink alcohol at some point. At least one in ten adults has had an STI. You do the maths.

DRUGS It's not called heroin chic for nothing. Courtesy of the 'diet pill', women have had a long-standing relationship with the use of amphetamines as a form of appetite suppressant, so the fact that prescription drugs, and class A drugs like coke, speed, ecstasy, heroin and anabolic steroids have pretty much the same effect hasn't gone unnoticed by middle-class housewives, students, high-flying businesswomen and hungry supermodels. It's clearly nuts to use drugs in an effort to lose weight or build muscle, but women who suffer from negative body image tend to take the health implications of self-abuse less seriously, and any drug that makes them feel more confident whilst simultaneously suppressing their nagging appetite appears to be something of a magic bullet. However, the long term consequences of swapping appetite for oblivion are pretty hideous. Research shows that women become addicted to drugs faster than men and doctors are often slow to consider substance abuse as a diagnosis for women, so treatment is often delayed. A 1998 report to the European Monitoring Centre for Drugs and Drug Addiction indicated that 46.1% of young women aged between 16 and 24 had used drugs at some point, 14.9% of them in the last month. In the US, a two-year study by the National Centre on Addiction and Substance Abuse indicates that 11% of women over the age of 59 are addicted to prescription psychoactive drugs.

Booze is my number one vice. I can't resist it really. A drink after work relaxes me and sometimes I just stay in the pub. I know they say it is really bad for you and sometimes I have terrible hangovers but I don't think anyone my age worries about stuff like that. I do worry that it will make me bloated. Sometimes I look a bit puffy in the morning though a heavy session leaves me dehydrated so I weigh less. The minute I eat or drink anything, the weight goes straight back on though.
Hattie, 22, UK

My boyfriend and I started using Ecstasy about two years ago. I used to get so wasted that I would throw up but that didn't really bother me. In fact, I quite liked it because I wanted to get thinner. The E made me lose my appetite and I knew I was losing weight really quickly. I would wake up about 5lb [2.2kg] lighter after a night on E. Over the last two years my weight has dropped by about 1½st [9.5kg]. I don't think the Es we take are as strong now because I take about four now if we go clubbing and I used to only take one.
Rebecca, 24, UK

Eating disorders

I looked great when I was 14 years old. I was 5' 8" and weighed 8st 1lb [51kg], but then I ballooned to 15st 1lb [96kg]. That was when my hell began. By the age of 18, I weighed 11st 3lb [71kg]. By the time I was 24 I was semi-bulimic. I hated myself, I didn't have a boyfriend for years and I was very lonely. Once I considered throwing myself off the balcony of my Hong Kong flat. The final straw came when I asked my flatmate if I could lock the kitchen door as he didn't go in there and I couldn't stay away. Even after a huge evening meal I would come home and stuff myself. He said I could throw everything away but I left out a large tub of rice, sugar and flour. I mean, what could I do with that? The next night I came home and I was so desperate that I mixed the flour and sugar with water and stuffed it into my face. It took four years to get better and another eight years before I walked away from the therapist. Why did it happen? I don't know except that my family wanted me to be thin and my father constantly offered me incentives to diet.
All I know is that I was miserable and had zero confidence in myself.
Annabel, 39, US

HOW BIG IS THE PROBLEM? It is thought that approximately 70 million people worldwide have an eating disorder. And 90% of them are women. The Eating Disorders Association estimates that the combined total for women with an eating disorder in the UK (diagnosed and undiagnosed), is about 1.15 million. And about 10% of those women will die if their eating disorder goes untreated. The most common eating disorders are bulimia (bingeing and purging), anorexia (starving), and binge-eating (just bingeing). But other disorders exist. Some women severely restrict the range of food they eat, often using medically unidentified allergies or intolerances as an excuse. Others fast, exercise compulsively, chew and spit food or suffer from night-eating syndrome. Some women eat non-foods, such as paper tissues, to fill themselves up and many misuse laxatives, diuretics, enemas or diet pills at some point. The number of eating disorders is believed to have doubled since the 1960s, but it is difficult to estimate figures accurately because most sufferers won't admit they have a problem and go to great lengths to disguise their behaviour. Bulimia was only officially recognized as a psychiatric illness in the 1970s but it is now thought to be two to three times more common than anorexia. About 90% of anorexics are female and only around 60% ever recover completely. According to a ten-year study, 86% of sufferers are ill by the age of 20 and, of these, 10% report they were anorexic by the age of ten or younger. Anorexia is estimated to cause death in 16–20% of cases after 20 years. It is thought that about 10–20% of people who are mildly obese and on a diet have binge-eating disorder (2% of all adults). Conventional dieting is thought to make matters worse for binge eaters and experts believe that there is a strong link between dieting and the onset of all eating disorders.

TRIGGERS Adolescence appears to be the most critical time but eating disorders can be triggered or recur during times of distress or major change. Everyone is different, but most women who develop an eating disorder share certain personality characteristics – low self-esteem, a need to please others, perfectionist tendencies and difficulty in communicating. Many come from families in which emotional and physical needs are not met in some way. Feelings may not be verbally expressed and communication skills may be lacking, so eating too much or not eating enough becomes a way of expressing or manifesting difficult feelings. Overachieving, overprotective and critical parents are more likely to have daughters with eating disorders, as are parents who diet obsessively or make derogatory remarks about weight. A familial emphasis on the importance of being thin can impact on a child who has concerns about size or seeks to maintain parental approval. Emotionally or physically absent fathers can also heighten insecurity and make adolescence and growing up a more alarming prospect. There may also be a family history of depression, alcoholism, drug abuse or eating disorders.

ANOREXIA Anorexia now claims the highest death rate of any psychiatric illness. It often begins as a normal diet that is carried to extremes. Anorexics basically eat as little as possible. They fill up on water and develop bizarre ritualistic eating behaviours, such as only eating very low calorie foods like frozen grapes or lettuce, or chewing anything from gum to pistachio nuts without swallowing. They deny that they feel hungry, though they often appear to be preoccupied with food and food preparation. Adolescence, when many young girls are disturbed by natural weight gain during puberty, is a critical point for its onset.

Anorexics are generally high achievers and perfectionists. They are controlled, fastidious and highly disciplined. They find it hard to allow themselves to be emotional and because they generally find it difficult to communicate their feelings, dramatic weight loss becomes a way of saying something with the body that they cannot say in words. By maintaining the body of a child, an anorexic postpones or avoids becoming an adult, which makes cutting ties, adult responsibility and sexual intimacy less likely. Though girls who have been abused may believe that physically disappearing and not developing curves will help them avoid the attention of their abuser, for a child who might otherwise be ignored in her family, shrinking actually makes her more visible. A skeletal appearance demands help and effectively generates desperately craved attention. However, the concern of family, friends and colleagues can sometimes serve to make an anorexic more determined to maintain their interest by losing even more weight. Losing weight when so many others can't, gives an anorexic a sense of control and accomplishment that she doesn't feel she gets from other aspects of her life. But eventually anorexics lose control of both their minds and their bodies as they become increasingly imprisoned by their obsessive behaviours and thought patterns.

The long-term health consequences are appalling. As the body starves, it tries to conserve energy. The menstrual cycles ceases and the muscles gradually waste away. Anorexics become increasingly feeble as their bodies give in under the strain of starvation. The skin and hair become dry and hair loss is common, though anorexics often experience the growth of a downy layer of hair all over the body, including the face, as the body struggles to retain heat. Severe dehydration can result in kidney failure. Lack of nutrition reduces the density of the bones causing osteoporosis (p.279). And the heart slows down abnormally, which leads to low blood pressure and eventually to heart failure. Over 25% of anorexics will require hospitalization at some point. Doctors can use force feeding once a person's bodyweight has fallen below a certain level, because they are no longer capable of making rational decisions, but it is only a temporary physical fix. Without psychiatric help the anorexic simply resumes dieting as soon as she is released from hospital.

Weborexia

Despite all attempts by web providers to ban them, there are currently about 400 pro-anorexia and pro-bulimia websites hiding on the Internet and anyone who tries hard enough will find them. They provide an unimaginably shocking list of 'thinspirations'such as; chew, but don't swallow; eat only sugar-free jelly; take up smoking; drink gallons of Diet Coke; punch your stomach when it rumbles; hide your weight loss by wearing baggy jeans with stretch pants underneath; put rolls of pennies in your waistband and drink 2 litres [3½ pints]of water before getting weighed at the doctor's office. The basic theme is how to starve and binge without getting caught and how to eat six 50-calorie meals a day (a daily total of 300 calories (1600 calories less than a young woman needs). Galleries of images of sufferers – living skeletons – are displayed beside pictures of celebrity role models who, in an ironic twist, actually look relatively well fed and healthy in comparison. And to keep visitors on track with their living suicide missions, the sites remind them that, 'Nothing tastes as good as being thin feels.'

BINGE-EATING DISORDER (BED) Binge eating is probably the most common eating disorder. It is characterized by episodes of uncontrollable eating, (usually carried out in private) but, unlike bulimics, binge eaters do not force themselves to vomit or take laxatives. As a result, BED inevitably leads to huge weight gain. People who suffer from BED find it difficult to cope with feelings of sadness, anger, depression or anxiety, so they literally eat them to make them go away. Many describe the process as almost trance-like and say they don't even taste the food they eat, they just shovel it in and swallow. About half of all obese binge eaters are depressed, while only 5% of obese people who don't binge eat are diagnosed with depression. Binge eaters often suffer from frustration and low self-esteem, and may connect other difficulties, for example, problems with relationships or employment, to their eating habits.

For a binge eater, food is an addiction – and in some ways it is the hardest addic-tion to treat because people with an alcohol or substance abuse problem can learn to completely avoid booze and drugs but it's impossible to totally give up food. When overeating becomes chronic, people with BED end up organizing their day around their bingeing. They may miss work or school or avoid people in order to eat and the secrecy involved means bingers often end up isolating themselves completely. The physical effects of overeating are blood sugar swings, cravings, stomach pain, intolerance to heat and cold, headaches, a messed-up metabolism and irregular menstruation. And with obesity comes the risk of a number of diseases: high blood pressure, high cholesterol, clogged blood vessels, heart attack, stroke, diabetes, osteoarthritis, chronic kidney problems or kidney failure and certain cancers.

BULIMIA Bulimics may appear to have an enormous appetite without putting on weight. Large amounts of food may disappear when they are around and you may find empty wrappers and containers in their room. Some bulimics specifically consume foods that are easier to throw up; fine grains, liquid sauces, milk shakes or ice cream are generally easier to purge than heavy solids, such as meat or bread. After meals, bulimics usually disappear to the bathroom and although most are expert at brushing teeth, there may be a smell of vomit in the bathroom or on their breath. Brushing teeth after vomiting causes tooth enamel to erode much more quickly than normal so bulimics may also have bad teeth (rinsing with a fluoride mouthwash is less corrosive).

Bulimics appear to be outgoing, confident and independent, but inside they are anxious and insecure. They fear criticism and avoid disagreements. Because they have difficulty processing and expressing their emotional needs, they literally throw

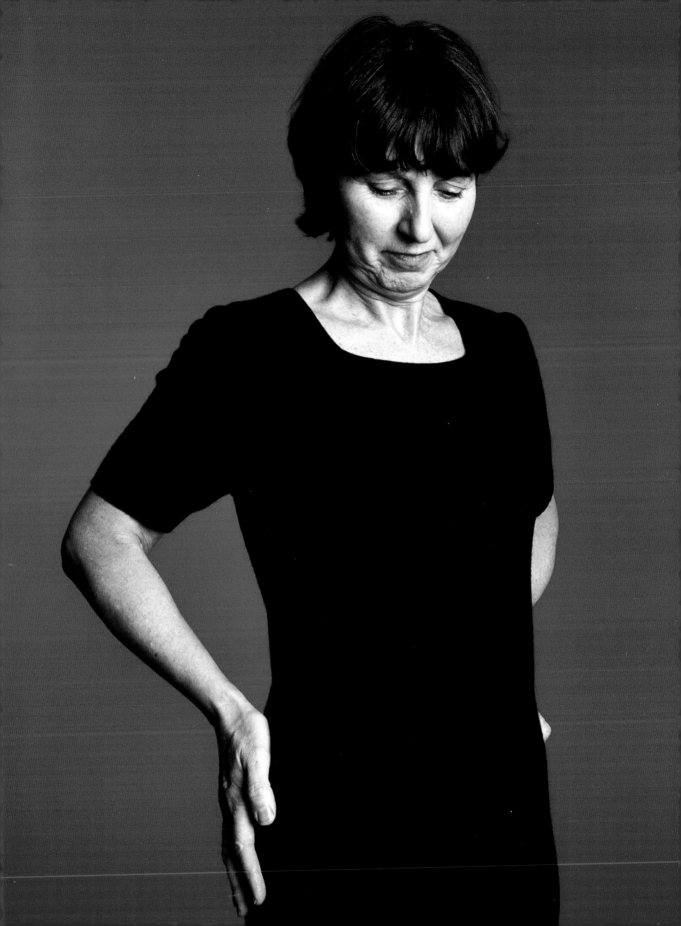

them up. Most bulimics have been preoccupied with eating and diet for years. This may derive from parental concerns with diet or the association between thinness and 'acceptability'. Many turn to purging when they have failed at a diet and fear that there is no other way for them to lose weight. Paradoxically, at this point the eating disorder can temporarily raise self-esteem due to a sense of undeserved success. A bulimic cheats. She appears to achieve the cultural ideal of thinness without having to diet. However, the comfort a bulimic derives from allowing herself to eat and the relief she feels when she purges herself, become a highly addictive method of controlling emotion. And once the binge/purge cycle becomes established, the physical and mental consequences erode any initial sense of self-worth and control.

Bulimia is falsely perceived as less dangerous than anorexia or addiction and, as such, it is particularly insidious. Although the fatality rate is lower, it has serious mental and physical consequences. Bulimics alienate themselves from friends and family, suffer confusion, mood swings, irritability and an inability to concentrate on anything other than the next binge/purge cycle. Constant vomiting causes unusual swelling of the cheeks and jaw area and bulimics may develop calluses on the back of their hands and knuckles from self-induced vomiting. Bulimics may have irregular periods or stop having periods at all. Constant vomiting leads to dehydration and a loss of potassium and sodium, which causes electrolyte imbalances in the body. This can lead to irregular heartbeats and possibly heart failure and death. Stomach acids released during vomiting can cause tooth decay, staining and bad breath. Vomiting also causes mouth ulcers, sore throats and stomach disorders. Chronic bulimics can also suffer from inflammation or rupture to the oesophagus or even gastric rupture.

TREATMENT FOR EATING DISORDERS Women with eating disorders usually need specialist professional help. However, self-help can also be effective. Cognitive behavioural therapy can be particularly helpful, especially if the patient is treated sooner rather than later, as can family counselling, psychotherapy, residential treatment and/or antidepressants. A UK pilot study that taught parents of anorexics psychotherapy skills lead to a much lower hospital re-admittance rate (10%) so larger clinical trials are now underway in both the US and the UK. However, since dysfunctional families are often the trigger for an eating disorder, it is unlikely that a scheme requiring enormous parental commitment will work for everyone. Education about health implications and nutrition can help but, ultimately, sufferers have to decide to get better themselves. They then need to learn how to modify their behaviour, to retrain their systems to recognize satiety, develop normal eating patterns and divorce themselves from what is essentially an addiction. Most importantly, they need to get rid of dysfunctional thoughts and feelings about the personal significance of body weight and address negative self-image.

Health after 50

MENOPAUSE One hundred years ago menopause didn't really exist because most women were dead by the age of 50 years. By the year 2008, post-menopausal women will comprise the largest demographic group in America, but despite the enormous number of women who have passed through this natural biological process unscathed, it continues to get more bad press than Saddam Hussein. 'The change' has become the fall guy for almost every aspect of female ill health in middle age. You name it – cardiovascular disease, osteoporosis, declining cognitive function, diminishing libido, even loss of attractiveness, and someone somewhere will have put a menopausal slant on it. In reality, much of the ill-health experienced by ageing women is a result of lifestyle issues dating back to their 20s and 30s and the fact that it begins to manifest during a woman's early 50s doesn't mean it should be automatically associated with a decline in oestrogen. Women currently in their 50s and 60s grew up during a period of relative affluence and unlike their mothers, they had a degree of financial independence. They drank (G&T), they smoked (Menthol), they ate (Black Forest Gateau) and some dabbled in prescription medicine (diet pills, Valium, barbiturates). Not many took exercise. Most did the Scarsdale diet. And all those behaviours have taken their toll. Menopause is also a time when women have to take on a number of significant and stressful new lifestyle changes. Children grow up and leave home. Elderly parents begin to fail and may need nursing. Or they may die. Older women find it harder to change jobs or move up in their career and some find themselves going through an unwanted mid-life divorce, which has an emotional and often financial impact. These factors can affect a woman's physical and mental wellbeing far more than hormonal changes do, but amorphous distress can't be cured with a pill so menopause gets blamed for the lot.

WHEN DOES IT HAPPEN? Menopause occurs when the ovaries finally stop producing the female sex hormones oestrogen and progesterone. It is estimated that in the first year of menopause the average drop in oestrogen levels is 80%, but until menopause is complete, you can still can become pregnant. (One in every 20 women between the ages of 40 and 55 who's seen their doctor to discuss missing periods will be pregnant.) While most women go through menopause around the age of 51, a small number experience menopause as early as age 40 and on rare occasions, menopause does not occur until the early sixties. Anorexics and smokers are more likely to hit menopause early, whereas women who are overweight may hit menopause later as oestrogen is produced by fatty tissue. This is not necessarily a good thing as women carrying excess weight are more likely to develop coronary heart disease. If you have had both ovaries removed (bilateral oophorectomy) or a full hysterectomy (removal of the uterus and ovaries), you will have the symptoms of menopause straight away, no matter

Supplements for symptoms

Approximately 16% of British women use alternative treatments to treat the symptoms of menopause. You must consult your doctor as supplements can react with other drugs you might be taking. Scientists speculate that the phytoestrogens in the soy-based diet of Japanese women play a role in preventing hot flushes. Try soya milk, tofu, tempeh or soy sauce. Natural vitamin E is labelled as d-alpha tocopherol. It is thought to alleviate depression. 200g+ daily may help minimize hot flushes. Herbal supplements such as Agnus Castus are also thought to help but ask your GP first. The amino acid Tryptophan is thought to help boost serotonin levels in the brain. A dose of 1g to 3g per day may alleviate depression or try 25mg to 50mg of vitamin B6 which has pretty much the same effect. St John's wort may help alleviate mild depression. Motherwort, calcium and B complex help anxiety, hawthorn, dandelion and celery seed help prevent fluid retention and melatonin or chamomile or Valerian help you sleep.

what your age. And your periods will stop completely if your uterus has been removed. However, many doctors leave healthy ovaries in place during a hysterectomy, which means the symptoms of menopause will occur normally.

PERIMENOPAUSE The build-up to menopause usually happens about three to five years before your last period (in your mid- to late 40s) and lasts until a year after your final period. Some signs or symptoms of menopause may appear during this time. Hormone levels may decrease in an erratic manner, causing irregular cycles, heavy bleeding and bleeding between periods. When your periods have stopped for a year, menopause is confirmed. A blood test for levels of follicle-stimulating hormone (FSH) can help to establish this. FSH normally rises to a high level at menopause and remains high. Other screening tests include blood pressure, cholesterol level and thyroid function. A mammogram and a PAP test also may be recommended. Some doctors also test for bone density, though women who are at risk of osteoporosis should probably be treated regardless of a bone-density test.

SYMPTOMS Up to 80% of women will experience one or more of the following symptoms, though only between 10 and 35% describe the impact as severly debilitating. There is no consensus as to why some women are more or less affected. In general, women who are unmarried and have never had children tend to have an easier time, whereas married mothers find it harder. Declining oestrogen levels cause changes in the way your blood vessels relax and contract. This leads to changes in circulation, which increase body temperature resulting in hot flushes, which can last from a few seconds to six minutes. They generally begin suddenly on the chest, neck and face and can occur up to several times a day. Hot flushes can be embarrassing and physically draining. Wearing several light layers of natural fibres can help you to respond more quickly to your changing body temperature. Some women find they are worse at night and waking up in a pool of sweat can interrupt sleep patterns, leading to tiredness and irritability. Make sure your bedroom is cool and use light layered blankets instead of a duvet. Other associated symptoms are headaches, nausea and difficulty with concentration.

Decreased oestrogen levels also affect the bladder. Women may need to pee frequently or suffer from fluid retention and vaginal irritation or stinging can occur during sex, making women more susceptible to infections such as thrush and cystitis (p.250). A lack of oestrogen thins the lining of the vagina and makes it less elastic. The amount of natural lubrication decreases which can make sex uncomfortable but a good lubricant will sort this out. Mood swings during the menopause can affect desire, libido and relationships, and depression is also common (women are twice as likely to experience major depression – p.267).

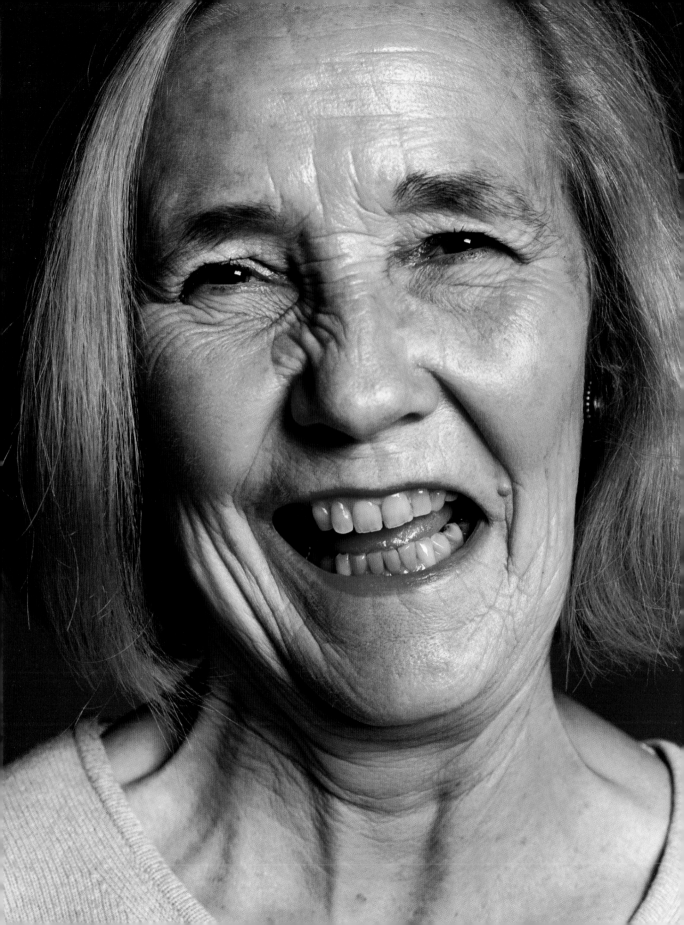

To HRT, or not to HRT...

In 1988, a study that reviewed menopause in the popular press (between 1981 and 1994) revealed that the experience was consistently presented in a negative light. Reflecting prevailing medical opinion, the frequency with which negative experiences were mentioned in the press increased steadily between 1981 and 1994 and so did the frequency with which menopause was said to be effectively treated with hormone replacement therapy (HRT). Thousands of studies have demonstrated that expectations impact experience (i.e. if you think something will be bad, it will be), which suggests that presenting menopause as an 'illness' or a 'deficiency' affects women's attitude towards it. The medicalization of menopause has lead many women to believe in HRT as a 'cure' and over the last twenty years fewer women have gone into menopause prepared to wait and see whether they need medical help or not. So, before asking a doctor for HRT, consider the fact that less oestrogen (i.e. not going on HRT) reduces the risk of uterine and breast cancer, shrinks fibroids and eliminates periods (you still bleed on HRT), PMS and menstrual migraines.

HRT was designed to replace the hormones that diminish as a woman ages, and counter symptoms such as hot flushes, night sweats and mood changes. Oestrogen therapy, the original HRT, became popular in the 1960s but by the 1970s, it became clear that oestrogen alone increased the risk of a cancer of the endometrium (lining of the uterus) six to eightfold. Since then, most doctors have prescribed a version that combines progestin with much lower doses of oestrogen to prevent the overgrowth of the endometrial lining. (The oral contraceptive pill is sometimes prescribed as an alternative to HRT because it contains both hormones.)

In the UK six million women take HRT every year to relieve the symptoms of the menopause. However, in 2002, a US study involving 16,608 women aged 50–70 years on oestrogen plus progestin which was scheduled to run until 2005, was stopped prematurely when researchers found a clear indication of an increase in the risk of breast cancer. Evidence was also found of an increase in coronary heart disease, strokes and pulmonary embolisms. UK doctors tried to dispel fears stressing that the exact combination of drugs used in the study were not available in Europe, but confidence in what was once seen as a wonder drug has been badly shaken. HRT had also been used to protect against osteoporosis but experts now feel that it doesn't provide enough protection to counter the other risks. The news has naturally created confusion and even panic among women. Doctors generally believe that short-term use (one year), which gets a woman through the worst of her symptoms is safe, though once she begins to withdraw from the drug, symptoms may begin again. If you have been on HRT for longer and are concerned, talk to your doctor. He may suggest that you stop taking HRT for two weeks and then have a mammogram to put your mind at ease.

Ten years ago I had a huge fibroid, which they shrunk with an injection but then they said they wanted to take everything out because I am prone to growing things. I had a hysterectomy through keyhole surgery and it went wrong. They shouldn't have done it that way and I haemorrhaged and nearly died. As a result, I am terribly against and terribly scared of surgery. After the operation I went straight onto HRT so menopause never happened and I never had any symptoms. I think HRT is great. I've been on it for ten years now and, if I came off it, I would go through menopause so I would rather chance my arm. My mum died from cancer when she was 36 so we are all a bit edgy about cancer in my family, but I am now an ostrich. I got a gallstone a few years ago and it was agony but it settled. I had a laparoscopy and they found that my gallbladder had a boulder in it and it wasn't functioning at all. It is worrying because if it flares up, it could be cancerous but I am so terrified of invasive surgery and I think I would rather just live well for as long as I can. I am an optimist!
Roseanne, 60, UK

Hearts, bones and bosoms

HEART DISEASE AND STROKE Though breast cancer and osteoporosis tend to get more publicity, coronary heart disease (CHD) is actually the number one killer of older women. Cancer is the second biggest killer and stroke is the third, but heart disease and stroke kill almost twice as many females each year as all forms of cancer combined. Heart and blood vessel diseases develop over time when deposits of cells, fat and cholesterol begin to clog the arteries that supply the heart or brain with blood. If a blood clot or other particle suddenly blocks blood flow in a narrowed artery, you can have a heart attack or stroke. Though young women generally have higher HDL (good cholesterol) levels than men, as women approach menopause, LDL (bad cholesterol) and total cholesterol levels in most women start to rise. It is not known whether this is due to declining oestrogen but the risk of CHD increases significantly after the age of 50 years. Though more men have heart attacks, women have lower chances of surviving them because they are older when heart attacks occur. Studies show that 38% of women die within a year of a heart attack compared with 25% of men. During the first six years following a heart attack, the rate of having a second attack is 35% for women compared with 18% for men. You can reduce your risk by paying attention to your diet (chapter 2), taking regular exercise (chapter 4), controlling high blood pressure, not smoking, having regular medical checkups and learning the warning signs of heart attack and stroke (see right) so you can recognize a stroke in progress and get medical attention if a stroke occurs. Immediate medical attention can often reduce disability from stroke.

OSTEOPOROSIS Osteoporosis causes thinning of the bones and increases the risk of fracture, particularly in the wrists, hips or spine. The first sign of the disease is usually when a minor bump or fall causes a bone fracture. Cumulatively, fractures can result in pain, imobility, loss of independence, even death. As women get older, osteoporosis also causes height loss and the development of the characteristic 'dowager's hump'. It is estimated that osteoporosis causes over 200,000 fractures in the UK each year. The condition affects 1 in 3 women and 1 in 12 men over the age of 50, but slender, light-skinned menopausal women have a higher risk of developing it. Long-term use of corticosteroid medication, maternal osteoporosis, smoking, heavy drinking, sedentary lifestyle, and low body weight also increase risk. Measures to prevent osteoporosis (a diet rich in calcium and regular exercise) must start well before menopause begins because women begin to lose bone mass as early as age 30. It's too late for the 3 million sufferers currently costing the NHS and the government over £1.7 billion each year (£5 million each day), but women who want to avoid the pain and immobility of osteoporosis should quit smoking, drink within safe recommended levels, take regular weight-bearing exercise (p.128), maintain an ideal weight and eat a diet that is rich in

Warning signs of heart attack

Discomfort in the centre of the chest that lasts more than a few minutes, or that goes away and comes back. It can feel like an uncomfortable pressure, squeezing, fullness or pain.

Pain or discomfort in one or both arms, the back, neck, jaw or stomach.

Shortness of breath. This often occurs with chest discomfort, but can occur beforehand.

Breaking out in a cold sweat, nausea or light-headedness.

Warning signs of stroke

Sudden numbness or weakness of the face, arm or leg, especially on one side of the body.

Sudden confusion, trouble speaking or understanding.

Sudden trouble seeing in one or both eyes or sudden severe headache.

Sudden trouble walking, dizziness, loss of co-ordination or balance.

If you or someone with you has one or more of these signs, call 9-9-9 immediately.

I am pleased I have got to 76 but I hope to go on a lot longer. I had a mastectomy four years ago so I won't know till next year if I am clear. I found the lump myself and rang my doctor straight away. When I first heard, it was very traumatic but I did it on the NHS and I couldn't have done it better. I didn't have any chemo or radiation because when he did the mastectomy there was no cancer in the nodes and he took them all away anyway. My friend who had it privately with chemo and radiation died. I didn't have a reconstruction because of my age but if I had been younger, I would probably have. If your partner is sympathetic and accepts it, it is very important for your self-esteem. My recovery was very good but I was upset a few months ago when I fell over. You mustn't get any damage to your arm because you get lymphodema drainage out of your arm. I get upset with my skin being dry but I take Tamoxifen and I think that makes it dry. The doctor gave me aqueous cream and emulsifying ointment but it doesn't work. I recently bought Boots No.17 for dry skin and I think it's worked.
Helen, 78, Uk

calcium, vitamin D and soya (p.80). Although HRT has long been prescribed for women at risk, there are a range of other drugs available to treat osteoporosis. Bisphosphonates are non-hormonal drugs, which help maintain bone density and reduce fracture rates. Calcium and vitamin D supplements can be of benefit for older people to reduce the risk of hip fracture. Selective Estrogen Receptor Modulators (SERMs) are drugs which act in a similar way to oestrogen, helping to maintain bone density and reduce fracture rates specifically in the spine. The anti-oestrogen drug Tamoxifen provides protection against osteoporosis and breast cancer, but it stimulates uterine tissue, slightly increasing the risk of uterine cancer.

BREAST CANCER Industrialized countries generally have higher rates of breast cancer than non-industrialized countries. The causes are not fully under-stood, but your risk increases if you have a family history of breast cancer, if you started your periods early or your menopause late (after the age of 55), if you take combined HRT, if you have never had children, had children later in life, smoke or drink a lot of alcohol. A fatty diet and obesity may also play a big part in increasing the incidence of breast cancer because fat stimulates the production of oestrogen, something the hordes of women on the Atkins diet might want to bear in mind.

Because no one knows exactly what causes breast cancer, there are no sure ways to prevent it. Eating healthily, exercising regularly and limiting the amount of alcohol you drink will decrease but not eliminate the possibility. The older a woman is, the more likely she is to get breast cancer. White women are more likely to get breast cancer than any other racial or ethnic group but they also have a better chance of survival, primarily because their cancer is usually detected earlier. Only about 5% of all breast cancers happen because of inherited mutations, but high-risk women can be given Tamoxifen as a preventative measure.

Most breast cancers are first discovered by women themselves. So for the last 30 years doctors have recommended that all women should check their own breasts monthly (women 39+ need a medical examination once a year). However, recent research by a Canadian task force on preventative health warns that self-examination for breast cancer shows 'fair evidence of no benefit and good evidence of harm'. Their concern is that women who find lumps that generate false alarm are more likely to undergo unnecessary biopsies, which cause scarring, deformity and emotional stress. Though the breast cancer mortality rates between women who self-examine and those who don't are virtually identical, a regular breast examination allows you to become familiar with the fluctuations your breasts go through each month, making unusual changes more easy to spot.

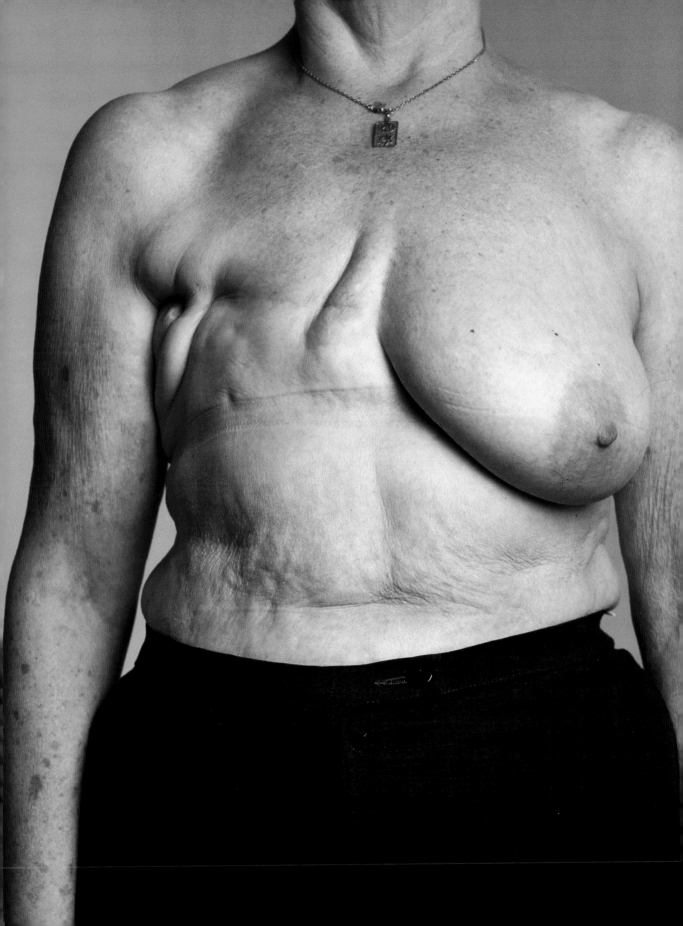

HOW TO EXAMINE YOUR BREASTS The best time to examine your breasts is about a week after the end of your periods. It is best done in the shower or in the bath because your fingers glide over wet skin more easily. With flat fingers, gently move over every part of your breasts from underneath up to your armpit. Check for lumps, knots or thickening. Next, stand in front of a mirror and raise your arms over your head. Then rest your palms on your hips and press down firmly to flex your chest muscles. Look for any changes in the contour of each breast and swelling, dimpled skin or changes in the nipple. Then lie on a bed and put a pillow or folded towel under your right shoulder. Raise your right hand and put it behind your head to distribute your breast tissue more evenly on your chest. With your left hand, using flat fingers, press gently in small circular motions around an imaginary clock face. Begin at the outermost top of your right breast, then move around the breast in a circle. A ridge of firm tissue in the lower curve of each breast is normal. Move in an inch, towards the nipple and keep circling to examine every part of your breast, including the nipple. Repeat the procedure on your left breast with a pillow under your left shoulder and left hand behind head. Finally, squeeze the nipple of each breast gently between thumb and index finger. If a lump, dimple or discharge is discovered, see your doctor as soon as possible but don't panic, eight out of ten lumps are nothing to worry about.

TREATMENT 80% of the time, breast lumps are not cancerous and do not need to be removed. Some go away on their own and some are caused by normal hormonal changes, occasionally appearing and disappearing throughout the menstrual cycle when the breasts can become fuller and possibly a little tender. Depending on your age, your risk factors and the features of the lump, your doctor might recommend further tests, such as an ultrasound, mammogram or biopsy. You have more choices of treatment and a better chance of surviving if your breast cancer is found early. The five-year survival rate for all women diagnosed with breast cancer is 86% and many women who are diagnosed with breast cancer do not have to lose a breast. Lab tests can measure how virulent the cancer is and whether it has spread to the lymph nodes or to other parts. In some women, breast cancer cells depend on female hormones (oestrogen and progesterone) for growth and this can be treated by removing your ovaries to stop your body producing natural hormones, or with the drug Tamoxifen, which helps to reduce the chances of recurrence in the treated breast by up to 40% but slightly increases the risk for cancer of the uterus. New research in the UK on the drug Anastrozole, which stops the production of oestrogen, has proved very successful and it appears to have fewer side effects than Tamoxifen. Trials are being carried out on 10,000 post-menopausal women and if the results are positive, this could be the first preventative option for women at a high risk of developing breast cancer.

Index

Recommended Reading

The Body Project : An Intimate History of American Girls by Joan Jacobs Brumberg (Vintage)

Fasting girls: The emergence of Anorexia nervosa as a modern disease by Joan Jacobs Brumberg (Harvard University Press)

Reviving Ophelia: Saving the Selves of Adolescent Girls by Mary Pipher (Ballantine Books)

Body Image: Understanding Body Dissatisfaction in Men, Women and Children by Sarah Grogan (Routledge)

Shame and Body Image: Culture and the Compulsive Eater by Barbara McFarland, (Baumann Health Communications)

Ways of seeing by John Berger (Penguin)

Fat Is a Feminist Issue by Susie Orbach (Arrow)

Backlash: The Undeclared War Against Women by Susan Faludi (Vintage)

Recommended Reading

The Perricone
Prescription by Nicholas
Perricone M.D.
(Harper Resource)

Eat, Drink, and Be
Healthy: The Harvard
Medical School Guide
to Healthy Eating
by Walter C. Willett,
P. J. Skerrett
(Free Press)

The Food Bible
by Judith Wills
(Quadrille)

The Complete Guide
to Sports Nutrition
by Anita Bean (A & C
Black)

Gender and Sport:
A Reader
Edited by Sheila
Scraton, Anne Flintoff
(Routledge)

Women, Sport
and Culture
by Susan Birrell PhD,
Cheryl L. Cole PhD
(Human Kinetics
Europe Ltd)

Fitness for Dummies
by Suzanne Schlosberg
(John Wiley & Sons Inc.)

The 21st Century
Beauty Bible
by Sarah Stacey and
Josephine Fairley
(Kyle Cathie Ltd)

Beauty Evolution
by Bobby Brown
(Aurum)

Recommended Reading

*Consciously Female :
How to Listen to Your
Body and Your Soul for
a Lifetime of Healthier
Living* by Tracey Gaudet,
Paula Spencer
(Bantam)

*Our Bodies, Ourselves
for the New Century: A
Book by and for
Women* by The Boston
Women's Health
Collective
(Touchstone)

*Taking Charge of Your
Fertility: The Definitive
Guide to Natural Birth
Control, Pregnancy
Achievement, and
Reproductive Health* by
Toni Weschler
(Quill)

*Women's Bodies,
Women's Wisdom*
by Christiane Northrup
(Bantam)

*The Wisdom of
Menopause*
by Christiane Northrup
(Bantam)

*The "Which?" Guide to
Understanding HRT and
the Menopause*
by Robert C.D. Wilson
(Which? Books)

*The Breast Cancer
Survival Manual: A Step-
By-Step Guide for the
Woman With Newly
Diagnosed Breast
Cancer* by John S. Link,
James Waisman Md.,
Cynthia Forstoff Md.